Aromatherapy *for* Bodyworkers

Jade Shutes, B.A., Diploma AT
Christina Weaver, LMT, NCTMB

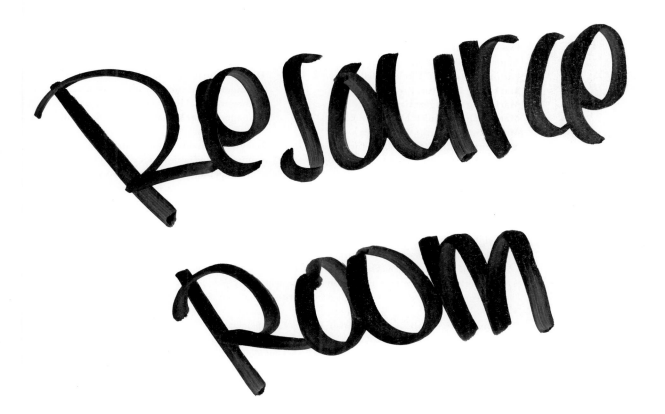

Resource Room

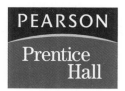

PEARSON
Prentice
Hall

Upper Saddle River, New Jersey 07458

Library of Congress Cataloging-in-Publication Data

Shutes, Jade.
    Aromatherapy for bodyworkers / Jade Shutes and Christina Weaver.
      p. ; cm.
    Includes bibliographical references and index.
    ISBN-13: 978-0-13-173737-2 (alk. paper)
    ISBN-10: 0-13-173737-6 (alk. paper)
    1. Aromatherapy. 2. Essences and essential oils—Therapeutic use.
    [DNLM: 1. Aromatherapy—methods. 2. Holistic Health. WB 925 S562a 2008] I. Weaver, Christina. II. Title.
    RM666.A68S42 2008
    615'.3219—dc22

                        2007020334

Publisher: Julie Alexander
Executive Editor: Mark Cohen
Associate Editor: Melissa Kerian
Editorial Assistant: Nicole Ragonese
Marketing Director: Karen Allman
Marketing Manager: Harper Coles
Marketing Specialist: Michael Sirinides
Marketing Assistant: Wayne Celia
Managing Editor Production: Patrick Walsh
Production Liaison: Christina Zingone
Manufacturing Manager: Ilene Sanford
Manufacturing Buyer: Pat Brown
Design Director: Maria Guglielmo

Cover Designer: Anthony Gemmellaro
Cover Images: Getty Images-Iconica; Getty Images-Westend 61
Director, Image Resource Center: Melinda Patelli
Manager, Rights and Permissions: Zina Arabia
Manager, Visual Research: Beth Brenzel
Manager, Cover Visual Research & Permissions: Karen Sanatar
Image Permission Coordinator: Ang'john Ferreri
Composition/Full-Service Project Management: GGS Book Services/Chitra Ganesan
Printer/Binder: Quebecor World Color Versailles
Cover Printer: Coral Graphics

Pearson Education LTD.
Pearson Education Singapore, Pte. Ltd
Pearson Education, Canada, Ltd
Pearson Education—Japan
Pearson Education Australia PTY, Limited

Pearson Education North Asia Ltd
Pearson Educación de Mexico, S.A. de C.V.
Pearson Education Malaysia, Pte. Ltd
Pearson Education, Upper Saddle River, New Jersey

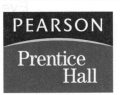

10 9 8 7 6 5 4 3 2 1
ISBN-13: 978-0-13-173737-2
ISBN-10: 0-13-173737-6

Dedication

For my son, my father, and my husband. . . thank you for your true understanding, continuous support, and never ending love. I AM grateful. (CW)

For all the students, practitioners, and teachers who embrace holistic aromatherapy and share the aromatic path with others. (JS)

BRIEF CONTENTS

CONTENTS

PART IV Integration with Bodywork   159

CHAPTER 8 Aromatic Applications and Techniques   159

PART V **Essential Oil Data Sheets**   **281**

CHAPTER 13 Exploring 48 Essential Oils   281

END MATTER

Aromatherapy is gaining popularity and is considered by many to be one of the leading complementary healthcare modalities of the twenty-first century. In recent years, rapid developments in aromatic medicine, neuroanatomy, stress-related disease, and complementary care have enormously expanded the boundaries of aromatherapy. This expansion of knowledge and application has been accompanied by an ever-increasing integration of aromatherapy and bodywork in a variety of settings, including spa, hospice, hospitals, complementary healthcare centers, and individual practices.

These developments have produced a need for high-quality education in aromatherapy. Aromatherapy encompasses a vast array of knowledge that has, until now, been generalized to a wide audience. Often, for the health professional, overly generalized books on aromatherapy can be discouraging. As aromatherapy continues to gain legitimacy as a complementary healthcare modality, it becomes essential for student success in integrating aromatherapy into traditional and nontraditional healthcare practices and settings to have a solid education in the application of essential oils.

Aromatherapy for Bodyworkers text could not be timelier and is of great value to all healthcare professionals—massage therapists, bodyworkers, estheticians, nurses, and others who utilize touch for patient/client care—with an interest in deepening their knowledge, understanding, and application of holistic aromatherapy. *Aromatherapy for Bodyworkers* is written in a very readable style, accompanied by numerous pedagogical aids that serve to support learning, to increase interest in the subject matter, and to provide motivation for the student to actively interact with and integrate the subject matter into their life and practice. To fully appreciate the benefits of aromatherapy and to understand how they work, we believe it is essential for a practitioner to have personal hands-on experience using essential oils.

ORGANIZATION

Thirteen chapters of *Aromatherapy for Bodyworkers* present the core material necessary for a massage therapist or bodyworker to successfully integrate aromatherapy into their practice. The selection of information has been based upon the National Association for Holistic Aromatherapy Core Curriculum requirements for a foundational education in aromatherapy as well as to reflect current trends in aromatherapy and massage integration. The introductory chapter explores the history of aromatherapy, the importance of language, modern uses in massage and bodywork, and the value of a holistic framework for practice.

The textbook is divided into four core parts: Part I: The Basics of Aromatherapy (Chapters 2 through 4) covers information from plant to essential oil; the necessary basics of essential oils, including pertinent information on purchasing essential oils, quality assurance, and safety, concluding with a basic exploration of the chemistry of essential oils. Part II: Blending (Chapter 5) addresses the dynamic aspects of blending, offering comprehensive methods in creating unique blends. Part III: Pathways into the Body (Chapters 6 and 7) explores the two core pathways into the body: the skin and olfaction. The chapter on skin includes valuable information on numerous vegetable and herbal oils as well as skin types and common disorders. The chapter on olfaction deals with the emotional benefits of essential oils, the impact of stress on health, and olfactory methods of application. Part IV: Integration with Bodywork (Chapters 8 through 12) is an exploration into the integration of aromatherapy with diverse massage applications and techniques, water and salt-based applications, special populations, and specific ailments a therapist may encounter. Chapter 12 concludes with some ideas on how to approach the business of aromatherapy, including supplies, cost accounting, and insurance needs as well as marketing ideas.

In Part V, Chapter 13 provides the Essential Oil Data Sheets that will be utilized through the textbook. Each full data sheet provides a full color image of the plant. We believe that the plant is essential to the very foundation of holistic aromatherapy and hope the images help to inspire you to further explore the living plant world. We recommend that 8 essential oils are covered during each chapter (except Chapter 1) until all 48 essential oils have been covered.

FEATURES

Each chapter contains a number of elements designed to facilitate learning, enhance interaction with the subject matter, and to enhance retention of information. To accomplish this, the text includes a variety of pedagogical features to enhance students' integration of course material into practice. These features include:

Chapter Learning Objectives

Each chapter opening page contains seven measurable objectives for the student. Each objective allows the student to identify what the key goals are and what information should be studied thoroughly.

Key Terms

When keywords are initially introduced and defined within the text, the keyword will be in boldface to highlight its importance.

Margin Notes and In Practice Boxes

Brief boxed inserts will appear as necessary to help make the material more interesting and to provide additional information on a particular subject matter. **In Practice** boxes include valuable information that enhances the actual application of aromatherapy, including case studies. Other In Practice boxes address specific issues about aromatherapy in practice.

Chapter Test

Objective-style true/false, multiple choice, and fill-in-the-blank questions have been designed to check the student's mastery of important subject matter contained within the chapter. Answers to all chapter tests are provided at the end of the text.

Review Questions

Subjective review questions at the end of each chapter will allow the student to describe what they have learned in the chapter. The key goal of review questions is to have students discuss information, voice opinions, and share experiences.

Chapter Summaries

Summaries at the end of each chapter provide a list of major topics and information discussed.

Worksheets

Worksheets are provided at the end of each chapter and contain experiential exercises such as integrating aromatherapy with massage, customizing a blend, performing mock case studies, making a salt glow treatment, and exploring essential oils. Each exercise has been designed to allow the student to interact with the information they have learned and the actual essential oils. Occasionally these exercises will include working with partners and performing aromatherapy massage treatments.

A FINAL WORD

Aromatherapy is an incredibly dynamic field to be involved with, and we encourage you to explore essential oils and their therapeutic benefits both at work and at home. Although essential oils have a wide range of therapeutic activity, they are not meant to take the place of traditional or orthodox medicine but rather to serve as valuable complementary tools for obtaining and maintaining health and well-being. Aromatherapy is blossoming and with this blossoming comes a responsibility to ensure that you are knowledgeable and competent in the application of genuine essential oils. Aromatherapy is so often confused with the use of synthetics or fragrances, and our hope is that this text facilitates a greater awareness and appreciation of the therapeutic benefits of authentic aromatherapy for psychological and physiological health. We hope you enjoy your journey in the world of aromatherapy.

ACKNOWLEDGMENTS

The writing of this book has been an incredible, and at times challenging, experience, one I could not have accomplished alone. It is with sincere gratitude that I thank the following individuals:

Anne Williams: for helping to create the opportunity to write this book and for believing in and supporting me throughout the years

Jan Kusmirek: for sharing his knowledge and creativeness with me and in so doing inspiring me to explore dynamic applications for aromatherapy

Elaine Shaughnessy: for being willing to review the material and offer invaluable insights

Gene Koselke: for providing me with ongoing support and a wonderful flat-screen monitor to stare at while writing this book

Joyce Benoit, Heidi Nielson, and Roxana Villa: for being the best of friends since the beginning of my career

My instructors, Marie Temmen, Zsuzsana Davidson, Michelle Thibert, and Cheryl Hoard: for their dedication and passion for education and aromatherapy

Christina Weaver: for her friendship, support, and willingness to take part in the writing of this book

All my students, friends, and clients: for teaching and inspiring me more than I could ever have foreseen or thought imaginable. Thank you!

And to my family who listened to me talk about this book for over two years and continued to support me throughout the entire process: Matt and our son Soren, and my Mom, Dad, and sisters, Gloria and Lisa

And finally, to Mark Cohen: for believing in me and supporting me throughout my journey

-JS

Jade Shutes, B.A., Diploma AT

Jade Shutes holds a Diploma in Holistic Aromatherapy, Holistic Massage, Anatomy and Physiology, and Reflexology from the Raworth College of Natural Medicine in Dorking, U.K., and a Diploma in Aromatherapy from the International Therapist Examining board (ITEC). She has studied with Jan Kusmirek of Fragrant Studies and has completed Part One of the Purdue University Advanced Studies of Essential Oils.

Jade has been practicing and studying forms of natural healing for nearly two decades and was one of the vanguard of professionals who helped introduce aromatherapy in the United States. She has been an aromatherapy educator for over seventeen years, opening her first aromatherapy school in the New England area in 1990. She has designed and taught aromatherapy courses for massage and bodywork therapists, estheticians, social workers, nurses, and other healthcare providers. Jade has taught at Bastyr University, Duke University (Continuing Education), Ashmead College, San Diego Hospice, and at various locations throughout the United States and Canada.

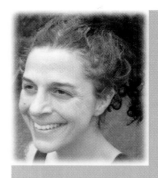

Jade Shutes

In addition to being a popular speaker, Jade has played an active role in the setting of standards for aromatherapy education in North America and has authored published articles on this and other aromatherapy issues. She is recognized for her leadership roles in the campaign to raise educational standards in the United States and has co-initiated the creation of the National Steering Committee on Educational Standards, now the Aromatherapy Registration Council. She served as president of the National Association for Holistic Aromatherapy (NAHA) from 2000 to 2003. She currently resides in Raleigh, North Carolina with her family.

Christina Weaver, LMT, NCTMB

Christina Weaver is the founder of Complementary Health Services, LLC and Archeiai Healing Arts in Tucson, Arizona where she has established a holistic healing center and hospital based, in-patient massage program. She also teaches prenatal massage and aromatherapy classes.

Christina moved to Tucson from the Seattle area in 2003 where prior to that she worked in various healing centers, spas and her own private practice both as a massage practitioner and aromatherapist. Christina is a graduate of the Brenneke School of Massage in Seattle, WA as well as the NW College for Herbal & Aromatic Studies. She holds a diploma in holistic aromatherapy and is a DONA certified birth doula, having completed training at Seattle Midwifery School. Christina has an advanced certification in prenatal massage and has also completed additional training in other areas of women's health including lymphatic based breast massage.

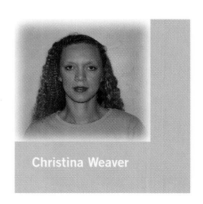

Christina Weaver

Most recently she has been studying CranioSacral therapy and looks forward to working with more pediatric clients in the future. Christina has always focused on therapeutic massage and bodywork for women as well as their families and is quite effective in the treatment of pain, recovery of injury and general wellness, but also includes the use of essential oils and all natural, holistic spa treatments amongst her skills and specialities.

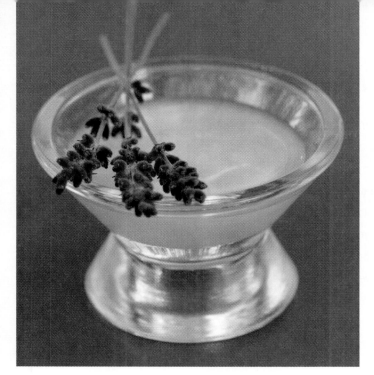

 LEARNING OBJECTIVES

After reading this chapter, you will be able to

1. Define the term aromatherapy.
2. Describe the general history of aromatic plant use for medicinal purposes.
3. Discuss the impact of Gattefosse, Valnet, and Maury had on the development of aromatherapy.
4. Describe traditional aromatherapy as practiced in England and list the top ten reasons the average person in England goes to see an aromatherapist.
5. Explain why language in aromatherapy is valuable and important.
6. Identify the therapeutic benefits of aromatherapy as a complement to bodywork and massage.
7. Describe the holistic framework for aromatherapy.

INTRODUCTION

Aromatherapy is often a misunderstood and undervalued holistic therapy in the United States, possibly due to its commercial exploitation. Aromatherapy is, however, an incredible holistic and complementary therapy that is gaining in recognition as more and more healthcare professionals incorporate it into their practice. This chapter is dedicated to shedding light on what genuine aromatherapy is, its history, modern development and practice, and why the language we use in describing it is crucial for the professional development of the field. From the birth of modern holistic aromatherapy, practitioners have been dedicated to a holistic framework of practice. The last section of this chapter will provide the student with an understanding of the philosophy of holism within the practice of aromatherapy.

↳ DEFINING AROMATHERAPY

"Is aromatherapy a nice smelling air freshener, a relaxing massage, a delightful beauty therapy, a useful home first aid tool, or a serious health care modality?" (Sheen and Stevens, 2002, p. 189). Aromatherapy continues to be one of the fastest growing complementary healthcare modalities of the twenty-first century and yet it continues to be one of the least understood, not only among healthcare practitioners but particularly within the mainstream. Defining aromatherapy, on the other hand, is a complex task and one that requires sensitivity to the diverse practices and philosophies that are encompassed by different practitioners. According to Sheen and Stevens (2002), "the 'misuse' of the term aromatherapy in the wider society could be an indication of the misunderstanding of what aromatherapy is, or an indication of aromatherapy's lack of a clear definition" (p. 190).

Aromatherapy is practiced by a diverse set of lay people and practitioners, including naturopaths, nurses, massage therapists, independent aromatherapy consultants, occupational therapists, social workers, psychologists, reflexologists, and, at times and in some countries, by medical doctors. Aromatherapy can be used to reduce anxiety and agitation, to heal skin ulcers, to reduce the impact of stress on the physical body, and to expectorate mucus from the lungs. Aromatherapy can be applied in hospice environments to increase quality of life, in maternity wards to support the delivery process and relieve postpartum stress, and in bodywork practices to enhance the therapeutic benefits of the bodywork technique itself. Aromatherapy has these therapeutic benefits and many more as will be discovered throughout this text.

Perhaps the best place to begin our understanding of the term aromatherapy is to go back in history and to its modern birth and the actual coining of the word.

↳ HISTORY OF AROMATIC PLANT USE

". . . there is virtually no people known to anthropology—however remote, isolated, or primitive—in which some form of doctoring with plants was not practiced."
BARBARA GRIGGS, GREEN PHARMACY

When we discuss the history of aromatherapy, we are really talking about the history of the use of aromatics or aromatic plants. Aromatherapy, as the profession we know today, is actually quite young and has a relatively short history. However, the history of medicinal and aromatic plants is indeed ancient, and aromatic plants did enjoy some similar uses as we have to this present day, albeit in different forms.

The history of aromatic substances could place us as far back as the origins of humankind, when he/she put material onto a fire or ate particular plants. Remember our sense of smell was quite powerful during these early stages of humanity. Primitive humans may have found the smoke, scents, and aromas affecting them in different ways. Some of the plant material would have made him/her feel restful, while others stimulated, and some would have gone to the chest, making breathing easier. Primitive humans discovered that leaves, berries, roots, etc. made sick people better. Also twigs thrown on the fire made people happy or excited, or they had spiritual experiences. Smudging or burning aromatic plant material to treat a patient is one of the earliest recorded forms of treatment with herbs, often used to drive out evil spirits or as a form of incense for protection and potential health benefit.

The ancient Egyptians, Greeks, and Romans are well known for their use of aromatic plants and aromatic extracts. The Egyptians used balsams, perfumed oils, scented barks and resins for medicine, food preservation, and religious ceremonies and for embalming the dead. It is thought that the Greeks learned much of their aromatic knowledge from the Egyptians. Hippocrates, the renowned Greek physician, is often quoted as having said "the way to health is to have an aromatic bath and scented massage every day." And, of course, the Romans are known to have popularized the use of the bathhouse as a place to use aromatic oils and other scented products for beautification and for health.

Aromatics were also used during the Middle Ages for defense against the bubonic plague. Aromatics were burned in the streets and in homes to ward off infection. It is commonly suspected that the perfumers and glove makers were mostly immune to the plague because they were constantly surrounded by aromatic essential oils.

During the eighteenth century we begin to find essential oils being used extensively, and much research was being carried out on their medicinal properties. Some apothecaries even had their own stills to produce essential oils. On the other hand, it was during this time that the growing specialization of medicine was occurring, which would eventually attempt to take medicine out of the hands of lay people.

In the nineteenth century the "family doctor" was established. Oils of chamomile, cinnamon, fennel, bay, juniper, rosemary, and thyme are recorded as official essential oils in William Whitla's *Materia Medica* (1882). In 1887, M. Chamberland published studies showing the antibacterial and antifungal properties of many essential oils (e.g., lavender, juniper, sandalwood, thyme, cinnamon, and cedar wood).

In many ways the history of aromatherapy is the history of herbal medicine, which enjoys a long and abundant history throughout the world. Plants, specifically aromatic plants, have been employed for thousands of years and are still considered to be an important source of medicine. Aromatherapy, as it is known today, however, is a modern development of how aromatic plants were used by these early cultures. To understand modern aromatherapy, we shall turn to Rene-Maurice Gattefosse, who coined the term in 1937.

AROMATHERAPY: MODERN DEVELOPMENT

This history has been compiled from the work of Marcel Gattefosse (1992) on writing about his father in the *International Journal of Aromatherapy*. Rene-Maurice Gattefosse was born in the French region of Lyon in 1881 (Figure 1-1). Gattefosse

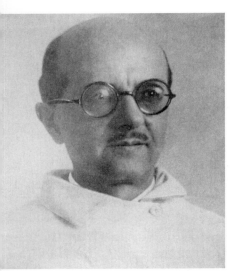

Figure 1-1 Rene-Maurice Gattefosse

Source: Elsevier Publishing

grew up around plants and aromas. His father, Louis Gattefosse, owned and operated the Gattefosse perfume business, which remains in business today. During Rene's youth, perfumes were still created from a mixture of natural essential oils, alcohol extracts, flower pomades, and some synthetic products. Louis and his two sons, Abel and Rene-Maurice, worked closely together to define the conditions under which perfume compositions were prepared so as to achieve constant levels of strength and odor. In 1906, they published a book entitled "Formulaires de Parfumerie de Gattefosse."

The Gattefosse family was active in many areas of the perfume business, from plant cultivation to formulating perfume compositions. In the early 1900s the Gattefosses initiated a campaign to promote lavender as well as to support its distillation for essential oil production. This campaign was in response to the need to increase trade in lavender to support economic conditions for local farmers within various areas of France. During the early 1900s Rene-Maurice assisted with the organization of mint and other herbs for culture in France. He also embarked on a systematic study of exotic essential oils and the creation of distillation units that would be easy to build on location.

Sometime between 1908 and 1910, Gattefosse joined forces with his younger brother Jean, a botanist and chemist, to pursue his research of exotic plants. Jean and Rene-Maurice spent time in Morocco compiling a large selection of new plants and establishing distillation in North Africa. It was during his stay in Morocco that Rene-Maurice began to learn of the ways in which the peasants used essential oils as popular medicines. This intrigued Rene-Maurice so much that he set to work to discover the medicinal properties of these essential oils and understand their efficacy in healing the body. From the peasants of Morocco, he learned the incredible healing properties of lavender essential oil, including its antiseptic, prophylactic, and vulnerary properties.

According to Marcel Gattefosse, it was July of 1910 when the famous laboratory explosion, so commonly referred to in most aromatherapy books and training courses, took place. Rene-Maurice sustained burns to his hands and scalp for which he treated himself with lavender. He was able to directly observe the medicinal benefits of lavender. The lavender seemed to have reduced the trauma to the skin from the burn and in fact was helping the skin to recover with great efficacy. This experience led Gattefosse to a lifelong passion and commitment for uncovering the therapeutic benefits of these aromatic substances, known as "essential oils."

The term "aromatherapie" was coined by Rene-Maurice Gattefosse in 1937 with his publication of a book by that name. His book, *Gattefosse's Aromatherapy*, contains early clinical findings for utilizing essential oils for a host of physiological ailments. It seems vital to understand what Gattefosse's intention for coining the word was, as he clearly meant to distinguish the medicinal application of essential oils from their perfumery applications. Gattefosse was already a perfumer and as such had a love and passion for the aromas they imparted. However, by 1918 he had become deeply involved with the study and application of the essential oils for medicinal purposes. He was to remain active throughout the 1930s, writing articles and working with hospitals and others to test the medicinal actions of essential oils.

So we can interpret his coining of the word "aromatherapie" to mean *the therapeutic application or use of aromatic substances* (essential oils). Since its origin, aromatherapy has implied a practice that encompasses human pathology and the treatment of different emotional and physical conditions with essential oils. As aromatherapy developed into a practice, it adopted a more holistic approach encompassing the body, the mind, and the spirit (energy).

Aromatherapy Cofounders

The following individuals also contributed greatly to the shaping of modern aromatherapy.

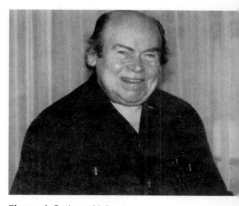

Figure 1-2 Jean Valnet
Source: Elsevier Publishing

Dr. Jean Valnet was trained as a traditional medical doctor at the University of Lyon in 1945 (Figure 1-2). According to Scott (1993), Valnet began his research into essential oils in 1953, and his focus was mainly on the best methods of application as well as dosage levels needed to attain maximum benefit without risk of side effects. Valnet successfully utilized essential oils as antiseptics in the treatment of war wounds during World War II. In 1964, Valnet's book, *The Practice of Aromatherapy,* was published and has since become a classic in aromatherapy. Over a period of ten years, Valnet created a number of effective remedies utilizing essential oils, including remedies for skin conditions, respiratory conditions, muscular aches and pains, and other things.

Marguerite Maury deserves special attention as her work with essential oils led to the creation of holistic aromatherapy practice as we know it today. Born in Austria in 1895, Maury led an interesting and passionate life. She was trained as a nurse and surgical assistant in Vienna and then moved to France, where she was given a book entitled "Les Grandes Possibilites par les Matieres Odoriferantes" (Ryman, 1989). This book was to provide Maury with a lifelong passion for researching and educating others on the applications of aromatherapy. Together with her husband, Dr. Maury, they explored numerous healing therapies, including homeopathy, naturopathy, acupuncture, yoga, meditation, and others.

Marguerite Maury pioneered the dermal application of essential oils and the recognition of both the psychological and physiological benefits gained through this pathway into the body. The popular application of essential oils to the skin has been attributed to the seminal work of Marguerite Maury entitled Marguerite Maury's Guide to Aromatherapy: *The Secret of Life and Youth,* published in France in 1961. In this book, Maury expands on her ideas about the secrets of staying young and shares her insights in using essential oils that provided the seeds for the modern development of holistic aromatherapy.

Her many contributions to the development of aromatherapy include the following:

▪ **Integrated massage and aromatherapy:** Maury (1989) states: "Massage of the conjunctive, neuro-muscular or soft tissue pave the way admirably for the penetration of the odoriferous substances, and the resultant rejuvenation" (p. 158). Maury not only pioneered the dermal application of essential oils but was one of the first to draw attention to the enhancing effects of essential oils on the already beneficial effects of massage itself.

"We had to find a method capable both of influencing the muscular tonus, the quality and aspect of the skin and the tissues, and to obtain a better functioning and a normalization of the individual's rhythm" (Maury, 1989, p. 108).

▪ **Recognized the importance of a holistic approach:** Throughout her book, Maury acknowledges the importance of maintaining health through nutrition, exercise, a healthy emotional and spiritual life, and massage or hydrotherapy. She draws on such philosophical traditions as traditional Chinese medicine and Tibetan and Ayurvedic medicine in providing an understanding of different approaches to health, disease, and healing.

■ **Emphasized the importance of the individual:** Perhaps her greatest contribution to the evolution of aromatherapy was her clear commitment to and recognition of the importance of treating the individual. The idea of treating the individual is one of the core principles for holistic aromatherapy practice.

> To reach the individual we need an individual remedy. Each of us is a unique message. It is only the unique remedy which will suffice.

> We must, therefore, seek odoriferous substances which present affinities with the human being we intend to treat, those which will compensate for his deficiencies and those which will make his faculties blossom. (Maury, 1989, p. 94)

■ **Recognized the dual effect of essential oils:** Maury was keen to observe that essential oils applied to the skin not only had a physiological effect but also a corresponding psychological effect.

> Applied to the skin these essences regulate the activity of the capillaries and restore vitality to the tissues. . . . But of the greatest interest is the effect of (aroma) has on the psychic and mental state of the individual. Powers of perception become clearer and more acute. . . . The use of odoriferous matter induces a true sentimental and mental liberation . . . the essential oils free us from the (challenging emotion) but leave our faculties unimpaired. (Maury, 1989, p. 82–83)

From these observations and applications, modern holistic aromatherapy was born. Based upon Maury's contributions to the practice of aromatherapy, we can then define aromatherapy more comprehensively:

> Aromatherapy is the holistic therapeutic application of genuine essential oils for enhancing the physical, emotional, mental, and spiritual health of the individual.

THE MODERN PRACTICE OF AROMATHERAPY

The aromatherapy industry is dynamic, diverse, and often divided in opinion and practice. This state of affairs is perhaps a reflection of the industries youth and seemingly constant growth. In general, aromatherapy can be used to enhance a client's well-being and encourage positive states of health. Clinical or medical aromatherapy was born of the medical tradition in France; holistic aromatherapy was born of the touch tradition in England and then throughout the world.

Holistic aromatherapy, also known as traditional aromatherapy, was popularized in England, where the standard aromatherapy program includes the following core subjects: essential oil therapeutics, anatomy and physiology, Swedish massage, basic pathology, basic counseling skills, reflexology (both as a diagnostic tool as well as a treatment approach), Touch for Health, and basic nutrition. Traditional aromatherapy is a hands-on approach to applying essential oils for stress reduction and other psychological benefits as well as to enhance overall health and well-being.

According to Harris (2003), the typical aromatherapy client is female and in her middle years. The top ten reasons the average person in the United Kingdom (U.K.) goes to see aromatherapists are:

1. stress/anxiety
2. headaches/migraines
3. insomnia

4. musculoskeletal problems
5. hormonal problems
6. respiratory problems
7. arthritis and rheumatism
8. skin problems
9. chronic fatigue
10. sinus problems

Traditional aromatherapy, as practiced in the U.K., has experienced many setbacks in its introduction and acceptance within the United States. The original introduction of aromatherapy into the U.S. mainstream was through the retail and gift industries rather than through the profession (such as occurred in England). With this original introduction came the additional problem of low-quality essential oils and synthetics being sold as the best and the most pure. Today, there are more and more educated consumers and practitioners seeking high-quality essential oils for their therapeutic application and potential. Unfortunately, there remains a plethora of synthetic fragrances and adulterants in products posing as natural aromatherapy, and this underlies the continued importance of educating the public and healthcare professionals on the value of genuine aromatherapy.

Aromatherapy, Bodywork, and Massage Therapy

The growth of the aromatherapy profession, both as a stand alone therapy and as a complementary therapy to such professions as nursing, bodywork, and massage practices, has been slow due to the aforementioned factors; however, it would appear that over the past five years the aromatherapy profession in the United States has been growing, becoming more popular with the mainstream. Even more interesting, it appears to be growing the most quickly within the bodywork/massage therapy, nursing, and cosmetology professions—the very same professions that tend to use aromatherapy in England.

Tisserand (1988), speaking about traditional aromatherapy practice in England (which combines aromatics with massage), defined aromatherapy as "a caring, hands-on therapy which seeks to induce relaxation, to increase energy, to reduce the effects of stress and to restore lost balance to mind, body, and soul. Aromatherapy works with the forces of nature, not against them, and so is capable of bringing about true healing" (p. 1).

Complementary and alternative medicine (CAM) practices include manipulative and body-based methods, such as bodywork and massage therapy, and mind-body practices, such as aromatherapy. Clinical research and empirical studies by massage therapists are showing that the use of massage and aromatherapy can dramatically increase the effects of the treatment. According to the AMTA (2005):

a massage therapist focuses on the normalization of soft tissues affected by stress, injury, and illness through the use of manual techniques that:

- improve circulation
- enhance muscular relaxation
- relieve pain
- reduce stress
- enhance immune function
- promote health and well-being

Bodywork and massage therapy techniques are being found to be beneficial for a wide range of conditions, including arthritis, immune function disorders, asthma and bronchitis, insomnia, carpal tunnel syndrome, myofascial pain, chronic and acute pain, circulatory problems, reduced range of motion, gastrointestinal disorders

IN PRACTICE

Case Study 1.1

Muscular Aches and Pains/Emotional Support

G. is a forty-three-year-old woman who is experiencing chronic neck and shoulder pain due to an automobile accident. She also reports that her boyfriend has just moved in, and she is planning her wedding which will take place in six months. She believes that she holds her emotional stress in her neck and shoulders, which increases the pain and reduces her range of motion. She is hoping that aromatherapy massage and home remedies will reduce her feelings of stress as well as reduce pain levels.

Massage Blend

Sore and Painful Muscles

Apricot Kernel oil 100%

Peppermint (*Mentha* x *piperita*) 5 drops

Bay Laurel (*Laurus nobilis*) 7 drops

Rosemary ct. camphor (*Rosmarinus officinalis*) 10 drops

Lavender (*Lavandula angustifolia*) 14 drops

2oz. glass bottle/ 3% dilution

Full body massage was given. She reported a reduced feeling of pain and feeling more relaxed. She took the remainder of the blend home with her to use as needed on her neck and shoulders.

Home Blend (bath and inhalation)

Emotional Support

Lavender (*Lavandula angustifolia*) 10 drops

Mandarin (*Citrus reticulata*) 10 drops

Neroli (*Citrus aurantium* var. *amara*: Flowers) 4 drops

1oz. bottle with 4% dilution in 100% Jojoba

A two-week follow-up was conducted. G. stated that she is enjoying the emotional support blend and feels it is helping her to relax more and that the sore muscle blend is helping to reduce pain and allowing more movement in the neck and shoulders. She will continue using the blends as well as having a massage every two weeks.

(including spastic colon, colic, and constipation), sports injuries, stress, headache, TMJ (temporomandibular joint) dysfunction and much more (AMTA, 2005).

Aromatherapy can serve as a valuable complementary tool to enhance many of the above physical benefits of massage. For instance, the essential oils of peppermint (*Mentha* x *piperita*), clary sage (*Salvia sclarea*) and lavender (*Lavandula angustifolia*) can further relieve muscle tension and stiffness, reduce muscle spasm, and reduce stress. The essential oil of rosemary (*Rosmarinus officinalis*) or black pepper (*Piper nigrum*) can be used to enhance circulation. And the essential oil of pine (*Pinus sylvestris*) or eucalyptus (*Eucalyptus globulus*) can stimulate deeper breathing. One recent study points to the potential benefit of combining aromatherapy and massage to strengthen the immune system and reduce psychological stress (Kuriyama et al., 2005). Integrating aromatherapy with massage also enhances the psychological benefits of massage by reducing stress and helping individuals cope with a variety of other emotional issues. The integration of massage with aromatherapy in a variety of settings will be discussed in greater depth in Chapters 8 and 11.

Other areas where aromatherapy can enhance therapeutic bodywork and massage work include:

> ▶ **Spa therapy:** Aromatherapy is being used in various spa treatments and is commonly employed for a general aromatherapy massage session, during hydrotherapy or balneotherapy.

> ▶ **Cancer care:** Aromatherapy is being introduced into complementary medicine for cancer patients to reduce stress, tension, anxiety, and fear as

well as for general comfort therapy. Aromatherapy is also being applied for its physiological benefits of healing radiation burns and reducing nausea.

▶ **Hospice care:** Aromatherapy is being used to reduce undesirable odors in the air, to enhance quality of life and mood, to support family members, and as a general comfort therapy.

▶ **Elderly care:** Aromatherapy is being used to enhance skin integrity, reduce stress, tension, anxiety, and fear, as well as to enhance quality of life.

Clinical research by nurses and massage therapists are supporting the use and introduction of aromatherapy into hospital and hospice settings throughout the United States. According to leading nurse aromatherapist, Jane Buckle, Ph.D. (2003), "Because health insurance is so expensive, one of the most acceptable ways of integrating aromatherapy into a hospital or health facility is to link research to reducing cost of care." Thanks to the dedication of individual nurses and massage therapists who utilize aromatherapy as a complementary therapy, hospitals and other healthcare centers are beginning to recognize that aromatherapy can be of great benefit.

Buckle (2003) reports that aromatherapy is increasingly being used in hospitals and other clinical environments:

▶ to relieve postsurgical pain and anxiety
▶ to promote sleep
▶ to reduce stress
▶ to reduce chronic pain
▶ to heal skin ulcers
▶ to relieve emotional distress

Aromatherapy promises to be a valuable complementary therapy for bodyworkers and massage therapists in a wide range of settings. This text will address many of the valuable ways in which aromatherapy can be introduced and integrated into all kinds of bodywork and massage practices.

THE LANGUAGE OF AROMAS

Aromatherapy appears to be suffering from an identity crisis and has been since its rapid growth within the retail industry throughout the late 1980s and into the present time. The average consumer is confused as to what aromatherapy is and if there is a difference between synthetic fragrances and genuine essential oils.

In aromatherapy, language becomes crucial in defining the profession as well as providing a clear identity for its practice and growth within the public and private sector. Language provides insight into a given subject and often defines a practice. The language we use in relation to the practice of aromatherapy is crucial in educating the general public on genuine aromatherapy. Since the vast majority of the public thinks of perfume when one uses the word "fragrance," one would like to put forth that aromatherapists begin to use a more specific language that more adequately describes aromatherapy as a holistic healing therapy. The following words relate to and express genuine aromatherapy:

Aroma: An odor arising from spices, plants, cooking, etc., especially an agreeable odor.

Aromatic: Having an aroma; fragrant or sweet-scented; odoriferous.

Aromaticity: The quality or state of being aromatic.

Fragrant: Having a pleasant scent or aroma.

Scent: A word derived from the French "*Sentir,*" which means to feel, smell. Also based on the Latin word "*Sentire*" meaning to feel or perceive (Classen, 1993).

However, many individuals, even aromatherapy practitioners, use the word "fragrance" when describing an essential oil or an aroma. Essential oils and aromas both have a reference back to plants and to natural scents or odors. Fragrance, on the other hand, has a reference back to perfume and cologne as can be seen in the very definition of "fragrance." It would seem that the use of the word "fragrance" furthers the misconceptions of what aromatherapy is, particularly among the general public. Therefore, it may be prudent for each person who practices genuine aromatherapy to refrain from using the term "fragrance," since it inadequately describes genuine aromatherapy and the essential oils (nature's aromas) that have been derived from medicinal plants.

Fragrance: Perfume, cologne, toilet water, or the like; the quality of being fragrant.

(All definitions, except for scent, have been taken from: *Webster's Encyclopedic Unabridged Dictionary of the English Language*. 1996. New Jersey: Random House.)

The language of aromas offers us a new vocabulary to work with. Although aromas contribute to our perception of the world and our own lives, we lack a true vocabulary for describing these individual aromas. This may be because aromas or odors do not get remembered as a word or even as a scent/odor, but rather an aroma will be remembered by its meanings and memory-based associations. Describing an aroma is a highly individual experience so we need a universal vocabulary to describe particular characteristics of an individual essential oil aroma. The following is a list of words gathered from a book, *Perfume and Flavor Materials of Natural Origin*, by Stephan Arctander, which is considered to be a definitive guide to odor descriptions.

Table 1.1 presents a list of words that can be used to describe various aromas:

TABLE 1.1

Potential Words Used to Describe Different Aromas

Balsamic	Green undertone	Pine-like	Spicy-peppery
Balsamic-woody	Haylike	Powerful	Sweet
Bitter	Heavy	Pungent	Sweet-fruity
Bittersweet	Herbaceous	Radiant	Sweet-spicy
Camphoraceous	Honeylike	Rancid	Tea leaflike
Citrusy	Intensely sweet	Reminiscent of	Tenacious
Clean	Leafy-woody	Resinous	Turpentine-like
Earthy	Light	Rich and tenacious	Vanillin-like
Floral	Meadow-like sweetness	Rosy	Warm
Floral-woody	Medicinal, reminiscent of cough	Rosy-leafy	Warm-woody
Fresh	preparations	Root-like	Woody
Fresh-fruity	Mild	Smokey	Woody-green
Fruity-sweet	Minty	Soft	Woody-resinous
Fruity-warm	Musky animal-like	Spicy	
Grassy	Penetrating	Spicy-herbaceous	
	Peppery		

As you begin your studies of individual essential oils, you may want to refer back to this list and use these words to help describe the aroma of a given essential oil.

HOLISTIC FRAMEWORK

Complementary and alternative medicine (CAM) practices differ from orthodox medicine in their philosophy and approach to health and healing. This difference in approach can be attributed to the belief that arises from philosophical and conceptual ideas regarding the role of the practitioner in supporting the client back to health and wellness. While orthodox medicine, focusing only on the disease, seeks out an agent (microbe) or malfunctioning organ to either kill or repair, holistic therapies focus on healing the patient by addressing the nature of the disease within the context of the whole person.

Holistic CAM therapies, such as aromatherapy and bodywork, foster a cooperative relationship between client and practitioner with the goal of attaining optimal physical, mental, emotional, social, and spiritual well-being. It emphasizes the need to look at the whole person, including an analysis of physical, nutritional, environmental, emotional, social, spiritual, and lifestyle values.

The aim of developing holistic principles for the practice of aromatherapy for bodyworkers is to provide a basis for one's therapeutic approach. With a holistic framework of principles, practitioners are able to act continuously and consistently through a particular mind-set that guides them in their treatment approach and applications.

The majority of aromatherapy practitioners, as they have developed over the past twenty to thirty years, have professed certain philosophical themes that, when pulled together, provide the practitioner with a holistic framework for practice.

These themes include the ideas that aromatherapy:

> ▶ stimulates and supports the body's own natural healing abilities
> ▶ encompasses the whole person
> ▶ attempts to address the underlying causes of an illness
> ▶ is a preventative healthcare approach
> ▶ is about educating client and self on the nature of essential oils and their benefits
> ▶ adopts the philosophy of Hippocrates: *First, Do No Harm*

These common themes can be utilized to create six philosophical principles of holistic aromatherapy:

1. Stimulate and support the body's own natural healing abilities.

It is known that humans have an incredible ability and potential to facilitate self-healing. In naturopathic medicine this process is described as *Vis Medicatrix Naturae*, and it recognizes the individual's capacity to "self-right" or "self-heal." Aromatherapy, as a complementary therapy to bodywork and massage, is able to support and enhance the body's own natural healing abilities during acute and chronic stages of "dis-ease."

According to the NCBTMB, a massage therapy or bodywork practitioner is *"one who employs a conceptual and philosophical framework and uses knowledge of various systems of anatomy, physiology, and contraindications to facilitate the optimal functioning of individual human beings through the manual application of various modalities. The practitioner assesses the client to develop a session strategy, applies relevant techniques to support optimal functioning of the human body, establishes a relationship with the client that is conducive to healing, and adheres to professional standards for practice and a code of ethics."*

http://www.ncbtmb.com/Newsletter/emerging/fall97.htm

Figure 1-3 Mind/Body/Spirit drawing

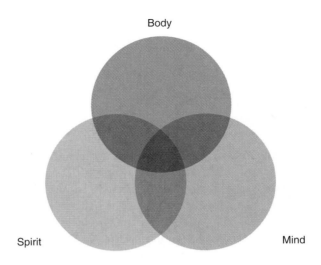

Body

Spirit

Mind

2. Encompass the whole (individual) person.

Holistic therapies recognize that an individual is a whole made up of interdependent parts, including the physical, mental, emotional, and spiritual (Figure 1-3). The integration of aromatherapy with bodywork and massage therapy practices creates a dynamic avenue which enables practitioners to work on each of these levels simultaneously. Aromatherapy and bodywork therapies recognize the uniqueness of the individual on all levels of being and treatment is customized according to individual needs and goals.

- **Mental/Emotional**
  Aromatherapy bodywork is able to affect the mental and emotional aspects of an individual via the power of touch as well as the olfactory link to the limbic system (the emotional brain).

- **Body (Physical)**
  Aromatherapy bodywork is able to affect the physical aspects of an individual via therapeutic benefits of massage as well as the therapeutic activity of essential oils (e.g., anti-inflammatory, antispasmodic, antimicrobial, etc.).

- **Spirit/Energy**
  Aromatherapy bodywork is able to affect the spiritual/energetic aspects of an individual via the power of touch as well as the energetic and spiritual impact of different aromas/essential oils.

3. Address the underlying cause of disease.

Tolle causum is the Latin expression for addressing the underlying cause of disease. While orthodox medicine seeks a diseased organ or invasive microbe, holistic aromatherapy seeks to find the imbalances that led to the manifestation of the disease state. As Hippocrates once said, "I would rather know the person who has a disease, than the disease a person has." Aromatherapists seek to understand the potential contributing factors of disharmony as well as the potential pathways for supporting the body in reaching its optimal state of being.

4. Practice aromacere (aromatherapist as teacher).

To be an aromatherapist, one must experience aromatherapy firsthand in all its therapeutic potential for healing. To teach is to share one's knowledge and experience of using aromatherapy within one's own life or within the lives of your clients, family members, or friends. To teach is to enhance and deepen one's understanding and awareness of the amazing effectiveness of aromatics by applying it within one's everyday life. The better your relationship is with aromatherapy the better you will be able to apply it with other individuals. This idea is reflected in bodywork and massage therapy education, where the therapist is trained by both receiving and giving treatments in order to better understand the benefits of the bodywork and massage technique being learned.

5. Use aromatherapy as preventative measure.

Aromatherapy can be used to reduce the likelihood of occurrence and/or prevent the manifestation of chronic degenerative disease when integrated into a whole health lifestyle. The use of aromatherapy for preventative measures often involves the reduction of stress as well as strengthening the immune system and uplifting a client's perception of their life, including stressors they may deal with on a day-to-day basis.

6. Practice *First, Do No Harm.*

The idea of *First, Do No Harm* is derived from the Hippocratic Oath of medicine. The idea is that the intervention used shall do more good than harm. In aromatherapy, this idea is expressed in our selection of essential oils, our understanding of their safety issues, as well as the understanding of the client's constitution. *You should always know about an essential oil prior to using it on a client.* This way you reduce the likelihood of an adverse reaction.

> As a healing tool combining both touch and smell or the physical and the non-physical, aromatherapy massage sits well in the holistic framework. The individual blends of oils mixed for the recipient's treatment are chosen to complement the person's physical and emotional state. Massage is the means of application, but, much more than that, it allows the giving of a caring and soothing touch, which helps to de-stress the system completely and sends deep messages of calm to the mind.
>
> —Jennie Harding (2005)

Adopting the above framework for the practice of aromatherapy would be of great benefit to bodywork and massage practitioners as it allows aromatherapy to be viewed as a holistic complementary therapy rather than a "treatment" approach to disease. It also keeps the practitioner from diagnosing and prescribing, which is outside the scope of practice for both the aromatherapist and bodywork practitioner. The holistic framework provides the therapist with a basis for a therapeutic approach that lays emphasis on supporting and enhancing the client's ability to reach health and well-being through facilitation utilizing bodywork and aromatherapy rather than through the treatment of a specific disease or illness.

Aromatherapy is indeed a dynamic profession with many potential applications in diverse settings. As this text unfolds, aromatherapy will be presented in a manner that is easy to understand and its application easy to integrate into any form of bodywork and massage therapy being practiced. I hope that this text inspires you to embrace genuine aromatherapy as a valuable complementary therapy that can deepen and expand your practice and life.

As aromatherapy bodywork and massage practitioners, we acknowledge that aromatherapy is a modality of healing and can serve as a complement to traditional or orthodox medicine. Aromatherapy practitioners are typically not qualified to diagnose, unless they are an M.D. or N.D., and hence the practice of aromatherapy is considered to be a complementary therapy.

In the words of the Associated Massage and Bodywork Professionals (AMBP) association (n/d): "Massage, bodywork and somatic therapies specifically exclude diagnosis, prescription, manipulation or adjustments of the human skeletal structure, or any other service, procedure or therapy which requires a license to practice orthopedics, physical therapy, podiatry, chiropractic, osteopathy, psychotherapy, acupuncture, or any other profession or branch of medicine."

SUMMARY

- Aromatherapy is one of the fastest growing complementary healthcare modalities of the twenty-first century and is practiced by a diverse set of lay people and practitioners, including naturopaths, nurses, massage therapists, independent aromatherapy consultants, occupational therapists, social workers, psychologists, reflexologists, and, at times and in some countries, by medical doctors.
- Aromatic plants and their aromas have been used throughout history and were popularized by the Greeks, Romans, and Egyptians. Aromatics have been used for their psychological impact as well as for medicinal purposes since early humanity.
- The term "aromatherapie" was coined by Rene-Maurice Gattefosse in 1937 and was meant to imply the therapeutic application of aromatic substances, specifically essential oils.
- Marguerite Maury made valuable contributions to the development of holistic aromatherapy. Her contributions include pioneering the dermal application of essential oils, being the first to integrate aromatherapy with massage, recognizing the importance of the individual, providing a holistic framework for the practice, and acknowledging the emotional/physical effects of essential oils when applied dermally.
- Aromatherapy is the holistic therapeutic application of genuine essential oils for enhancing the physical, emotional, mental, and spiritual health of the individual.
- The integration of aromatherapy with massage can effectively and holistically enhance the overall benefits of the massage or bodywork technique employed.
- The use of the term "fragrance" should be discouraged in the practice of aromatherapy as this may lead to misconceptions by the general public and clientele as to what genuine aromatherapy is and what a true essential oil is as differentiated from synthetic or adulterated fragrances.
- A holistic framework of aromatherapy bodywork includes the following ideas: stimulates and supports the body's own natural healing abilities, encompasses the whole person, attempts to address the underlying causes of an illness, is a preventative healthcare approach, is about educating client and self on the nature of essential oils and their benefits, and adopts the philosophy of Hippocrates: First do no harm.
- Diagnosing and prescribing are outside the scope of practice for both the aromatherapist and bodywork practitioner.

NEW TERMINOLOGY

Aromatherapy

Aroma

Aromatic

Aromaticity

Fragrant

Fragrance

Scent

⟶ REFERENCES

AMBP. (n/d). *Introduction to Massage*. Retrieved June 20, 2006, from http://www.massagetherapy.com/learnmore/index.php.

AMTA. (2005). *Massage Therapy: Facts for Physicians*. Retrieved March 10, 2006, from http://www.amtamassage.org/pdf/FactsForPhysicians.pdf.

Arctander, S. (1994). *Perfume and Flavor Materials of Natural Origin*. Carol Stream, Illinois: Allured Publishing Corp.

Buckle, J. (2003). Aromatherapy in the USA. *International Journal of Aromatherapy 13* (1), 9–17.

Classen, C. (1993). *Worlds of Sense*. London: Routledge Publishing.

Gattefosse, M. (1992). Rene-Maurice Gattefosse. *International Journal of Aromatherapy 4* (4), 18–19.

Griggs, B. (1991). *Green Pharmacy*. Rochester, VT: Healing Arts Press.

Harding, J. (2005). *Total Aromatherapy Massage*. London: Duncan Baird Publishers, Ltd.

Harris, R. (2003). Anglo-Saxon Aromatherapy: Its Evolution and Current Situation. *International Journal of Aromatherapy 13* (1), 9–17.

Kuriyama, H., Watanabe, S., Nakaya, T., Shigemori, I., Kita, M., Yoshido, et al. (2005). Immunological and Psychological Benefits of Aromatherapy Massage. *Evidence Based Complementary and Alternative Medicine 2* (2): 179–184. Oxford University Press.

Maury, M. (1989). *Marguerite Maury's Guide to Aromatherapy: The Secret of Life and Youth*. Essex, England: C.W. Daniel Company.

Ryman, D. (1989). Introduction to *Marguerite Maury's Guide to Aromatherapy: The Secret of Life and Youth*. Essex, England: C.W. Daniel Company.

Scott, C. (1993). In Profile: Dr. Jean Valnet. *International Journal of Aromatherapy 5* (4), 10–13.

Sheen, J. G., and Stevens, J. (2002). Aromatherapy as a Profession. *International Journal of Aromatherapy 12* (4), 189–191.

Tisserand, R. (1988). *Aromatherapy, To Heal and Tend the Body*. Wilmont, WI: Lotus Press.

Further Recommended Reading

Gattefosse, R. (1993). *Gattefosse's Aromatherapy*. Essex, England: C.W. Daniel Company.

Valnet, J. (1990). *The Practice of Aromatherapy*. Rochester, VT: Healing Arts Press.

1. The word "aromatherapy" was coined by:

    a. Marguerite Maury

    b. Jean Valnet

    c. Rene-Maurice Gattefosse

    d. Robert Tisserand

2. Which essential oil did Gattefosse use to heal his burns from a laboratory explosion?

    a. clary sage

    b. lavender

    c. ginger

    d. eucalyptus

3. List five conditions and/or types of clients that would benefit from the integration of aromatherapy with massage or bodywork.

    a.

    b.

    c.

    d.

    e.

4. Marguerite Maury is recognized for pioneering the dermal application of essential oils via massage.

    _____ True   _____ False

5. Marguerite Maury emphasized the importance of treating the _____.

    a. individual

    b. language used

    c. wound healing

    d. mind

6. List five top reasons an individual in the U.K. might visit an aromatherapist.

    a.

    b.

    c.

    d.

    e.

7. Aromatherapy is a useful complementary therapy for bodywork and massage because it can enhance the therapeutic benefits of the techniques applied.

    _____ True   _____ False

8. Aromatherapy affects the mind via which of the following pathways?

   a. olfaction

   b. inhalation

   c. dermal application

   d. the energetic body

9. The goal of a philosophical framework is to provide a practitioner with a basis for one's therapeutic approach.

   _____ True   _____ False

10. "First, do no harm" means that people can use essential oils even if they know nothing about them.

    _____ True   _____ False

REVIEW QUESTIONS

1. Discuss the importance of language in the practice of aromatherapy.

2. Discuss the contributions of three individuals to the development of aromatherapy.

3. Discuss how the use of aromatherapy can be a valuable complementary therapy in a wide range of bodywork and massage therapy settings.

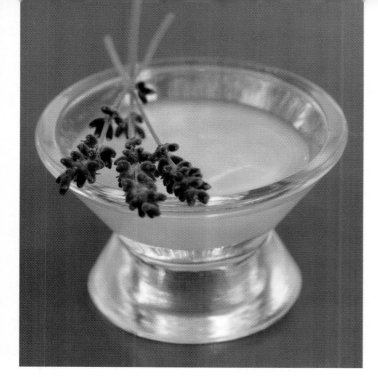

From Plant to Essential Oil

LEARNING OBJECTIVES

After reading this chapter, you will be able to

1. Discuss the importance of plants in relation to aromatherapy.
2. Describe four biological roles of essential oils within plants.
3. Describe the storage of essential oils within the plant.
4. Draw, label, and explain the general distillation process.
5. Define what an essential oil and a hydrosol are.
6. Briefly describe at least two other processes of extracting odoriferous substances from plants.
7. Discuss the difference between an expressed and a distilled citrus oil.

INTRODUCTION

You may be wondering why, as a massage therapist, you need to learn about plants? Aromatherapy depends upon pure, unadulterated, and genuine essential oils derived specifically from the living world of plants. You won't have to become a botanist or anything of that sort, but many aromatherapists or individuals who utilize aromatherapy products may never actually interact with the plants they are derived from. It is, however, important to have an appreciation for the plant world since without it genuine and authentic aromatherapy would not be possible. Genuine and authentic aromatherapy utilizes only essential oils derived directly from plants, avoiding, at all cost, the use of synthetics, reconstructions, perfumes, and other adulterated versions. The importance of this chapter is to develop an appreciation for our interconnected and symbiotic relationship with plants, how and why they produce essential oils, how essential oils are extracted, and how we put them to use once extracted.

↪ WHAT IS A PLANT?

"Plants mean nothing in isolation; they are a life-form rooted in and identified by their community, by their relationships to and interactions with all other life on Earth."
STEPHEN HARROD BUHNER, 2002, P. 177

Defining what a plant is has its difficulties. One could say that plants are green, have stems and roots, and normally produce flowers, resins, and/or fruits. However, this definition does not adequately define all plants nor does it convey an idea of the variations found within the plant world. There are many kinds of plants, ranging from tiny mosses and ferns to giant sequoias and eucalyptus trees. In aromatherapy, we will be studying two groups within the plant kingdom: the **angiosperms** or flowering plants, which include the vast majority of essential oils, and the **gymnosperms**, plants that lack flowers but produce seeds such as the conifers. Tables 2.1 and 2.2 outlines the botanical families and essential oils of the angiosperm and gymnosperm groups.

TABLE 2.1

Angiosperm/Flowering Plants Botanical Families and Essential Oils

Botanical Family	Essential Oils
Annonaceae	Ylang ylang
Betulaceae	Birch
Burseraceae	Elemi, Frankincense, Myrrh
Asteraceae/Compositae	Roman chamomile, German chamomile, Helichrysum, Inula, Yarrow
Geraniaceae	Geranium, Rose geranium
Gramineae	Lemongrass, Palmarosa
Lamiaceae/Labiatae	Basil, Catnip, Clary sage, Hyssop, Lavender, Melissa, Oregano, Patchouli, Peppermint, Rosemary, Sage, Thyme

TABLE 2.1 *(Continued)*

Botanical Family	Essential Oils
Lauraceae	Bay laurel, Cinnamon, Ravensara, Rosewood
Myristicaceae	Nutmeg
Myrtaceae	Clove, Eucalyptus, Myrtle, Tea tree
Piperaceae	Black pepper
Rosaceae	Rose
Rutaceae	Bergamot, Grapefruit, Lemon, Lime, Orange, Tangerine/Mandarin
Santalaceae	Sandalwood
Apiaceae/Umbelliferae	Angelica, Caraway, Carrot seed, Celery, Dill, Fennel, Parsley
Zingiberaceae	Cardamom, Ginger

TABLE 2.2

Gymnosperm Botanical Families and Essential Oils

Botanical Family	Essential Oils
Pinaceae	*Abies* (firs), *Cedrus* (cedar), Larix (larch), *Picea* (spruce), *Pinus* (pine), *Pseudotsuga* (Douglas fir), *Tsuga* (hemlock)
Cupressaceae	*Cupressus* (cypress), *Juniperus* (juniper), *Libocedrus* (incense cedar), *Thuja* (arborvitae)

Of the over 400,000 known species of plants, over half are members of the angiosperm group. The angiosperms and gymnosperms were the first groups in the plant kingdom to begin widespread production of essential oils. Early evolved plants, such as the bryophytes (e.g., mosses and liverworts) and seedless vascular plants (e.g., ferns), contained little to no essential oil. It is believed that as plant life evolved they began producing secondary metabolites, such as essential oils, in response to an increasingly changing environment.

Plants are structured in a physical body, and they depend on the soil, water, air, and sunlight to sustain life and perform complex chemical activity. This complex chemical activity produces **primary metabolites**, meaning they are vital to the plant's life, such as enzymes, protein, lipids, carbohydrates, and chlorophyll, and **secondary metabolites**, constituents that are not considered necessary for life, such as alkaloids, flavonoids, and essential oils.

Plants are **photoautotrophs**, which means they depend on the sun in order for photosynthesis to occur thereby producing complex organic compounds necessary to sustain life. All plants need sunlight to grow, with the exception of parasitic plants that are able to grow with or without sunlight. Humans, on the other hand, are considered **heterotrophs**. Humans depend on the release of oxygen from plants to provide the necessary energy to sustain life. Plants are responsible for their own growth and molecules by utilizing carbon dioxide, water, and various nitrates, sulfates, and other minerals found on earth and its atmosphere. Photoautotrophs are the only form of life that can transform radiant energy into chemical energy (photosynthesis).

↪ PLANTS AS MEDICINE

In her widely acclaimed book, *Green Pharmacy*, Griggs (1991) reminds us that "there is virtually no people known to anthropology—however remote, isolated or primitive—in which some form of doctoring with plants was not practiced" (p. 5). Plants have been used throughout history for medicine, food, clothing, and shelter. Plants provide a variety of active components including: fatty acids, essential oils, gums, resins, alkaloids, and steroids, all of which have found their way into medicine.

One example of plant-based medicine would be the *Eucalyptus* species, which is used to isolate the active constituent eucalyptol (syn. 1, 8 cineol) for its expectorating action. Eucalyptol is one of three essential oil compounds that makes up the famed chest rub, Vicks™ VapoRub. The other compounds include camphor from rosemary or camphor tree and menthol from peppermint. All three oils are used for the treatment of muscular aches and pains as well. Another example is the active constituent of birch (*Betula* ssp.), methyl salicylate, used for its analgesic properties; it is the active ingredient in BenGay™.

Other examples of important medicinal constituents from plants include the active compound salicin from the willow tree (*Salix* species), which is used as an anti-inflammatory and analgesic compound for treating headaches; the active compound digitoxin from foxglove (*Digitalis purpurea*), which is used to treat heart conditions; steroids from yams (*Dioscorea* species), which are used to create cortisone, oral contraceptives, and hormone-based drugs; and morphine from the opium poppy (*Papver somniferum*). Approximately 80 percent of the world's population still depends on medicinal plants for their primary healthcare, and approximately 20 percent of modern drugs have either been extracted from plants or are synthetically reproduced based upon isolated chemicals from plants (De Silva and Atal, n/d).

Our environment of plants is important. Indeed humans and plants have a crucial symbiotic relationship based upon an interconnectedness and interdependence with the natural world. This relationship is crucial not only for our own survival but for the survival of the plant world. Exploring the biological role of essential oils within plants sheds light on some of the very same reasons humans use essential oils. Historically and in modern times, humans have utilized essential oils to attract and even repel other beings (consciously or unconsciously), to protect against microbial agents, to support respiration, and to defend against pests and insects such as mosquitoes.

↪ THE BIOLOGICAL ROLE OF ESSENTIAL OILS WITHIN PLANTS

While essential oils are in the plant, they are constantly changing their chemical composition, helping the plant to adapt to the ever-changing internal and external environment. Recent scientific research has shown that plants produce essential oils for a variety of purposes including:

▪ **To attract pollinators and dispersal agents:** Insects have been pollinating flowers for over 200 million years. Insects, like humans, are attracted to specific plants for one of three possible reasons: its aroma, its color, or its morphology or physical structure. According to Shawe (1996), scent appears to be more ancient than flower color as an attractant to insects (p. 25). Various insects, including bees, butterflies, and even beetles, are known to be attracted to the aroma of a plant.

■ **To play a role in allelopathy, a type of plant-to-plant competition:** **Allelopathy** occurs when a plant releases chemicals to prevent competing vegetation from growing within its area or zone. An often cited example is in southern California, home to the dominant shrubs *Salvia leucophylla* (sage bush) and *Artemisia californica* (a type of sage). Both species release allelopathic terpenoids, eucalyptol and camphor, into the surrounding area, which effectively prevents other plant species from growing around them. This is allelopathy. Chemicals that deter competing growth (terpenes, for example), are referred to as **allelochemics**.

■ **To serve as defense compounds against insects and other animals:** Plants, like other living things, need to protect themselves from various types of predators. Plants use terpenoid compounds to deter insects and other animals from approaching them. Shawe (1996) pointed out that "insects are very rarely found on peppermint plants and the presence of linalol in the peel of citrus fruits confers resistance to attack by the Caribbean fruit fly" (p. 26). The Douglas fir tree releases a complex mixture of volatile oils, or terpenes, from their needles to defend against the spruce budworm. Even more fascinating is that the Douglas fir trees "will vary the composition and production of terpenes each year thus decreasing the ability of the budworm to develop widespread immunity to specific compounds" (Buhner, 2002, p. 160).

■ **To protect the plant by their antifungal and antibacterial nature:** Resins and complex combinations of terpenes are released by some plants and trees, such as evergreens, to act as antimicrobial, antifungal, and antibacterial agents against a wide range of organisms that may threaten the survival of the plants or tree. Compounds such as sesquiterpene lactones found in plants such as feverfew, yarrow, and blessed thistle, have been found to play a strong antimicrobial role as well as a protective role from herbivores.

THE STORAGE OF ESSENTIAL OIL WITHIN THE PLANT

Plants store essential oils either in **external secretory structures**, which are found on the surface of the plant, or **internal secretory structures**, which are found inside the plant material. Usually with plants having external secretory structure, you just have to lightly touch them and you will notice an aroma imparted to your skin. With plants having internal secretory structures, you will need to break the leaf, seed, or other plant material in order to get to the aroma/essential oil.

External Secretory Structures

Glandular Trichomes

External secretory structures in plants are called **glandular trichomes**. They can be found on the surface of the plant (such as herbaceous leaves) and are thought to be responsible for the production of chemicals that deter or attract pests or pollinators.

Figure 2-1 Trichome from *Origanum dictamnus*
Source: Jennifer Forman Orth

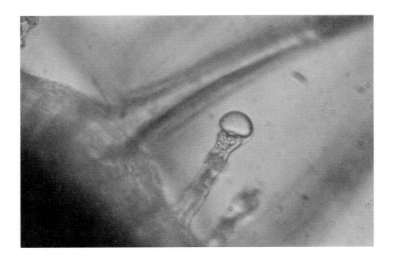

Figure 2-2 Trichome from *Rosmarinus officinalis*
Source: Jennifer Forman Orth

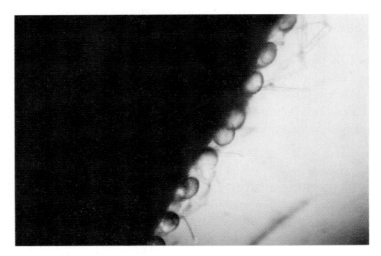

Glandular trichomes are most commonly found in the Lamiaceae (syn. Labiatae) family. The oil storage capacity varies from species to species and also between trichomes. Biochemical experiments have shown that these volatile oils are synthesized by highly refined enzyme reactions taking place within the plant. See Figures 2-1 and 2-2 for images of glandular trichomes.

Common essential oils that have glandular trichomes: Basil, Lavender, Marjoram, Melissa, Oregano, Peppermint, Rosemary, and Spearmint

Internal Secretory Structures

Secretory Cavities and Ducts

"**Secretory cavities and ducts** consist of large, intercellular spaces that are formed either by the separation of the walls of neighboring cells, or by the disintegration of cells" (Svoboda, 1996, p. 26). Cavities occur as spherical spaces and are most commonly found in the Myrtaceae and Rutaceae families. Ducts are more elongated spaces and are most commonly seen in the Asteraceae (syn. Compositae), Pinaceae, Apiaceae (syn. Umbelliferae), and Coniferae families.

Common essential oils with secretory cavities: Citrus oils: Bergamot, Grapefruit, Lemon, Lime, Orange, and Tangerine; Eucalyptus species; Clove bud; and Resin trees: Benzoin, Frankincense, and Myrrh.

Common essential oils with secretory ducts: Angelica, Caraway, Carrot seed, Dill, Fennel, Fir, Cedar, Pine, Spruce, Juniper, and Cypress.

Essential Oil Cells

Essential oil cells are found within the plant tissue and are unique from other cells in content and size. They can often be found throughout the plant and are most commonly seen in the Lauraceae, Piperaceae, Gramineae, and Zingiberaceae families.

> **Common essential oils with cells:** Bay Laurel, Black pepper, Cardamon, Cinnamon, Citronella, Ginger, Lemongrass, Nutmeg, Palmarosa, and Patchouli.

⤳ METHODS OF EXTRACTION

It is common in the mass market to refer to just about anything that is liquid in a brown bottle and smells as an essential oil. Even within the aromatherapy profession, many call absolutes and CO_2 extracts as essential oils. Technically, however, only distilled or expressed substances are essential oils. The International Organization for Standardization (ISO) in their Vocabulary of Natural Materials (ISO/D1S9235.2) defines an **essential oil** as a product made by distillation with either water or steam or by mechanical processing of citrus rinds or by dry distillation of natural materials. Following the distillation, the essential oil is physically separated from the water phase.

According to Dr. Brian Lawrence (2000) "for an essential oil to be a true essential oil, it must be isolated by physical means only. The physical methods used are distillation (steam, steam/water and water) or expression (also known as cold pressing, a unique feature for citrus peel oils). There is one other method of oil isolation specific to a very limited number of essential oil plants. This is a maceration/distillation. In the process, the plant material is macerated in warm water to release the enzyme-bound essential oil. Examples of oils produced by maceration are onion, garlic, wintergreen, bitter almond, etc." (p. 8).

For our purposes, we shall summarize the above within the context of aromatherapy and therefore define **essential oils** as highly concentrated aromatic extracts that are distilled or expressed from a variety of aromatic plant material, including flowers, flowering tops, fruits/zests, grasses, leaves, needles and twigs, resins, roots, seeds, and woods.

> *A pure essential oil is a vibrant, dynamic liquid which almost seems to have a life quality of its own. An essential oil destined for aromatherapy should come from an organically grown, properly tended plant source, and certain standards are also required during distillation.*
>
> —Robert Tisserand (1988)

NOTE: GUMS AND RESINS

Resins, such as frankincense, myrrh, and benzoin, are very thick and sticky when extracted from the tree. In aromatherapy, resins such as frankincense and myrrh are distilled, resulting in an essential oil that is more fluid and easier to pour. Benzoin, although an uncommon oil, cannot be distilled and remains a thick resinoid. Often benzoin will be diluted down with a perfume grade alcohol to make it more usable. Resins are used in perfumes as fixative agents to prolong the fragrant effects of perfumes. Frankincense and myrrh are the most commonly used resins for a wide range of therapeutic benefits in aromatherapy.

The two methods of extracting an essential oil include:

> ▶ **Distillation:** Produces essential oils and hydrosols (hydrolats).
> ▶ **Expression:** Produces citrus oils, which can also be called essential oils.

Other methods that are used to produce other aromatic products include:

▶ **Solvent extraction:** Produces absolutes.
▶ **Enfleurage:** Produces absolutes.
▶ **CO_2 extraction:** Produces CO_2 extracts.

The Practice of Distillation

Distillation appears to have been practiced throughout ancient times. According to Schnaubelt (2002), "Based upon the current interpretation of Paolo Rovesti's discovery of an earthenware distillation apparatus, the production or extraction of aromatic oils by means of steam distillation has been known for 5000 years" (p. 81). During the fifth century AD, the famed writer, Zosimus of Panopolis, refers to the distilling of a divine water and panacea. Throughout the early Middle Ages and beyond, a crude form of distillation was known and was used primarily to prepare floral waters or distilled aromatic waters. These appear to have been used in perfumery, as digestive tonics, in cooking, and for trading.

Although an extensive trade of odoriferous material has been shown to have occurred in the ancient Orient and ancient Greece and Rome, the oils used were not essential oil, "rather they were obtained by placing flowers, roots, and other plant material into a fatty oil of best quality, submitting the glass bottles containing these mixtures to the warming influence of the sun and finally separating odoriferous oil from the solid constituents" (Guenther, 1982, p. 9). In 900 AD, Avicenna, the famous child prodigy from Arabia who wrote many documents on plants and their uses and also instructions for massage, was accredited with refining the process of distillation by improving the cooling system. Today distillation is still the most common process of extracting essential oils from plants. The advantage of distillation is that the volatile components can be distilled at temperatures lower than the boiling points of their individual constituents and are easily separated from the condensed water. See Figure 2.3 for Vetiver and geranium distillation unit.

Preparation of Plant Material

Some types of plant material require preparation prior to distillation. Since essences are stored in a variety of locations within the plant, such as glandular trichomes, oil cavities, ducts, and cells, it is sometimes necessary to crush, open, or in some other manner prepare the plant material in order for the plant to release its essence during the distillation process. Plants, such as those in the Lamiaceae/Labiatae family, tend not to need much preparation. However, woods, roots, and seeds do need preparation. Seeds are crushed to release their aromatic essence prior to distillation. Woods are often cut into shorter lengths in order to expose the oil glands. The main purpose of preparing plant material is to allow easier access to the volatile constituents as the steam passes through the material. Immediately after the plant material has been prepared, it must be distilled. If the plant material is not distilled immediately, two things may occur: (1) the total quantity yielded will be reduced, and (2) the composition and hence the aroma will be altered by evaporation of some of the constituents.

Once the plant material has been prepared, it then enters the distillation process. The three types of distillation include:

■ **Water distillation:** The plant material comes into direct contact with the water. This method is most often employed with flowers (rose and orange blossoms), as direct steam causes these flowers to clump together making it difficult for steam to pass through.

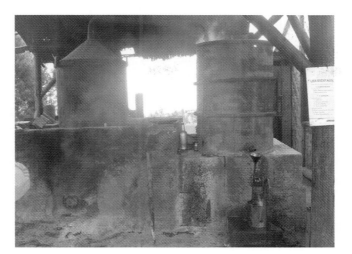

Figure 2-3 Vetiver and geranium distillery
Source: David Monniaux

■ **Water and steam:** This method can be employed with herb and leaf material. During this process, the water remains below the plant material, which has been placed on a grate while the steam is introduced from outside the main still (indirect steam).

■ **Steam distillation:** This method is the most commonly used. During this process, steam is injected into the still, usually at slightly higher pressures and temperatures than the above two methods.

> **NOTE ON BOILING POINT**
>
> The boiling point represents the temperature at which a liquid is converted to a gas at a specified pressure.
>
> The fundamental nature of steam distillation is that it enables a compound or mixture of compounds to be distilled (and subsequently recovered) at a temperature substantially below that of the boiling point(s) of the individual constituent(s). Essential oils contain substances with boiling points up to 200°C or higher, including some that are solids at normal temperatures. In the presence of steam or boiling water, however, these substances are volatilized at a temperature close to 100°C at atmospheric pressure (Food and Agriculture Organization of the United Nations, 1995).

The Distillation Process

During distillation the plant material is placed upon a grid inside the still. Once inside, the still is sealed, and, depending upon the above methods, steam or water/steam slowly breaks through the plant material to remove its volatile constituents. These volatile constituents rise upward through a connecting pipe that leads them into a condenser. The condenser cools the rising vapor back into liquid form. The liquid is then collected in a vehicle below the condenser. Since water and essential oil do not mix, the essential oil will be found on the surface of the water where it is siphoned off. Occasionally an essential oil is heavier than water and is found on the bottom rather than the top, such as clove essential oil.

Percolation or Hydro-Diffusion

This is a relatively recent method and is very similar to steam distillation except that the steam comes in through the top rather than the bottom, and there is a shorter

Figure 2-4   Distillation

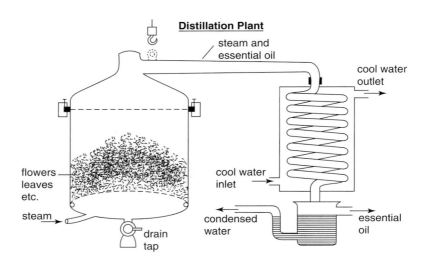

distillation time. It is useful in extracting essential oils from woody or tough material or seeds such as fennel and dill.

Expression

Expression, also referred to as **cold pressing**, is a method of extraction specific to citrus essential oils, such as tangerine, lemon, bergamot, sweet orange, and lime. In older times, expression was done in the form of sponge pressing, which was literally accomplished by hand. The zest or rind of the citrus would first be soaked in warm water to make the rind more receptive to the pressing process. A sponge would then be used to press the rind, thus breaking the essential oil cavities, and absorb the essential oil. Once the sponge was filled with the extraction, it would then be pressed over a collecting container, and there it would stand to allow for the separation of the essential oil and water/juice. The essential oil would finally be siphoned off. (See Figure 2-4.)

A more modern method of extraction, and less labor-intensive, has been termed the **ecuelle a piquer** process that involves a prodding, pricking, sticking action to release the essential oil. During this process, the rind of the fruit is placed in a container having spikes that will puncture the peel while the device is rotated. The puncturing of the rind will release the essential oil that is then collected in a

HYDROSOLS: A BY-PRODUCT OF DISTILLATION

Hydrosols, also known as hydrolats, are the by-product of the distillation process. Hydrosols contain the *water-soluble constituents* of the aromatic plant and retain a small amount of essential oil. According to Catty (2001), "every liter of hydrosol contains between 0.05 and 0.2 milliliter of dissolved essential oil, depending on the water solubility of the plant's components and the distillation parameters (p.12). The therapeutic benefits of utilizing hydrosols will be discussed in Chapter Nine.

*Please Note: The addition of essential oils to water is not at all the same as true hydrosols, and it is recommended that you read the ingredients label on products to ascertain whether or not you are getting a true hydrosol. When water and essential oils are mixed together with or without a dispersant, this is called a "spritzer" or "aromatic spritzer," and this product should not be confused with a true hydrosol.

small area below the container. The end process is the same as above. The majority of modern expression techniques are accomplished by using machines using centrifugal force. The spinning in a centrifuge separates the majority of essential oil from the fruit juice.

EXTRACTION TECHNIQUES FOR ABSOLUTES AND CO_2 EXTRACTS

The following methods of extraction, enfleurage, solvent extraction, and CO_2 extraction, will only be briefly discussed. This textbook does not cover the therapeutic use of CO_2 extracts or absolutes.

Enfleurage

Flowers were being processed via enfleurage in the Grasse region of Southern France long before the modern method of solvent extraction. In the early days of perfumery, many flower scents were extracted via enfleurage, now considered an ancient art that is passed down from father to son or from generation to generation. Enfleurage is a cold-fat extraction process that is based upon the principles that fat possesses a high power of absorption, particularly animal fat. The fat used must be relatively stable against rancidity. It is a method used for flowers that continue developing and giving off their aroma even after harvesting (e.g., jasmine and tuberose). Today, Grasse continues to be one of the few areas in the world that continues to employ enfleurage as a method of extraction, although it is rare in the aromatherapy market due to the expense. If one finds a jasmine enfleurage on the market, this would typically be considered an absolute.

Solvent Extraction

Some plant material is too fragile to be distilled and an alternative method must be employed. **Solvent extraction** is the use of solvents, such as petroleum ether, methanol, ethanol, or hexane, to extract the odoriferous **lipophilic** material from the plant. The solvent will also pull out the chlorophyll and other plant tissue, resulting in a highly colored or thick/viscous extract. The first product made via solvent extraction is known as a concrete. A **concrete** is the concentrated extract that contains the waxes and/or fats as well as the odoriferous material from the

WHAT IS THE DIFFERENCE BETWEEN EXPRESSED AND DISTILLED CITRUS OILS?

Some aromatherapy companies sell both a distilled and an expressed citrus essential oil from the same species. The main differences between a distilled and an expressed citrus essential oil have to do with their toxicity, volatility, and aroma. Distilled citrus oils deteriorate more quickly and are considerably more unstable than the expressed oils. According to Williams (1996), distilled citrus oils are not recommended for aromatherapy use. The one exception would be for distilled lime essential oil, which is considered to be superior in aroma to its expressed counterpart.

Both the expressed and distilled essential oil of bergamot (*Citrus bergamia*) contains the phototoxic furanocoumarin, bergaptene. The aroma of the distilled oil is considered to be of lower quality than the expressed.

plant. The concrete is then mixed with alcohol, which serves to extract the aromatic principle of the material. The final product is known as an **absolute**.

Solvent extraction is used for jasmine, tuberose, carnation, gardenia, jonquil, violet leaf, narcissus, mimosa, and other delicate flowers. Neroli and rose can be distilled or solvent-extracted. The name *neroli* typically implies the essential oil, whereas the name orange blossom is commonly used for the absolute or hydrosol of neroli. The name *rose* is used to describe either the essential oil or the absolute. Companies selling essential oils should clarify whether the product you are purchasing is an essential oil or absolute. This information should be on the label and in the product catalog.

After the solvent extraction process has been completed, the resulting absolute will have an extremely low concentration of solvent residue, approximately 5 to 10ppm (parts per million). According to Guba (2002), "the current European Union standards are for less than 10 parts per million solvent residues in a finished absolute" (p. 124). However, even with such a potentially small residue (less than .0001%), many aromatherapists disagree with the use of absolutes for individuals with a compromised immune system due to the potential effect of the residual solvent. However, absolutes do have therapeutic value and are often used for psychological purposes and for animals, particularly horses. Many therapists incorporate absolutes, such as rose absolute, jasmine, and tuberose, as a valuable part of their therapeutic applications of aromatherapy. Ultimately the decision to use absolutes is up to the practitioner and his/her own personal preferences.

Absolutes are highly concentrated aromatic substances and are obtained from delicate flowers by either enfleurage or solvent extraction. Absolutes will most often resemble the natural aroma of the plant and are normally more colored and viscous than essential oils. Absolutes are used extensively in the cosmetic and perfume industries due to their strong aromas. There are also different grades of absolutes. The top grade is the uncut, which can be a thick or semisolid substance, making them difficult to work with. Less expensive grades are diluted with alcohol to make them more user-friendly, although often the strength of aroma is slightly diminished.

CO_2 Hypercritical Extraction

Hypercritical carbon dioxide (CO_2) extraction is a relatively new process used for the extraction of aromatic products. The basic concept is that CO_2 under pressure will turn from a gas into a liquid that can then be used as an inert liquid solvent. This liquid solvent is able to diffuse throughout the plant material thus extracting its aromatic constituents. CO_2 extracts contain most of the same constituents as their essential oil counterparts, although they can contain some elements not found in essential oils. For instance, the essential oil of ginger (*Zingiber officinale*) does not contain the bitter principles, however the CO_2 extract does. Also, the CO_2 extract of frankincense (*Boswellia carterii*) has immune enhancing and anti-inflammatory activity not found in the essential oil. CO_2 extracts are known for their strong similarity in aroma to the actual plant aroma.

According to Guba (2002), the three main disadvantages for this process are cost, potential pesticide residue, and the lack of information regarding their safety and therapeutic benefits. With regard to pesticide residue, Guba comments that "carbon dioxide extraction has been demonstrated to concentrate from 7 to 53 times more pesticide residues in the final extract." Therefore, it seems pertinent to only use organic plant material for CO_2 extraction. Perhaps as more CO_2

extracts become available and more practitioners use them, further details regarding their applications will become apparent. Two of the most common essential oils available via CO_2 extraction include frankincense and ginger.

ESSENTIAL OILS IN MODERN TIMES

Essential oils are produced for a variety of purposes, and they are distilled all over the world. They are utilized by a wide range of industries, including the cosmetic, pharmaceutical, tobacco, food and flavoring, and perfume industries. They are used as preservatives in cosmetics, flavors in food, insect repellants, fragrance compounds for perfumes and body care products, antimicrobial compounds in such products as mouthwashes, and masking agents for unpleasant odors. Essential oils and their isolated constituents have been the focus of research for their antimicrobial activity and other medicinal benefits. They offer a plethora of uses within the above industries as well as others.

This would lead one to wonder, are the essential oils used in all the above industries the same essential oils we use in aromatherapy? Most of the industries listed above are not necessarily concerned with the purity and wholeness of the essential oil, and in fact many will have fragrance oils made in a lab to maintain consistency in aroma or to reduce the cost of making a product. For genuine aromatherapy and effective applications, the purity and wholeness of the essential oil cannot be understated. We will be addressing this issue in the next chapter.

In the words of Schnaubelt (2004), "Genuine and authentic essential oils from plants are necessary conditions of wholistic aromatherapy. They are fundamentally different from the industrial, semi-natural oils which are commonly offered on the market. As semi-natural or synthetic oils are materially different from authentic oils it is logical that their physiological effects are also different. Most importantly, authentic oils are much less allergenic and irritant than their industrial counterparts.(p.33)"

SUMMARY

- Holistic therapeutic aromatherapy must utilize the most genuine and authentic essential oils extracted from known botanical sources in order to maintain its efficacy and safety. The use of synthetics, reconstructions, perfumes, or cheap adulterated essential oils reduces the effectiveness of the therapy and may lead to adverse reactions.
- Plants produce essential oils for a variety of purposes, including to attract pollinators and dispersal agents, to play a role in allelopathy (plant-to-plant competition), to serve as defense compounds against insects and other animals, and to protect the plant by their antifungal and antibacterial nature.
- Plants store essential oils either in external (found on surface of plant) secretory structures, known as glandular trichomes, and internal (found within the plant) secretory structures, known as cavities and ducts or essential oil cells.
- Genuine and authentic essential oils are produced from aromatic plants via distillation or expression. Odoriferous substances extracted via enfleurage or

solvent extraction are known as absolutes, and aromatic substances extracted via CO_2 extraction are known as CO_2 extracts.

■ The fundamental nature of steam distillation is that it enables a compound or mixture of compounds to be distilled (and subsequently recovered) at a temperature substantially below that of the boiling point(s) of the individual constituent(s).

■ True hydrosols are a by-product of the distillation process and are not a mixture of water and essential oil. A combination of water and essential oils would correctly be called an aromatic spritzer.

■ Expression, also referred to as cold pressing, is a method of extraction specific to citrus essential oils, such as tangerine, lemon, bergamot, sweet orange, and lime.

■ Solvent extraction is the use of solvents, such as petroleum ether, methanol, ethanol or hexane, to extract the odoriferous lipophilic material from the plant.

■ Hypercritical carbon dioxide (CO_2) extraction utilizes CO_2 under pressure, which then turns from a gas into a liquid and can be used as an inert liquid solvent. CO_2 extracts contain most of the same constituents as their essential oil counterparts, although they can contain some elements not found in essential oils.

NEW TERMINOLOGY

Absolutes	External secretory structures
Allelochemics	Glandular trichomes
Allelopathy	Gymnosperm
Angiosperm	Heterotrophs
CO_2 extraction	Internal secretory structures
Cold pressing	Lipophilic
Concrete	Percolation
Distillation	Photoautotrophs
ecuelle a piquer	Primary metabolites
Enfleurage	Secondary metabolites
Essential oil	Secretory cavities and ducts
Essential oil cells	Solvent extraction
Expression	

REFERENCES

Arctander, S. (1994). *Perfume and Flavor Materials of Natural Origin*. Carol Stream, Illinois: Allured Publishing Corporation.

Buhner, S. (2002). *The Lost Language of Plants*. White River Junction, Vermont: Chelsea Green Publishing.

Catty, S. (2001). *Hydrosols: The Next Aromatherapy*. Rochester, VT: Healing Arts Press.

De Silva, T., and Atal, C.K. (n/d). *Processing, refinement and value addition of non-wood forest products*. Retrieved August 18, 2005, from http://www.fao.org//docrep/V7540e/V7540e18.htm.

Food and Agriculture Organization of the United Nations (1995). *Basic Principles of Steam Distillation*. Retrieved August 18, 2005, from http://www.fao.org/docrep/V5350e/V5350e13.htm.

Griggs, B. (1991). *Green Pharmacy*. Rochester, Vermont: Healing Arts Press.

Guba, R. (2002). The Modern Alchemy of Carbon Dioxide Extraction. *International Journal of Aromatherapy 12* (3), 120–126.

Guenther, E. (1982). *The Essential Oils*. Melbourne, Florida: Krieger Publishing.

Lawrence, B. (2000). Essential Oils: From Agriculture to Chemistry. *NAHA's World of Aromatherapy III Conference Proceedings*, 8–26.

Schnaubelt, K. (2002). *Biology of Essential Oils*. San Rafael, CA: Terra Linda Scent.

Schnaubelt, K. (2004). *Aromatherapy Lifestyle*. San Rafael, CA: Terra Linda Scent.

Shawe, K. (1996). The Biological Role of Essential Oils. *Aromatherapy Quarterly 50*, 23–27.

Simpson, B.B., and Ogorzaly, M.C. (1995). *Plants in Our World*. United States: McGraw-Hill, Inc.

Svoboda, K. (1996). The Biology of Fragrance. *Aromatherapy Quarterly 49*, 25–28.

Tisserand, R. (1988). *Aromatherapy, To Heal and Tend the Body*. Wilmont, WI: Lotus Press.

Tisserand, R., and Balacs, T. (1995). *Essential Oil Safety*. New York: Churchill Livingstone.

Williams, D. (1996). *The Chemistry of Essential Oils*. Dorset, England: Micelle Press.

Experiential Exercise for Secretory Structures

In Class: Your instructor will pass around four different types of plant material: rosemary (leaves), orange (peel), fennel (seed), and ginger (root).

Experiencing internal and external secretory structures can be accomplished by interacting with different plant material. Rub some rosemary between your hands and experience how the aroma is imparted onto your skin; break open the peel of an orange and/or fennel seed and smell the aroma; cut open a fresh piece of ginger to release its essential oil.

Compare the aroma that accompanies the actual plant with the aroma of the essential oil. Describe any differences or similarities and make notes below. Also comment on your perception of the aroma from the plant and how it affected you.

Rosemary:

Orange:

Fennel:

Ginger:

CHAPTER TEST

1. Essential oils are products of _____ within the plant.
   a. primary metabolism
   b. photoautotrophs
   c. secondary metabolism
   d. steroids

2. One of the active components of Vicks VapoRub is:
   a. gingerol
   b. terpenol
   c. eucalyptol
   d. linalyl acetate

3. The most ancient plant attractant for insects is:
   a. size
   b. aroma
   c. morphology
   d. color

4. When a plant releases chemicals to prevent the growth of competing vegetation, this is called:
   a. heterotroph
   b. photosynthesis
   c. allelopathy
   d. pollination

5. _____ are considered external secretory structures.
   a. Cells
   b. Citrus cavities
   c. Resin ducts
   d. Glandular trichomes

6. Which essential oil is derived from a secretory cavity?
   a. spearmint
   b. tangerine
   c. cardamom
   d. lemongrass

7. Citrus oils extracted via expression are considered to have a superior aroma when compared to the distilled oil, with the exception of _____.

   a. tangerine

   b. bergamot

   c. lime

   d. lemon

8. Solvent extraction produces:

   a. an absolute

   b. an essential oil

   c. a citrus oil

   d. a pomade

9. The following is an example of plant material that is commonly found either as a distilled essential oil or absolute:

   a. peppermint

   b. rose

   c. lemon

   d. ginger

10. Frankincense and myrrh are most commonly produced via:

    a. enfleurage

    b. solvent extraction

    c. distillation

    d. expression

REVIEW QUESTIONS

1. Why are plants an important aspect of aromatherapy?

2. Describe two methods of extraction specifically for essential oils.

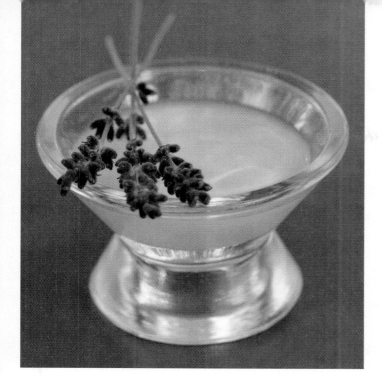

LEARNING OBJECTIVES

After reading this chapter, you will be able to

1. List and describe eight pieces of information to look for in purchasing an essential oil.
2. Describe the optimal storage conditions for an essential oil.
3. List and describe seven general characteristics of essential oils.
4. Discuss the importance of utilizing high-quality, unadulterated organic essential oils.
5. Perform four basic purity tests and discuss the value of a GC/MS analysis.
6. Describe potential dermal reactions and apply knowledge of safety information when using essential oils.
7. List and describe five general safety precautions and three safety measures.

INTRODUCTION

Holistic aromatherapy begins with the quality and authenticity of the essential oils to be utilized. Optimal therapeutic and safe applications can only truly be derived from the use of whole, genuine, authentic essential oils. The use of low-quality, cheap, or inexpensive adulterated essential oils increases the likelihood of an adverse response and/or reduced therapeutic activity. Companies selling a wide range of essential oils seem to be a dime-a-dozen these days. An internet search on aromatherapy will produce over 10,000 links to this plethora of "aromatherapy" businesses. So how does one choose? What information should you look for? How do you know if it is adulterated? How should essential oils be stored? How safe are essential oils? These are important questions, and by the end of this chapter you will be able to answer each one accurately with knowledge and experience.

ESSENTIAL OIL INFORMATION

When looking for essential oils to purchase and from what company, there are a number of factors to consider. Aromatherapy companies should provide uniform information on each essential oil they sell. This information is often found on the essential oil label and/or in their product catalog. This information should include:

■ **Common name:** The common name is the most widely accepted name for a given plant species within a given culture or regional area. Common names, however, do not always correctly identify an exact botanical species because these names are often used generally for all hybrids or cultivars that belong to that species. Common names can also vary from region to region as well as in various countries throughout the world.

For aromatherapy purposes, one must be able to identify the exact essential oil being used. For instance, if one were to say "I used lavender in the blend", almost everyone would think of the type of lavender they are familiar with. Lavender in this context could be *Lavandula angustifolia* or a cultivar, such as *L. angustifolia* "Maillette" or the hybrid Lavendin (*L.* x *intermedia*). Each of these essential oils has a slightly different chemical composition and is applied for different therapeutic purposes. The common name is great for the general public, but for the practitioner, it is best to document and identify each essential oil used during a session by its Latin name.

■ **Latin name: botanical specificity:** The Latin name is the internationally recognized identity of a given plant and is often referred to as the plant's scientific name. When referring to the botanical specificity of an essential oil, the Latin binomial is used. The **Latin binomial** refers to one kind of plant, critically distinguished from all others, and identifies a biological species name consisting of two terms: **genus** and **species**.

The **genus** refers to a group or category of plants that are similar in botanical structure. The genus name is the first word and is always italicized and capitalized, for example, *Lavandula*. The **species** name identifies the exact plant within a specific genus. Species has to do with direct characteristics of the plant, including leaf structure, flower structure, reproduction, and other characteristics within a family of plants. The species name is technically the full Latin binomial but is represented in the second name, for example, *angustifolia*. Species names are always italicized and in lower case. The full Latin binomial of lavender would then be *Lavandula angustifolia*.

To appreciate the importance of the Latin binomial, we will look at the eucalyptus species. There are over 250 species of the eucalyptus genus, of which 6 to 8 are commonly found within the aromatherapy industry. These may include *Eucalyptus globulus, Eucalyptus dives, Eucalyptus citriodora, Eucalyptus smitthi, Eucalyptus camaldulensis, Eucalyptus polybractea, Eucalyptus stageriana,* and *Eucalyptus radiata*. Although there are many common therapeutic benefits to all eucalyptus species, each one also has its own unique chemistry and therefore therapeutic applications. Another example of a genus with numerous species is the chamomile plant. Chamomile has three unique species, including *Chamaemelum mixtum, Matricaria recutita*, and *Chamaemelum nobile*.

A variation of a Latin binomial you may come across in your study and use of essential oils regarding botanical nomenclature is a **hybrid**. A hybrid is the result of a cross-fertilization between two different plant species and/or two varieties within a species. Hybrids are symbolized through the use of a multiplication sign ($\times$), for example, *Lavandula $\times$ intermedia* is a hybrid between *Lavandula angustifolia* and *Lavandula spica*.

■ **Country of origin:** The country of origin reflects the country where the essential oil is either indigenous or where it is cultivated or harvested in the wild. The country of origin can have an effect on the chemical composition of a given essential oil due to differences in environmental conditions, such as light, soil, temperature, moisture, climatic influence, and altitude as well as geographic area. Essential oils from the same botanical species but different countries may also have vastly different aromas, and often essential oils from a specific country may be considered superior to those from other countries. For instance, lavender (*Lavandula angustifolia*) from France is commonly considered to be a superior oil than the same oil from other countries.

■ **Part of plant used: morphological specificity:** Some plants produce essential oils from more than one part, such as from the seed and root or the flower, fruit, and leaf. These are known as **morphological structures** (e.g., leaf, fruit, etc.). One such botanical species that bears essential oils from three different morphological structures is the bitter orange tree, *Citrus aurantium* var. *amara*. From the bitter orange tree we obtain petitgrain from the leaves, neroli from the orange blossoms, and bitter orange from the zest of the fruit.

This is not a chemotype or a species difference. It is simply one botanical species that bears three separate essential oils from three different parts of the plant. Petitgrain and neroli are commonly used for their antidepressant and stress-relieving properties; however, each one has a unique aroma and a slightly different chemical composition. When a plant produces essential oils in more than one of its parts, differences in aroma and chemical composition occur.

Another example is the essential oils obtained from the cinnamon tree, *Cinnamomum zeylanicum*. Cinnamon bark essential oil has the characteristic "cinnamon" aroma, is rich in cinnamic aldehyde, and is considered to be a major skin irritant when used undiluted or in high dosages. Cinnamon leaf, on the other hand, has a cinnamon-clovelike aroma, is rich in the phenol, eugenol, and is less irritating to the skin. Both oils have a wide range of antimicrobial activity, although cinnamon leaf tends to be more commonly employed by aromatherapists.

The parts of a plant an essential oil can be extracted from include:

Berries: Juniper

Buds: Clove

Flowering tops (flower and top leaves): Clary sage, Geranium, Lavender, Rosemary

Flowers: Roman and German chamomile, Jasmine, Lavender (English), Rose, Ylang ylang

Fruits/Zests: Bergamot, Grapefruit, Lemon, Lime, Mandarin, Orange

Grasses: Lemongrass, Palmarosa

Leaves: Basil, Eucalyptus, Melissa, Patchouli, Petitgrain, Peppermint, Tea tree, Thyme

Needles and twigs: Cypress, Fir, Pine

Resins: Benzoin, Elemi, Frankincense, Myrrh

Roots/Rhizomes: Angelica, Garlic, Ginger, Vetiver

Seeds: Angelica, Black pepper, Cardamom, Celery, Coriander, Dill, Fennel

Wood/Trees: Cedarwood, Cinnamon, Sandalwood

■ **Biochemical specificity:** **Biochemical specificity** refers to the identification of a chemotype of a specific essential oil. Many factors influence the chemical composition of any given essential oil, including environmental conditions such as light, soil, temperature, moisture, climatic influence, and altitude as well as geographic area.

The term "**chemotype**" is used to describe essential oils that have been extracted from one botanical species yet vary in chemical compositions (Bowles, 2003). Catty (2001) defines a chemotype as follows: "A chemotype occurs when a plant of a specific genus and species produces a particular chemical in a higher than normal amount because of geographic location, weather, altitude, insect and environmental interactions, and the like. A chemotype is not a different species or genus, nor is it a type of chemical; it is merely a chemical anomaly within the plant that occurs naturally" (p. 67).

Not all essential oils have chemotypes nor are all chemotypes available in the market. Rosemary (*Rosmarinus officinalis*) and thyme (*Thymus vulgaris*) are the most common chemotypes available within the aromatherapy industry. A chemotype will be noted as follows: Rosemary **ct**. verbenon or Thyme ct. linalol.

Rosemary is one botanical species that produces three well-known chemotypes. Bowles (2003) states: "Rosemary oil from Spain is known as CT1 and has higher levels of camphor, whereas Rosemary from Tunisia is known as CT2 and contains higher levels of 1,8 cineole (eucalyptol). A third rosemary chemotype, CT3 from France, has higher levels of verbenone, which is thought to be a less toxic ketone than camphor." According to Barker (1996), it is vitally important that the most suitable chemotype of rosemary oil be chosen for clinical use.

The full essential oil datasheet is provided for Rosemary ct. camphor and following is a synopsis of the core applications for Rosemary ct. 1,8 cineol and ct. verbenon.

Rosemary ct. 1,8 Cineole

Therapeutic Actions

Mild analgesic, antidepressant, anti-inflammatory, antirheumatic, antiseptic, antispasmodic, **antiviral**, carminative, **cephalic**, digestive, **expectorant**, **mucolytic, stimulant**.

Core aromatic applications:

▷ has a direct correlation with the respiratory and pulmonary systems of the body
▷ expectorant, respiratory decongestant
▷ excellent mucolytic, anticatarrhal applications
▷ antifungal agent (Barker, 1996)
▷ antibacterial agent (e.g., *Staphylococcus aureus, staph. alba*) (Barker, 1996)
▷ analgesic for headaches and the pain of rheumatoid arthritis
▷ cerebral tonic, stimulates mental functions
▷ bronchitis, sinusitis, flu, common cold (Haas, 2004)

Rosemary ct. Verbenon

Therapeutic Actions

Mild analgesic, antiviral, expectorant, **mucolytic**, **stimulant**, **vulnerary**

Core aromatic applications:

▷ mucolytic and cell regenerating, skin care (Haas, 2004)
▷ endocrine regulator; effective in treating postmenopausal syndrome especially hot flashes, useful for postnatal depression (Barker, 1996)
▷ general and nerve stimulant, restores psychological balance (Goeb, 1996)

■ **How it is grown:** Typically an aromatherapy supply company should be able to tell you how the plant was grown. There are four main types of ways a plant can be grown:

Ethical wild-crafted: Plants that have been collected in the wild or in their native environment. Ethically wild-crafted means that a company or individual has taken care to insure that the "species can withstand harvesting and still proliferate" (Catty, 2001).

Cultivated: Plants that are specifically grown to be distilled for essential oils.

Traditional/Conventional: Plants that have been grown with the use of pesticides.

Organic: Plants that have been grown without the use of pesticides and usually fulfill organic guidelines set out by independent agencies. Organic farming is not just the absence of pesticides, but the presence of an agricultural system that protects croplands, supports biodiversity, and respects the balance of nature rather than attempting to control it with powerful, often toxic synthetic chemicals. The Organic Trade Association (1995) defines organic agriculture as "an ecological production management system that promotes and enhances biodiversity, biological cycles and soil biological activity. The primary goal of organic agriculture is to optimize the health and productivity of interdependent communities of soil life, plants, animals and people."

■ **Batch number:** Some aromatherapy companies supply a **batch number**. This batch number is used to identify a specific batch or drum of essential oil, from a specific supplier, during a specific year. The batch of essential oil will be accompanied by a specific independent GC/MS (Gas chromatography/Mass spectrometry, see Quality Assurance section below for further details) analysis for that batch.

■ **Standard safety warning on essential oils:** The standard safety note on the vast majority of essential oils is *Not for internal use. Keep away from children.* Essential oils are not commonly used internally and are not recommended for internal application without the supervision or advice of an individual qualified to do so. The internal use of essential oils is beyond the scope of this textbook and further education is highly recommended. It is important to keep all essential oils out of reach of children as some can be highly toxic, especially if taken internally. Many aromatherapy companies will note in their catalog and/or on their website that caution should be taken when utilizing essential oils during pregnancy. This issue is addressed later in the section on safety in this chapter.

■ **Size of bottle/essential oil content:** Most essential oil companies use the metric system for describing the amount of essential oil within a bottle. The most common sizes found within aromatherapy are:

> 5 milliliters (mls) is the equivalent of 1/6 of an ounce
> 10 mls is the equivalent of 1/3 of an ounce
> 30 mls is equal to 1 ounce
> 120 mls is equal to 4 ounces
> 240 mls is equal to 8 ounces

↪ STORAGE INFORMATION

Essential oils have a general shelf life of two to five or more years depending on the individual oil and the manner in which they are stored. For instance, citrus oils tend to have a much shorter shelf life than more viscous essential oils such as vetiver or patchouli. It is wise to replace citrus essential oils every six to twelve months to avoid adverse reactions caused by oxidation of compounds found within them. Adhering to the following guidelines will enhance the longevity of essential oils.

■ **Essential oils are stored in amber or blue bottles:** Essential oils are volatile organic compounds that are sensitive to heat and light. It has been an accepted part of the aromatherapy industry that essential oils need to be in a dark-colored glass to protect them from ultraviolet rays from the sun and other similar light.

■ **Bottles must have an appropriate orifice reducer:** To reduce the impact of oxygen on essential oil degradation, all essential oil bottles must have an appropriate orifice reducer. This is a small dropper insert that fills the opening of the bottle. Eyedroppers *should not be used* as these are porous and hence allow oxygen to enter into the essential oil. Essential oils will also slowly dissolve the plastic on an eyedropper leading to plastic (rubber) in the essential oil as well as disintegration of the dropper.

Orifice reducers serve two other important purposes in addition to reducing oxidation. These purposes include:

1. to prevent excessive/large amounts of the oil coming from the bottle in case a child has gotten a hold of the oil and
2. to allow the practitioner to count the appropriate number of drops

■ **Essential oils are best stored away from sunlight and direct heat:** Essential oils are susceptible to heat and light and hence are best stored in a relatively cool area and away from direct light. Tisserand (1995) recommends that essential oils be stored in the refrigerator to increase shelf life (p. 10). Some aromatherapists follow this guideline while others simply choose to store their essential oils in a cool area. The most important essential oils to refrigerate are the citrus oils.

■ **Move essential oils to smaller bottles:** If you are purchasing essential oils in 1, 2, 4, 8, 16 or 32-ounce sizes, then it is important to pour essential oils into a smaller container once a certain amount has been used. As you use an essential oil from a larger bottle, the headspace of air between the top of the bottle and the essential oil increases, which can increase oxidation of the oil. It is therefore prudent to pour the essential oil into a smaller bottle to decrease the headspace and thereby reduce to some extent the potential for oxidation.

↪ GENERAL CHARACTERISTICS OF ESSENTIAL OILS

Essential oils display a set of general physical characteristics that give them their identity. In general, essential oils are:

■ **Highly concentrated:** This means that the therapeutic effect is considerably magnified. The fact that essential oils are highly concentrated makes them powerful agents, and often, due to their concentration, it is typically necessary to dilute them prior to use. Many aromatherapists believe that it is due to their incredibly high concentration that only a small amount is necessary to have therapeutic effects.

■ **Volatile substances: Volatility** refers to the ability of an essential oil to turn from liquid to vapor. An essential oil as a whole is volatile, and individual chemical constituents within an essential oil will volatize more or less quickly than others. For example, lemon is more volatile than vetiver, and limonene (a hydrocarbon terpene) is more volatile than borneol (an oxygenated hydrocarbon alcohol).

■ **Light and nongreasy:** The name essential oil can be deceptive. Essential oils are not vegetable or fatty oils, rather they are light, volatile substances that are referred to as "oils." They have a consistency more like water (although they are insoluble in water) than oil and lack the oily texture of vegetable oils (with the exception of viscous essential oils, such as sandalwood, vetiver, and myrrh).

■ **Mostly clear in color:** Most oils have a slight hint of color from clear to light yellow. A few essential oils do have some color, for example, German chamomile, tansy, and yarrow are all a deep rich blue; patchouli can be dark brown; and bergamot can have a light green tint. Absolutes tend to be richer in color due to the chlorophyll and other plant pigments drawn out by the solvent. Resinoids, such as benzoin, myrrh, and frankincense, tend to be dark in color unless they are distilled.

■ **Lipophilic:** Essential oils are **lipophilic** substances, which means they are attracted to and soluble in fatty substances. Essential oils have a strong affinity for lipids and are therefore soluble in:

Vegetable oils: Sweet almond, Sunflower, Apricot kernel, etc.
Herbal oils: Calendula, St. John's wort, Comfrey, and Arnica
Full fat milk, cream, or honey
Essential oils are also soluble in alcohol and ether.

■ **Viscosity: Viscosity** is the measurement of an essential oil's thickness. Viscous essential oils are less volatile than low-viscosity oils. Viscosity of an essential oil may slow down absorption through the skin. Viscous essential oils also tend to have a heavier aroma. For example, vetiver essential oil is very viscous compared to tangerine essential oil.

■ **Highly complex chemically:** Essential oils are made up of different combinations of a variety of chemical constituents. Some essential oils are considered to be simple in their chemistry, such as wintergreen or birch that contain up to 99 percent of one active constituent. Other essential oils are highly complex and contain over 100 different main constituents and hundreds more trace components. According to Schnaubelt (2004), "the therapeutic potential of essential oils arises from the synergistic action of the complex mixture of all its components" (p. 10).

■ **Dynamic substance that exhibits a wide range of therapeutic activity:** Essential oils exhibit a wide range of therapeutic activity, including psychological, physiological, spiritual, and energetic. One of the most researched aspects of essential oils is their antimicrobial and antiseptic activity. It is beyond doubt that essential oils are effective antifungal, antiviral, and antibacterial agents and that their natural aroma has an impact on our emotions, spirituality, perception, and behavior.

↳ QUALITY ASSURANCE

The concept of pure and natural or genuine and authentic within the aromatherapy profession is perhaps one of the most difficult concepts to ascertain. A pure essential oil is one that has been produced from a specified botanical source and has not been modified in any way whatsoever. According to Schnaubelt (2004), a genuine essential oil means it is completely unaltered and authentic means it is from a specified plant only. The adulteration of an essential oil may alter its unique therapeutic benefits as well as lead to increased risk of adverse reactions.

The aromatherapy industry worldwide has adopted terms such as: pure and natural, genuine and authentic, aromatherapy grade, true aromatherapy grade, therapeutic grade, and probably some others I am not yet familiar with. These terms are used by both discerning and non-discerning companies making it difficult to judge an essential oil merely by the marketing material a company puts forth. All the terms above are loosely defined, and there are absolutely no regulations at this time that govern the aromatherapy essential oil industry. (See Appendix 3 for reliable sources of genuine and authentic essential oils.)

Common Adulterations of Essential Oils

A number of methods may be employed to stretch, reconstruct, or otherwise alter an essential oil, and this is what is meant by adulteration. Adulterated essential oils pose a number of potential problems for aromatherapy such as: the potential increase in adverse dermal reactions (dermal irritation or sensitization) and the potential decrease in therapcutic benefits. Melissa, rose, sandalwood, and birch offer examples of essential oils that are commonly adulterated.

According to Burfield (2003–2005), "As far as adulteration is concerned, producers and distributors of essential oils are frequently painted as 'the bad guys,' but it should be pointed out that their oil customers frequently demand oils below the market price while still wanting to be told that they are authentic. In this climate, the honest oil trader may find it virtually impossible to survive on the margins he is allowed to make (many have already gone bust). For example, in the late 20th Century, lavender oil (*Lavandula angustifolia*) was being sold almost as a lost leader by many French producers as the market was unwilling to pay a realistic price; currently, the aroma industry is dominated by a handful of large and powerful

IN PRACTICE 3.1

Signs of Poor Quality

Signs of poor quality to watch for when purchasing essential oils include:

1. Essential oils are being sold at unreasonably low prices or all at the same price.

2. Rose, jasmine, sandalwood and melissa being sold in ½ to 1-ounce sizes. The average price of ½ ounce of rose otto essential oil is $195–200 and an ounce would be $400 or more. This makes it almost impossible to retail these oils in such a large quantity.

Due to the expense of all of these essential oils, most aromatherapy companies will offer them either by the drop or in 1ml, 2ml, or 5ml quantities.

international houses whose corporate buyers often attempt to drive raw material prices to impossibly low levels, not allowing workable profits to be made. This sets the scene for unethical practices."

Common adulterations to essential oils include such techniques as:

▶ Alcohol or a vegetable oil is added to stretch the volume of essential oil.
▶ A synthetic chemical constituent is added to the main oil to increase its volume. Arctander (1994) reports that bergamot and lavender are commonly adulterated by adding synthetic linalyl-acetate or synthetic linalol, respectively.
▶ A cheaper essential oil is added to or distilled with the main essential oil. According to Arctander (1994), melissa (*Melissa officinalis*) essential oil is often distilled with lemon, verbena, lemongrass, or citronella essential oil to increase the overall quantity of commercial melissa essential oil (p. 412). The plant, melissa or lemon balm, contains less than .01 percent essential oil so it takes a vast amount of plant material to produce a small amount of melissa, making it an expensive oil to purchase.
▶ A completely synthetic product is produced in a laboratory and can be marketed as natural. This is common for both wintergreen and birch essential oils that are typically 100 percent synthetic methyl salicylate.
▶ A cheaper essential oil is substituted, for example, lavendin for lavender.

BASIC PURITY TESTS

There are a number of ways in which you can test your essential oils for *basic* purity. The following are four basic tests you can do at home.

1. Place a drop of essential oil on a clean white sheet of blotting or watercolor paper. The essential oil should evaporate completely within a twenty-four to forty-eight-hour period, leaving no stain (unless the essential oil is colored, such as with some citrus oils and German chamomile) or reminiscent aroma. This method should not be employed with viscous essential oils, such as vetiver and sandalwood, as the more viscous the essential oil the longer evaporation will take. Citrus oils and others with a relatively high volatility are best suited to this basic test.

2. Place a drop of essential oil in a clear glass of water. If the water becomes discolored or turns milky, then the essential oil has been diluted with water and an emulsifier has been used to keep the essential oil and water together.

3. Place a drop of essential oil between two fingers on one hand and a drop of carrier or base oil between two fingers on the other hand and compare viscosity. There should not be the same oily texture to the essential oil as there is to the base oil. If it feels the same, then it is possible that the essential oil has been extended in a carrier or base oil. This process must be done by comparison and should not be utilized with the more viscous essential oils.

4. Our sense of smell is often underrated as a tool in determining the quality of an essential oil, but it is perhaps the most powerful tool we have, particularly once it has been trained and exercised. We are not typically accustomed to paying attention to our sense of smell so sometimes it takes practice and attention to strengthen it. In order to be able to effectively smell the quality of an essential oil,

one could spend time smelling diverse aromas in the environment and a range of qualities of essential oils. For instance, first smell an excellent quality essential oil (such as one from a company listed in Appendix 3), then immediately smell a questionable or low-quality essential oil (such as one sold for cheap in grocery stores or on-line). There should be a distinct difference in the quality and effect of the aroma. In time and with practice, your nose will become a great tool in determining the quality of an essential oil.

How to Smell an Essential Oil

Always approach essential oils with the awareness that they are very powerful. It is best to begin by holding the bottle or smell strip approximately four to five inches away from your nose and then move it upward toward your nose, depending on how much you can smell and how close you need it to be in order to enjoy its aroma.

As you hold the smell testing strip or the bottle of essential oil below your nose, gently move it back and forth from the left nostril to the right. This way you receive the full spectrum of aroma the oil has to give. The aroma will expand as you continue to smell, with several layers to the aroma. Natural, high-quality, genuine essential oils will be pleasant to the nose, whereas synthetics tend to attack the nose with a strong odor and then die off. Genuine essential oils continue to expand and develop as you smell them.

CHEMICAL ANALYSIS

The four basic tests for purity that you can practice at home are not considered full-proof methods by any means. Instead, essential oil buyers and sellers alike depend on a variety of scientific analysis to determine the composition and purity of an essential oil. We will discuss the two most common tests that are used to ensure the basic purity of essential oils via a chemical analysis of what the oil contains quantitatively and qualitatively.

Gas Chromatography

A **gas chromatography** (GC) is a chemical analysis instrument used to separate and identify individual constituents found within a given essential oil (Figure 3-1). Each chemical constituent of an essential oil will pass through the gas chromatograph instrument at different times and speeds. As each chemical is registered, it will produce some type of peak, from very short to very tall.

A gas chromatography report reveals the peaks of different chemical constituents within a given oil; it does not, however, name the specific chemical constituent (e.g., linalol); for this a mass spectrometry must be used.

Mass Spectrometry

Mass spectrometry (MS) is a technique that allows for the detection of compounds (chemical constituents) by separating ions by their unique mass. Mass spectrometry is utilized to identify specific compounds registered on the gas chromatography report. A typical mass spectrometer has three basic parts: an ion source, a mass analyzer, and a detector. Different molecules have different masses, and this fact is used to determine what molecules are present in a sample. An individual trained in reading GC/MS data will then clearly identify the exact

Figure 3-1 Gas Chromatography Report of Juniperus communis
Source: Dr. Robert S. Pappas

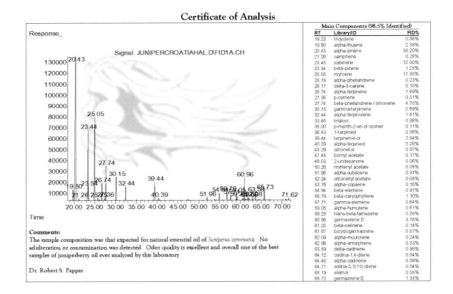

constituents and their quantity (e.g., 5% linalol, 25% camphor, and so on) present within a given essential oil sample.

According to Burfield (2005), "aromatherapists should not be too over-awed by the claims of essential oil traders, to the effect that GC-MS is the ultimate analytical tool. This simply is not true. When properly used it is certainly a powerful technique, but when used sloppily by untrained operators, the interpretation of results may be of limited value."

Interpretation of the information gained depends on the skill, experience, and knowledge of the individual who does the analysis. A GC-MS report may fail to reveal the age and quality of an essential oil, particularly in relation to the quality an aromatherapist is looking for. So, in general, although a GC-MS report on a given essential oil is incredibly helpful, it should not be used as the sole definitive guide to purchasing a high-quality, pure, unadulterated essential oil. Instead, it should be used along with an olfactory appraisal, confidence in the supplier and their intentions as a supplier (e.g., are they selling inexpensive essential oils to a general market or are they selling high-quality, typically high-priced essential oils specifically to practitioners of genuine aromatherapy?).

→ SAFETY AND ESSENTIAL OILS

Safety involves a state of being free from risk or occurrence of injury, harm, or danger. Individuals who practice aromatherapy need to be aware of the safety issues involved with using essential oils in order to avoid potential adverse effects. According to Burfield (2004), "Although many essential oils are potentially hazardous materials, if handled in the appropriate manner, the risks involved in their use can be very small. So therefore, most commercially offered essential oils are safe to use for the purpose intended in a domestic/professional or clinical environment." Schnaubelt (2004) states that the "informed use of essential oils may create occasional irritation or minor discomfort, but it is extremely unlikely to create serious injury or lasting physical problems," particularly when basic guidelines are followed.

Factors which influence the safety of essential oils include:

1. Quality of essential oil being utilized

As stated in the beginning of this chapter, adulterated essential oils increase the likelihood of an adverse response and hence the need for pure, authentic, and genuine essential oils is of the utmost importance.

2. Chemical composition of the oil

Essential oils rich in aldehydes (e.g., citronellal, citral) and phenols (e.g., cinnamic aldehyde, eugenol) may cause skin reactions. Oils rich in these constituents should always be diluted prior to application to the skin. According to Schnaubelt (2004), "diluting such oils so that the resulting solution becomes non-irritant, may require diluting them to concentrations much lower than in normal circumstances. Another option is to blend such irritant oils asymmetrically with other essential oils, which mitigate their irritant effects" (p. 45). For further details, see Chapter 4: The Chemistry of Essential Oils.

3. Method of application

Essential oils may be applied on the skin (dermally), inhaled, or taken internally. The potential safety concerns with dermal application will be discussed below. With regard to inhalation, Tisserand and Balacs (1995) state: "Inhalation, from a safety standpoint, presents a very low level of risk to most people. Even in a relatively small closed room, and assuming 100% evaporation, the concentration of any essential oil (or component thereof) is unlikely to reach a dangerous level, either from aromatherapy massage, or from essential oil vaporization" (p. 32). They further point out that "the only likely risk would be from prolonged exposure (perhaps 1 hour or more) to relatively high levels of essential oil vapor which could lead to headaches, vertigo, nausea and lethargy" (p. 32).

With regard to internal use, this method of application is not discussed in this textbook and further training is recommended prior to using essential oils internally.

4. Dosage/dilution to be applied

Most aromatherapy blends for massage and bodywork will be between 1 and 5 percent dilutions, which typically does not represent a safety concern. As one increases dilution, potential dermal (skin) reactions may take place depending on the individual essential oil, the area in which the oil is applied, and other factors related to the client's own sensitivity levels. Schnaubelt (2004) comments: "Any excessive usage of essential oils may cause irritation or other undesired effects due to their lipophilic nature" (p. 42).

5. Integrity of skin

Damaged, diseased, or inflamed skin is often more permeable to essential oils and may be more sensitive to dermal reactions. According to Tisserand and Balacs (1995), "It is potentially dangerous to put undiluted essential oils on to damaged, diseased or inflamed skin. Under these circumstances the skin condition may be worsened, and larger amounts of oil than normal will be absorbed. Sensitization reactions are also more likely to occur" (p. 77).

Possible Dermal Reactions

Of primary importance to the massage therapist and bodyworker is the safety of application to the skin. According to Tisserand and Balacs (1995), "skin reactions take three forms: irritation, sensitization and phototoxicity" (p. 77).

Dermal Irritant

A dermal irritant will produce an immediate effect of irritation on the skin. The reaction will be represented on the skin as blotchy or redness, which may be painful to some individuals. The severity of the reaction will depend on the concentration (dilution) applied.

General safety guidelines include: avoid application of known dermal irritant essential oils on any inflammatory or allergic skin condition; avoid undiluted application; avoid application on open or damaged skin; and dilute known dermal irritants with appropriate vegetable oil or other carrier. If you suspect a client has sensitive skin, perform a skin patch test (see below).

Table 3.1 lists some common essential oils considered to be dermal irritants.

Dermal Sensitization

Tisserand and Balacs (1995) define sensitization as "a type of allergic reaction. It occurs on first exposure to a substance, but on this occasion, the noticeable effect on the skin will be slight or absent. However, subsequent exposure to the same material, or to a similar one with which there is cross-sensitization, produces a severe inflammatory reaction brought about by cells of the immune system (T-lymphocytes)" (p. 78). The reaction on the skin will be red, irritated, and potentially raised patches, which may be painful to some individuals.

The problem with dermal sensitization is that once it occurs to a specific essential oil the individual is most likely going to be sensitive to it for many years and perhaps for the remainder of his/her life. The best way to prevent sensitization is to avoid known dermal sensitizers and avoid applying the same essential oils every day for lengthy periods of time. Tisserand and Balacs (1995) note that "sensitization is,

TABLE 3.1	
Dermal Irritants	
Essential Oil	**Latin Name**
Bay	*Pimento racemosa*
Cinnamon bark or leaf	*Cinnamomum zeylanicum* (Bark is more irritating than leaf)
Clove bud	*Syzygium aromaticum*
Citronella	*Cymbopogon nardus*
Cumin	*Cuminum cyminum*
Lemongrass	*Cymbopogon citratus*
Lemon verbena	*Lippia citriodora* syn. *Aloysia triphylla*
Oregano	*Origanum vulgare*
Tagetes	*Tagetes minuta*
Thyme ct. thymol	*Thymus vulgaris*
All citrus oils have the potential to be skin irritants if used in high dosages or undiluted.	

HOW TO PERFORM A SKIN PATCH TEST

Wash area to be used for testing. Best locations for testing include the outer arm or lower back. According to Clarke (2002), "a typical patch test is performed using the chosen essential oils at twice the concentration you intend to use in the massage" (p. 192). Place the blend to be used onto a Band-Aid and place inside of the appropriate location. Buckle (2003) recommends leaving the Band-Aid in place for twenty-four hours before assessing for any adverse reactions. Others have recommended that the test be carried out over a forty-eight-hour period. Once the Band-Aid is removed, check for signs of irritation.

Irritation will show as redness on the skin, burning itchy sensations, or raised skin as in blistering. If irritation should occur, gently wash the area with an unscented castile soap and place an unscented cream on the dry skin; also leave the skin open to the air for a while.

to an extent, unpredictable, as some individuals will be sensitive to a potential allergen and some will not" (p. 79).

According to Burfield (2004), the following oils listed in Table 3.2 are considered to be dermal sensitizers and are not recommended for use in aromatherapy massage.

Photosensitization

An essential oil that exhibits this quality will cause burning or skin pigmentation changes, such as tanning, on exposure to sun or similar light (ultraviolet rays). Reaction can range from a mild color change through to deep weeping burns. Do not use or recommend the use of photosensitizing essential oils prior to going into a sun tanning booth and for at least twenty-four hours after treatment if photosensitizing essential oils were used. Certain drugs, such as tetracycline, increase the

TABLE 3.2

Dermal Sensitizers

Essential Oil	Latin Name
Cassia	*Cinnamomum cassia*
Cinnamon bark	*Cinnamomum zeylanicum*
Peru balsam	*Myroxylon pereirae*
Verbena absolute	*Lippia citriodora*
Tea absolute	*Camellia sinensis*
Turpentine oil	*Pinus spp.*
Backhousia	*Backhousia citriodora*
Inula	*Inula graveolens*
Oxidized oils from Pinaceae family (e.g., Pinus and Cupressus species) and Rutaceae family (e.g., citrus oils)	

photosensitivity of the skin, thus increasing the harmful effects of photosensitizing essential oils under the necessary conditions.

Table 3.3 lists some common essential oils considered to be photosensitizers. The following citrus essential oils in Table 3.4 do not appear to be phototoxic.

Idiosyncratic Irritation or Sensitization

Idiosyncratic irritation or sensitization is an uncharacteristic or unusual reaction to a commonly used essential oil. This type of reaction is difficult to predict and rarely occurs but is a possibility.

Mucous Membrane Irritant

A mucous membrane irritant will produce a heating or drying effect on the mucous membranes of the mouth, eyes, nose, and reproductive organs. It is recommended

NOTE

To err on the side of caution, it may be prudent to advise clients to avoid sunbathing and tanning booths if a citrus essential oil has been used during a session.

TABLE 3.3

Photosensitizers

Essential Oil	Latin Name
Angelica root	*Angelica archangelica*
Bergamot	*Citrus bergamia*
Cumin	*Cuminum cyminum*
Distilled grapefruit	*Citrus paradisi*
Expressed lemon	*Citrus limon*
Expressed lime	*Citrus medica*
Distilled orange	*Citrus sinensis*
Distilled tangerine	*Citrus reticulata*
Verbena	*Lippia citriodora*

TABLE 3.4

Non-Phototoxic Citrus Oils

Essential Oil	Latin Name
Bergamot: Bergapteneless (FCF: Furanocoumarin Free)	*Citrus bergamia*
Expressed grapefruit	*Citrus paradisi*
Distilled lemon	*Citrus limon*
Distilled lime	*Citrus medica*
Expressed sweet orange	*Citrus sinensis*
Expressed tangerine	*Citrus reticulata*

TABLE 3.5 Mucous Membrane Irritants	
Essential Oil	**Latin Name**
Bay	*Pimento racemosa*
Caraway	*Carum carvi*
Cinnamon bark or leaf	*Cinnamomum zeylanicum*
Clove bud or leaf	*Syzygium aromaticum*
Lemongrass	*Cymbopogon citratus*
Peppermint	*Mentha x piperita*
Thyme ct. thymol	*Thymus vulgaris*

that mucus membrane irritating essential oils not be used in a full body bath unless placed in a dispersant first (e.g., milk, vegetable oil). Bay, clove, cinnamon bark, lemongrass, and thyme ct. thymol essential oils should be avoided in baths completely.

Table 3.5 lists some common essential oils considered to be mucous membrane irritants.

Other Safety Considerations

Safety During Pregnancy

The use of essential oils during pregnancy is a controversial topic and one that is yet to be fully understood. The main concern during pregnancy appears to be the risk of essential oil constituents crossing over into the placenta. According to Tisserand and Balacs (1995), "crossing the placenta does not necessarily mean that there is a risk of toxicity to the fetus; this will depend on the toxicity and the plasma concentration of the compound" (p. 105). Burfield (2000) states "it is probable that essential oil metabolites cross the placenta due to the intimate (but not direct) contact between maternal and embryonic or fetal blood" (p. 25). He goes on to say, "to my thinking the responsible attitude is to discourage the use of essential oils completely during the first few months of pregnancy" (p. 25).

Buckle (2003) comments that "the use of essential oils in pregnancy is a contentious subject, especially during the vital first 3-month period. It is extremely unlikely that a nightly bath containing a few drops of essential oils will cause any problems for the unborn child" (p. 95–96) and later states "there are no records of abnormal fetuses or aborted fetuses due to the 'normal' use of essential oils, either by inhalation or topical application" (p. 323).

According to Wildwood (2000), "A common myth in aromatherapy is that massage oils containing essential oils such as Clary sage, rose or even rosemary can cause a miscarriage and hence should be avoided throughout pregnancy. Authors such as Ron Guba, Kurt Schnaubelt, and Chrissie Wildwood have all pointed out that there have been 'no recorded cases of miscarriage or birth defect resulting from aromatherapy massage using therapeutic applications of any essential oil'" (p. 12).

Guba (2000) points out that toxicity during pregnancy is "almost exclusively due to pregnant women taking large, toxic doses of essential oils, notably pennyroyal (rich in the ketone, pulegone, which is metabolized to the highly toxic furan epoxide, menthofuron) and parsley seed (rich in the dimethyl ether, apiol) in an attempt to abort the fetus" (p. 40). And Battaglia (2002) shares this insight: "the judicious use of essential oils together with appropriate forms of massage by a skilled therapist can help ease the discomforts of pregnancy and provide a sense of nurturing that will comfort the mother at times she is likely to be feeling rather fragile" (p. 443).

Due to the lack of clear information regarding the toxicity of essential oils during pregnancy, it would be best to adhere to general safety guidelines. According to Tisserand and Balacs (1995), the following essential oils should not be used during pregnancy: wormwood, rue, oak moss, *Lavandula stoechas*, camphor, parsley seed, sage, and hyssop.

Essential oils that appear to be safe include cardamon, German and Roman chamomile, frankincense, geranium, ginger, neroli, patchouli, petitgrain, rosewood, rose, sandalwood, and other nontoxic essential oils (Tisserand and Balacs, 1995, p. 111). It would also be prudent to avoid the internal or undiluted application of essential oils throughout pregnancy. Aromatic applications during pregnancy will be discussed further under Prenatal/Postpartum massage in Chapter 11.

General Safety Precautions

1. Keep all essential oils out of reach of children.
2. Avoid use of photosensitizing essential oils and other citrus oils at least twenty-four hours prior to going sunbathing or into a tanning booth.
3. Avoid prolonged and/or daily use of the same essential oils, blends, or other fragrance products.
4. Avoid the use of essential oils you know nothing about on your clients. Research and get to know the oil prior to using it on others.
5. Avoid the use of undiluted essential oils on the skin, unless otherwise indicated.
6. If you suspect your client may be sensitive to specific essential oils or if your client has known allergies or sensitivities, it may be wise to perform a skin patch test.
7. Know the safety data on each essential oil to be used.
8. Use caution when treating a female client who suspects she is pregnant or has been trying to become pregnant.
9. Keep essential oils away from the eyes.
10. Essential oils are highly flammable substances and should be kept away from direct contact with flames, such as candles, fire, matches, cigarettes, and gas cookers (Buckle, 2003, p. 97).
11. Make sure your treatment room has good ventilation.
12. Do not use essential oils internally unless trained to do so.
13. Reduce or slow oxidation of essential oils by storing properly and limiting air exposure.

Safety Measures

1. According to Schnaubelt (2004), "if essential oils droplets accidentally get into the eye (or eyes) a cotton cloth or similar should be imbued with a fatty oil, such as olive or sesame, and carefully swiped over the closed lid" (p. 46). Then irrigate/flush eye with water.

Material Safety Data Sheets (MSDS)

The U.S. Occupational Safety & Health Administration requires that the "hazards of all chemicals produced or imported are evaluated, and that information concerning their hazards is transmitted to employers and employees. This transmittal of information is to be accomplished by means of comprehensive hazard communication programs, which are to include container labeling and other forms of warning, material safety data sheets and employee training."

Safety guidelines for essential oils can be found on a Material Safety Data Sheet (MSDS). MSDS sheets are required on all essential oils used within a healthcare facility and should also be kept in a massage or bodywork clinic employing essential oils as part of their treatment services. A sample MSDS sheet can be found in Appendix 2.

2. If an essential oil causes dermal irritation, apply a small amount of vegetable oil or cream to the area affected.

3. According to Buckle (2003), "if a child appears to have drunk several spoonfuls of essential oil, contact the nearest poison control unit (often listed in the front of a telephone directory). Keep the bottle for identification and encourage the child to drink whole milk. Do not try to induce vomiting (p. 96)."

SUMMARY

- For each essential oil in one's repertoire of oils, it is important to have the following information: common and Latin name, country of origin, part of plant used, biochemical specificity, how it is grown, and a batch number (if possible).
- Essential oils should be stored in amber or blue bottles, have an orifice reducer, and be stored away from sunlight or direct heat.
- Essential oils have a number of general characteristics: they are highly concentrated, volatile, mostly clear in color, lipophilic, light and nongreasy, highly complex chemically, and are diverse in their potential therapeutic applications.
- The importance of utilizing high-quality, pure, authentic, and genuine essential oils is crucial in holistic aromatherapy, not only to optimize the therapeutic benefits but also to reduce the likelihood of any adverse reactions.
- Factors that influence the safety of essential oils include the quality and purity of the essential oil, its chemical composition, the method of application, the dosage/dilution rate to be applied, and the integrity of the skin.
- Three possible dermal reactions to essential oils include dermal irritation, dermal sensitization, and photosensitization. Occasionally an individual reacts to a commonly used nontoxic essential oil; this is termed either idiosyncratic irritation or idiosyncratic sensitization.

NEW TERMINOLOGY

Batch number

Biochemical specificity

Botanical specificity

Chemotype

Dermal irritant

Dermal sensitizer

Gas chromatography

Genus

Hybrid

Idiosyncratic irritation

Latin binomial

Lipophilic

Mass spectrometry

Morphological structures

Mucous membrane irritant

Photosensitizer

Species

Viscosity

Volatility

⟶ REFERENCES

Arctander, S. (1994). *Perfume and Flavor Materials of Natural Origin*. Carol Stream, Illinois: Allured Publishing Corporation.

Battaglia, S. (2002). *The Complete Guide to Aromatherapy*. Brisbane, Australia: International Centre of Holistic Aromatherapy.

Bowles, E.J. (2003). *The Chemistry of Aromatherapeutic Oils*. Australia: Allen & Unwin.

Buckle, J. (2003). *Clinical Aromatherapy*. Philadelphia: Elsevier Science.

Burfield, T. (2000). Safety of Essential Oils. *International Journal of Aromatherapy 10* (1/2).

Burfield, T. (2004). *Opinion Document to NAHA: A Brief Safety Guidance on Essential Oils*. Retrieved October 2, 2005, from http://www.naha.org/articles/brief_safety%20guidance%20.htm.

Burfield, T. (2003–2005). *The Adulteration of Essential Oils and the Consequences to Aromatherapy & Natural Perfumery Practice*. Retrieved October 2, 2005, from http://www.naha.org/articles/adulteration_1.htm.

Burfield, T. (2005). *A Note on Gas Chromatography-Mass Spectrometry (GC-MS)*. Retrieved October 2, 2005, from http://www.naha.org/articles/adulteration_1.htm.

Catty, S. (2001). *Hydrosols: The Next Aromatherapy*. Rochester, VT: Healing Arts Press.

Clarke, S. (2002). *Essential Chemistry for Safe Aromatherapy*. Edinburgh, UK: Churchill Livingstone.

Guba, R. (2000). Toxicity Myths. *International Journal of Aromatherapy 10* (1/2)

Organic Trade Association (1995). *Definition of Organic*. Retrieved March 20, 2006, from http://www.ota.com/organic/definition.html.

Schnaubelt, K. (2004). *Aromatherapy Lifestyle*. San Rafael, CA: Terra Linda Scent.

Tisserand, R., and Balacs, T. (1995). *Essential Oil Safety*. New York: Churchill Livingstone.

U.S. Occupational Safety and Health Administration. (n/d). *Hazard Communication.* - 1910.1200. Retrieved October 2, 2005, from www.osha.gov/pls/oshaweb/owadisp.show_document?p_table=STANDARDS&p_id=10099.

Wildwood, C. (2000). Of Cabbages & Kings Aromatherapy Myths, part II. *Aromatherapy Today 14*, p. 12–14.

WORKSHEET

Exercise 1: Olfactory Exercise

The left and right sides of your nose will pick up different aroma qualities of the essential oils. To test this theory, simply occlude the right nostril and smell only with your left. Note below the qualities you observe. Then do the same by occluding the left nostril and smelling only with the right. Again, write down your observations. The final step is to smell the oil using the full spectrum of your sense of smell. Pass the aroma back and forth from your left to your right nostril and note the full spectrum of the aroma.

Notes

Left side perceptions:

Right side perceptions:

Perceptions using full range of smell of whole essential oil:

Exercise 2: Comparing Two Oils

Your instructor will share two essential oils from the same plant but of differing qualities, EO-A and EO-B. You will not be told which oils they are until the exercise is complete. After smelling each essential oil, answer the following questions:

Can you tell the difference between them?

Does one feel stronger? More potent?

Which one would you prefer to use?

Exercise 3: Basic Purity Test

Compare the viscosity between a vegetable oil and an essential oil. How does an essential oil differ from the vegetable oil? Write down your observations below.

CHAPTER TEST

1. The Latin binomial is made up of:

    a. the common name

    b. genus and species

    c. the chemotype

    d. the part of the plant an oil is extracted from

2. Biochemical specificity refers to:

    a. the Latin binomial

    b. the way a plant is grown

    c. specific chemotypes

    d. the common name

3. Viscosity refers to:

    a. the aroma of an oil

    b. the ability of an oil to evaporate

    c. the toxicity of an oil

    d. the thickness of an oil

4. A GC/MS analysis helps to determine:

    a. purity and chemical composition of an oil

    b. the origin of the oil

    c. the Latin binomial

    d. the quality of an oil

5. Dermal irritation is a reaction that:

    a. is an immediate reaction to an essential oil

    b. involves the immune system

    c. is a reaction from the sun

    d. is difficult to predict

6. Which of the following essential oils is considered a photosensitizer?

    a. lavender

    b. clary sage

    c. bergamot

    d. lemongrass

7. Which of the following essential oils is considered a dermal irritant?

   a. ginger

   b. cinnamon bark

   c. lavender

   d. clary sage

8. A GC/MS analysis is the sole definitive tool to determine the purity, quality, and age of an essential oil.

   _____ True   _____ False

9. Photosensitization is most commonly experienced by individuals with multiple sensitivities.

   _____ True   _____ False

10. It is perfectly safe to apply any essential oil during the early stages of pregnancy.

    _____ True   _____ False

REVIEW QUESTIONS

1. Discuss the importance of the Latin binomial in identifying an essential oil.

2. Discuss safety information and how to apply in practice.

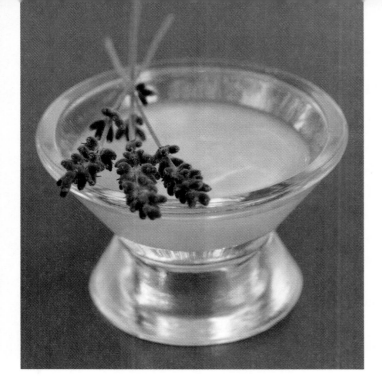

4

Basic Chemistry of Essential Oils

 LEARNING OBJECTIVES

After reading this chapter, you will be able to

1. Discuss the importance of studying organic chemistry in relation to the use of essential oils.

2. Define organic chemistry.

3. Explain the structure energy system and its value in understanding chemical families.

4. List ten chemical families found within essential oils.

5. List and discuss the general therapeutic actions for each of the ten families.

6. Discuss the potential toxicity of phenols, ketones, and furanocoumarins.

7. Apply your knowledge of the chemistry of essential oils in understanding their therapeutic benefits and actions as well as safety.

INTRODUCTION

The increasing role of science in complementary and alternative healthcare professions has been pivotal for those studying aromatherapy to better understand the chemistry of essential oils. It is this knowledge that allows a therapist to not only communicate more effectively with individuals in the medical or health professions but also to apply essential oils for their optimal therapeutic purpose. The chemistry of essential oils can often feel overwhelming for the beginner; however, it is an important aspect of developing a more complete picture of how and why essential oils have the therapeutic benefits that they have and how to apply them safely and effectively. The chemistry of essential oils can be compared to the anatomy and physiology of the body, for in understanding the framework of an essential oil one can come to understand how it works.

The goal of this chapter is to provide the basic vocabulary and framework for developing an understanding of essential oil chemistry. It is written using the common names for chemicals rather than the IUPAC (International Union of Pure and Applied Chemistry) system, which could be considered daunting at this stage of learning. For those seeking a greater understanding of the chemistry of essential oils, additional recommended reading is provided at the end of the chapter.

ORGANIC CHEMISTRY

Chemistry is the study of matter, its chemical and physical properties, the chemical and physical changes it undergoes, and the energy changes that accompany those processes. Compounds derived from plants fall into the realm of **organic chemistry** which is defined as: the study of matter composed principally of carbon and hydrogen. Organic chemistry was once known as the study of living organisms and/or substances which were derived from living organisms. It was believed to be impossible to synthesize an organic compound due to the 'life force' which emanated from the 'living' or 'once having lived' organism or substance. In the early half of the nineteenth century, however, a significant event occurred that forever altered the landscape of organic chemistry. In 1828, Friedrick Wohler, a German chemist, was able to successfully synthesize the organic compound urea from the inorganic compound ammonium carbonate. This achievement effectively broke the barrier between organic and inorganic within the context of its earlier definition and from this point on organic chemistry became the study of chemical compounds of carbon and hydrogen.

ORGANIC COMPOUNDS FOUND IN ESSENTIAL OILS

There are thousands of organic compounds biosynthesized within plants. Biosynthesis means that a plant creates diverse organic compounds. These compounds can be grouped into two major classes: primary metabolites, such as proteins, carbohydrates, and fats, and secondary metabolites such as essential oils, tannins, and alkaloids. The biochemical pathway leading to the creation of most terpenoid compounds is the mevalonate (mevalonic) acid pathway or the DOXP/MEP (deoxyxylulose

	TABLE 4.1

Synopsis of Terpenoid Compounds Found in Essential Oils

Family	Functional Group
Monoterpenes	Hydrocarbon
Sesquiterpenes	Hydrocarbon
Monoterpene Alcohols	Hydroxyl group (–OH)
Sesquiterpene Alcohols	Hydroxyl group (–OH)
Phenols	Hydroxyl group (–OH) attached to benzene ring
Phenylpropanoids	Basic 3-carbon chain attached to benzene ring
Esters	Carboxyl group (COOH)
Aldehydes	Carbonyl group (C=O)
Ketones	Carbonyl group (C=O) with only carbons attached directly to it
Oxides	Oxygen molecule situated between two carbon molecules
Sesquiterpene Lactones	Lactone ring structure derived from farnesyl pyrophosphate
Furanocoumarins	A type of coumarin; have 5-membered furan ring attached to a lactone ring adjoined to a benzene ring (Bowles, 2003)

phosphate/methylerythritol) pathway (Theis and Lerdau, 2003). Phenylpropanoids are formed via the shikimic acid pathway.

Essential oils contain simple hydrocarbons in the form of terpenes and more complex terpenoids called oxygenated hydrocarbons, or substituted hydrocarbons, in the form of alcohols, phenols, phenylpropanoids, esters, aldehydes, ketones, oxides, sesquiterpene lactones, and furanocoumarins (see Table 4.1).

Physical Characteristics of Organic Compounds

While reading about the families of chemicals found within essential oils, information on their physical characteristics and general therapeutic activity will be provided. Physical characteristics are those we can usually perceive through the senses. Physical properties include everything about a substance that can be observed, including color, odor, solubility in water, boiling point, and physical state.

■ **Polarity:** Each family is made up of either polar or nonpolar compounds. Polar compounds have a covalent bond made up of unequally shared electron pairs, with one end of the bond having more electrons and the other end having less electrons. Nonpolar compounds, on the other hand, have a center of both positive and negative charge and hence do not exhibit the two poles found in polar compounds.

■ **Volatility:** Volatility refers to the ability of the substance to turn from liquid to vapor. Some essential oil constituents are more readily volatile than others.

■ **Boiling point:** The boiling point represents the temperature at which a liquid is converted to a gas at a specified pressure.

■ **Solubility:** Solubility can be defined as the ability of a substance to dissolve in another. Essential oils are known to be soluble in vegetable oil, alcohol, ether, and other organic solvents. Essential oils, as a whole, are insoluble in water; however, the individual constituents making up the oil may or may not be more water soluble than the whole. Essential oils are considered to be lipophilic, meaning they are attracted to fatty substances.

General Therapeutic Actions

Each chemical family has been provided a section on the general therapeutic actions attributed to its family. These general therapeutic actions have been derived from the popular work of Daniel Penoel, Pierre Franchomme, and Kurt Schnaubelt. The system of attributing general therapeutic properties to each chemical family has been called the **structure effect (energy) system**. The system can be learned in more depth in *Advanced Aromatherapy, Aromatherapy Lifestyle* and *Medical Aromatherapy* by Kurt Schnaubelt. For the purpose of this text, a summation of the general therapeutic actions is provided (see Table 4.2).

It is important to note, however, that these general therapeutic actions are just that: general. Individual essential oil compounds have their own activity, which is often greater than the general actions given to them. Individual essential oil compounds must be understood on their own as much as within the whole. The goal of this section is simply to shed light on the generally accepted activity of various constituents found within essential oils so as to provide the basic framework necessary for developing an understanding and an appreciation for the chemistry behind the activity of essential oils.

→ HYDROCARBONS

The simplest organic compounds and the basic backbone of essential oils are **hydrocarbons**, consisting solely of hydrogen and carbon. Essential oils contain simple hydrocarbons in the form of **terpenes**. Terpenes make up the largest chemical group of natural products with over 30,000 known terpene compounds. Terpenes are classified according to the number of **isoprene units** that their molecules contain. The isoprene unit is technically referred to as 2-methyl-1,3-butadiene and is the molecular structural unit from which hydrocarbons are derived. Each isoprene unit contains five carbon atoms (Figure 4-1).

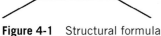

Figure 4-1 Structural formula for isoprene unit

Monoterpenes

Monoterpenes are unsaturated (molecules contain at least one double bond) hydrocarbons formed by the joining of two isoprene units and have ten carbon atoms. In general, monoterpenes are colorless and highly volatile, are insoluble in water, have low boiling points, and are prone to oxidation. They generally lack aroma. Monoterpenes are nonpolar compounds. Essential oils rich in monoterpenes (such as citrus oils) can be skin irritants. **Monoterpenes have names that end in-*ene*.**

TABLE 4.2

Synopsis of Major Chemical Families and Their General Therapeutic Actions

Family	General Therapeutic Actions
Monoterpenes	• Antiseptic • Antiviral • Stimulating; Energizing • Mild expectorants/Decongestants • Drying/dehydrating effect on skin
Sesquiterpenes	• Antiseptic • Antibacterial • Powerful anti-inflammatory • Antispasmodic • Calming and soothing to the nervous system
Monoterpene Alcohols	• Strong antimicrobial • Gentle to the skin • Antibacterial, antiviral • Immune system support
Sesquiterpene Alcohols	• Anti-inflammatory • Immune supportive
Phenols	• Strong antibacterial activity, antiseptic • Warming • Stimulant immune system • Strengthening yet stimulating to the nervous system
Phenylpropanoids	• Strong antibacterial activity, antiseptic • Stress-modulating (Schnaubelt, 2004) • Stimulant immune system • Strengthening yet stimulating to the nervous system • Antispasmodic
Esters	• Relaxing to CNS • Balancing • Antispasmodic • Nervous system tonic • Soothing to dermal inflammations
Aldehydes	• Strong antiviral • Calming and sedative to CNS • Anti-inflammatory • Skin irritants
Ketones	• Strong mucolytics • Promote skin/tissue regeneration • Wound healing agents • Calming to nervous system, sedative
Oxides	• Antiviral • Expectorant • Respiratory stimulant
Sesquiterpene Lactones	• Mucolytic and expectorant • Anti-inflammatory • Smooth muscle relaxant • Antimicrobial
Furanocoumarins	• Photosensitizers • Antifungal, antiviral (Clarke, 2002)

Greek Letters

Greek letters are used to denote isomer (when two chemicals have the same molecular formula but different molecular structure) compounds.

Alpha	α
Beta	β
Gamma	γ
Delta	δ

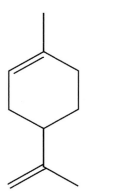

Figure 4-2   Limonene

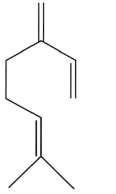

Figure 4-3   Myrcene

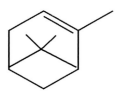

Figure 4-4   Alpha-pinene

General therapeutic actions of monoterpenes include:

- ▶ antiseptic; antibacterial; antiviral
- ▶ chemopreventative
- ▶ stimulating; energizing
- ▶ mild expectorants/decongestants (specifically needle oil, such as pine)
- ▶ drying/dehydrating effect on skin and mucous membranes

> **NOTE**
>
> All terpene compounds react easily to oxygen and can degrade quickly. This degradation can make certain essential oils potential irritants and/or sensitizers. To avoid oxidation, it is important to store essential oils correctly and to insure that the individual essential oil has not expired. Monoterpene and linalol-rich essential oils (Lavender, Thyme ct. linalol) should be preserved with Vitamin E or alpha-tocopheral to extend their shelf-life.

Examples of Monoterpenes

limonene	Citrus fruits, e.g., Lemon, Tangerine, Bitter and Sweet orange, Neroli, Caraway, Dill, Fir, Mint, Pine (Figure 4-2)
myrcene	Pine, Juniper, and many other oils (Figure 4-3)
α-pinene	Pine and many other oils
β-pinene	Pine and many other oils (Figure 4-4)
β-ocimene	Basil
_d_-limonene	Bergamot, Citronella, Lemongrass, Palmarosa
terpinoline	Eucalyptus, Tea tree
α-phellandrene	Dill, Fennel, Black pepper
β-phellandrene	Angelica seed, Dill, Pine, Fir, Cypress
α-terpinene	Marjoram, Cardamon, Lemon, and some _Ocimum_ species (Basil)
(-)-car-3-ene	Pine, Black pepper

Essential Oils Rich in Monoterpenes

Angelica root, Bergamot, Black pepper, Grapefruit, Juniper, Lemon, Lime, Mandarin, Orange, Pine

Sesquiterpenes

Sesquiterpenes have fifteen carbon atoms and are based upon the joining of three isoprene units. In general, sesquiterpenes are colorless (with the exception of chamazulene, which is blue), are insoluble in water, and are more aromatic, less volatile, and have higher boiling points than monoterpenes. Sesquiterpenes are non-polar compounds that oxidize slower than monoterpenes. **Sesquiterpenes have names that end in-_ene_.**

General therapeutic actions of sesquiterpenes are:

- ▶ antiseptic
- ▶ antibacterial
- ▶ powerful anti-inflammatory

▷ antispasmodic
▷ calming and soothing to the nervous system

Examples of Sesquiterpenes and Oils They Are Found In

bisabolene	German chamomile, Myrrh
β-cadinene	Juniper
β-caryophyllene	Clove, Lavender, Ylang ylang
chamazulene	German chamomile, Yarrow, Wormwood
α-cedrene	Cedarwood oil, Juniper
α-curcumene	Ginger
α-farnesene	German chamomile, Rose (Figure 4-5)
β-santalene	Sandalwood
β-selinene	Celery seed
α-ylangene	Ylang ylang
α-vetivene	Vetiver
zingiberene	Ginger (Figure 4-6)

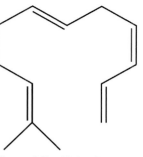

Figure 4-5   Alpha-farnesene

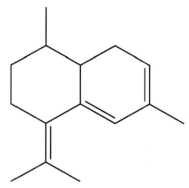

Figure 4-6   Zingiberene

Essential Oils Rich in Sesquiterpenes

German chamomile, Ginger, Helichrysum, Myrrh, Patchouli, Vetiver

OXYGENATED HYDROCARBONS: FUNCTIONAL GROUPS

The following constituents are hydrocarbons with the addition of oxygen. Each family of oxygenated hydrocarbons is governed by a functional group that provides the family with general physical and chemical attributes. A **functional group** is an atom or group of atoms that imparts specific chemical and physical properties to a molecule. For example, alcohols have the functional group hydroxyl or (−OH).

Alcohols

Alcohols are organic compounds that contain a hydroxyl group (−OH) attached to a saturated carbon. **Saturated** is when a carbon is bonded to other atoms only through single bonds, no double or triple bonds. Alcohols are polar molecules and have higher boiling points than terpenes of similar molecular weight. They typically have pleasant aromas and are slightly soluble in water. Essential oils rich in alcohols are considered to be generally nontoxic, safe for children and the elderly, and are typically used for skin care applications. Alcohols in essential oils are derived from terpenes and are categorized as either monoterpene alcohols (monoterpenols) or sesquiterpene alcohols (sesquiterpenols). **Alcohol compounds have names that end in −*ol*.**

Monoterpene Alcohols

General therapeutic actions of monoterpene alcohols:

▷ strong antimicrobial
▷ gentle to the skin

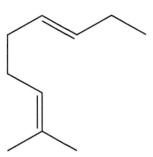

Figure 4-7   Geraniol

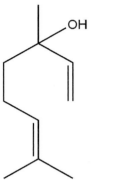

Figure 4-8   Linalol

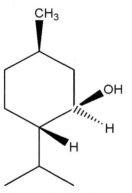

Figure 4-9   Menthol

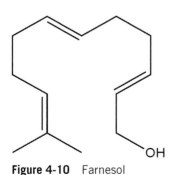

Figure 4-10   Farnesol

Figure 4-11   Beta-santalol

> ▶ antibacterial, antiviral
> ▶ immune system support

Examples of Monoterpene Alcohols Found in Essential Oils

borneol	Spike Lavender, Rosemary, Thyme
citronellol	Rose, Geranium, *Eucalyptus citriodora*
geraniol	Palmarosa, Citronella, Lemongrass, Geranium (Figure 4-7)
lavandulol	Lavender
linalol	Lavender, Bergamot, Orange, Rosewood (Figure 4-8) (**NOTE:** Linalol has sedative properties.)
menthol	Peppermint (Figure 4-9)
nerol	Neroli, Bergamot, Petitgrain, Rose
terpin-4-ol	Tea tree, Juniper berry

Essential Oils Rich in Monoterpene Alcohols

Geranium, *Lavandula angustifolia*, Lavendin, Sweet marjoram, Neroli, Palmarosa, Peppermint, Petitgrain, Rose, Tea tree, Thyme ct. linalol

Sesquiterpene Alcohols

According to Schnaubelt (1995), sesquiterpene alcohols "tonify the muscles and nerves, reduce congestion in the veins as well as in the lymphatic system and have moderate antimicrobial activity" (p. 29).

General therapeutic actions of sesquiterpene alcohols:

> ▶ anti-inflammatory
> ▶ immune supportive

Examples of Sesquiterpene Alcohols Found in Essential Oils

α-bisabolol	German chamomile
carotol	Carrot seed
daucol	Carrot seed
farnesol	Rose (Figure 4-10)
α-santalol	Sandalwood
β-santalol	Sandalwood (Figure 4-11)
zingiberol	Ginger

Essential Oils Rich in Sesquiterpene Alcohols

Carrot seed, German chamomile, Ginger, Patchouli, Sandalwood, Vetiver

Phenols

Phenols contain an —OH group attached to the carbon of a benzene ring (Figure 4-12), also known as an aromatic ring. Tisserand and Balacs (1996) point out that the —OH group attachment to the benzene ring makes phenols more reactive, which possibly creates more irritating compounds (p. 17). Phenols are polar compounds, have higher boiling points, and are somewhat more water soluble than alcohols. **The**

names of phenol compounds, like alcohols, end in *–ol*. Since there are fewer phenol compounds and to avoid confusion with alcohols, it is recommended that students memorize the name of phenols commonly found within essential oils.

> **NOTE**
>
> According to Tisserand and Balacs (1995), phenol or carbolic acid is "a disinfectant derived from coal tar" (p. 18). This phenol is not found in nature. Phenol or carbolic acid was popularized as an antiseptic by Joseph Lister who utilized it to reduce postsurgical infections and as an agent to clean surgical instruments. Phenol is no longer used as a disinfectant due to its damaging effects on the skin.

Figure 4-12   Benzene ring

Phenol Toxicity and Safety Information

Phenol compounds found within essential oils are a group of chemicals that have been found to be potentially liver toxins when taken internally in high doses or over lengthy periods of time. Phenol compounds have also exhibited skin irritating properties. Essential oils rich in phenols, such as thyme, clove, basil ct. methyl chavicol, and oregano, should be used in low dilutions and should always be applied diluted in a carrier oil prior to applying to the skin. A good way to remember this is to notice that the beginning of the word phenol sounds like "F", "F" for fire! Phenol compounds can burn like fire when in contact with mucous membranes or broken skin. Use with caution and always dilute. Phenol compounds can be irritating to the skin and are potential hepatotoxins.

General therapeutic actions of phenols:

▶ strong antibacterial activity, antimicrobial
▶ warming
▶ stimulant to the immune system
▶ strengthening yet stimulating to the nervous system

Examples of Phenols Found in Essential Oils

carvacrol	Wild marjoram, Oregano, Thyme
thymol	Thyme (Figure 4-13)
eugenol	Clove bud, Cinnamon (Figure 4-14)

Essential Oils Rich in Phenols

Basil, Thyme, Oregano, Cinnamon, Clove, Tarragon

Phenylpropanoids

Mills and Bone (2000) describe phenylpropanoids as having a "basic 3-carbon chain attached to a benzene ring" (p. 28). Phenylpropanoids are biosynthetically derived from the cinnamic acid or shikimic acid pathway rather than the mevalonic pathway. Phenylpropanoid compounds are rare in essential oils, although they have considerable and noteworthy actions. **Phenylpropanoid compounds have names that end in** *–ole* **or** *–ol*.

General therapeutic actions of phenylpropanoids:

▶ strong antibacterial activity, antiseptic
▶ stress-modulating (Schnaubelt, 2004)
▶ stimulant immune system

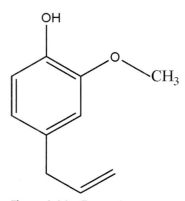

Figure 4-13   Thymol

Figure 4-14   Eugenol

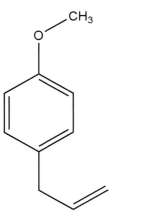

Figure 4-15 Methyl chavicol

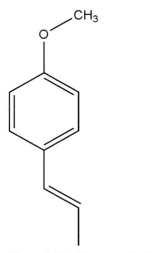

Figure 4-16 Trans-anethole

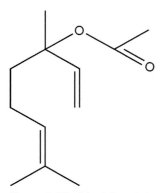

Figure 4-17 Linalyl acetate

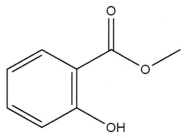

Figure 4-18 Methyl salicylate

▶ strengthening yet stimulating to the nervous system
▶ antispasmodic

Examples of Phenylpropanoid Found in Essential Oils

cinnamic aldehyde	Cinnamon bark
cis-anethole	Anise (up to 2.5%)
methyl chavicol syn. Estragole	Basil, Fennel, Tarragon (Figure 4-15)
safrole	Camphor, Sassafrass
trans-anethole	Anise (up to 80%), Fennel (up to 90%) (Figure 4-16)

Essential Oils Rich in Phenylpropanoids

Basil ct. methyl chavicol, Fennel, Cinnamon bark, Sassafras

> **NOTE**
>
> Cis-anethole has been found to be highly toxic, whereas trans-anethole is considered to be relatively nontoxic and safe for use. Sweet fennel is predominantly trans-anethole. To avoid toxicity, proper identification of the essential oil is crucial. Companies selling essential oils should clearly state the full Latin binomial as well as the chemotype constituent (e.g., Thymus vulgaris ct. thymol) to insure essential oil is used with appropriate safety precautions.

Esters

Esters are the product of a chemical reaction that occurs between an alcohol and an organic acid. Organic acids have a terminal carbon that shares electrons with both a carbonyl group and a hydroxyl group. This entire unit, COOH, is called a carboxyl group. Esters are mildly polar compounds with characteristically intense fruity aromas. They have a similar boiling point as alcohols or ketones of similar molecular weight and are somewhat soluble in water. **Esters have names that end in –*ate* or *ester*.**

An example of an ester forming would be: Acetic acid + Linalol = Linalyl acetate + molecule of water

General therapeutic actions of esters:

▶ relaxing to the central nervous system (CNS)
▶ balancing
▶ antispasmodic
▶ nervous system tonic
▶ soothing to dermal inflammations

Examples of Esters Found in Essential Oils

bornyl acetate	Pine and fir species, Rosemary, Thyme
geranyl acetate	Geranium (leaves), Lemon, Rose, Lavender, Marjoram
linalyl acetate	Lavender, Bergamot, Clary sage, Petitgrain, Neroli (Figure 4-17)
menthyl acetate	Peppermint and other mint species
methyl salicylate	Wintergreen, Birch (Figure 4-18)
thymol acetate	Thyme

Additional Esters		
benzyl acetate	citronellyl acetate	citronellyl butyrate
eugenyl acetate	lavandulyl acetate	methyl benzoate
sabinyl acetate	terpineol acetate	vetiverol acetate

Essential Oils Rich in Esters

Birch, Roman chamomile, Clary sage, Lavender, Neroli, Petitgrain, Wintergreen

> **NOTE**
>
> Birch and wintergreen essential oils contain up to 95 to 98 percent methyl salicylate and are commonly adulterated with synthetic methyl salicylate. Methyl salicylate is a highly toxic compound that easily passes through the skin into the bloodstream. Tisserand and Balacs (1995) report that internal doses as small as 4ml have caused death in infants and that numerous cases of methyl salicylate poisoning have been reported. According to Merck pharmaceuticals, "The most toxic form of salicylate is oil of wintergreen (methyl salicylate); death has been reported from ingestion of 1 tsp in a young child. Any exposure to methyl salicylate (found in liniments and in solutions used in hot vaporizers) is potentially lethal."

Do not use birch or wintergreen on infants, on damaged skin, or with individuals on other salicylate-based medication. Do not use with individuals who are taking warfarin. Tisserand and Balacs (1995) report that topically applied methyl salicylate can potentiate the anticoagulant effects of warfarin, causing side effects such as internal hemorrhage (p. 195).

The U.S. Environmental Protection Agency (1997) reports: "Besides its use as a flavoring agent in foods, methyl salicylate has been used in mouthwash, suntan lotions, and in U.S. Pharmocopeia (U.S.P.) preparations as a counterirritant and analgesic for painful muscles or joints, in liniments, ointments, and other preparations. An FDA Advisory Review Panel has concluded that methyl salicylate is safe for use up to a concentration of 0.4% in the form of a rinse or mouthwash. The compound is extensively used in foods, beverages, pharmaceuticals, lotions and perfumes and has wide distribution in commerce with no reports of adverse outcomes associated with intended uses."

Methyl salicylate is the active ingredient in BenGay™ and Deep Heat products for muscular aches, pains, and sprains. One should note that both these products tend to be in a petroleum base, which would minimize skin absorption.

Aldehydes

Aldehydes contain the polar carbonyl group (C=O) with the carbonyl group directly attached to at least one hydrogen atom and a second attached directly to a hydrogen or carbon atom. Aldehydes are considered to be some of the most aromatic molecules within essential oils and have a slightly fruity aroma when smelled as isolated chemicals. Aldehydes are mildly polar compounds and have a lower boiling point than alcohols, yet a higher boiling point than hydrocarbon molecules. They are also slightly more soluble in water than alcohols. Aldehydes readily oxidize into carboxylic acids, thus exhibiting more irritating effects. **Aldehyde compounds have names that end in −al**.

> **NOTE**
>
> Many aldehyde compounds are skin irritants and may initiate an allergic reaction when used undiluted. Essential oils rich in aldehydes should always be used diluted or as airborne antiseptics that are not being placed on the skin.

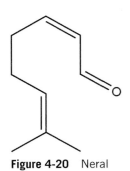

Figure 4-19   Geranial

Figure 4-20   Neral

General therapeutic actions of aldehydes:

- ▶ strong antiviral; antimicrobial
- ▶ calming and sedative to CNS
- ▶ anti-inflammatory
- ▶ skin irritants

Examples of Aldehydes Found in Essential Oils

citral	Lemongrass, Lemon verbena
citronellal	Citronella, *Eucalyptus citriodora*, Melissa
geranial	Lemon, Lemongrass, Lime, Melissa (Figure 4-19)
neral	Ginger, Lemon, Lemongrass, Melissa (Figure 4-20)

Other Aldehydes		
acetaldehyde	benzaldehyde	cuminic aldehyde
nonanal	perillaldehyde	piperonal

Essential Oils Rich in Aldehydes

Citronella, *Eucalyptus citriodora*, Lemongrass

Ketones

Ketones are similar to aldehydes with the exception that only carbons are directly attached to the carbonyl group (C=O). Ketones are moderately polar compounds and are considered to be stable and not prone to oxidation. Ketones, like aldehydes, have a lower boiling point than alcohols, yet a higher boiling point than hydrocarbon molecules. Ketones are slightly more soluble in water than alcohols. **Ketone compounds have names that end in** *–one*, **except for camphor**.

Ketone Toxicity and Safety Information

Ketone compounds found within essential oils are considered to be the more highly toxic components found within essential oils, particularly when taken internally. Specifically, ketones exhibit a potential for neurotoxicity and may initiate epileptic-like seizures in large dosages. Thujone, an ingredient of absinthe, has been subject to much research for its toxicity to the nervous system when taken internally. Overdose with thujone internally has resulted in brain damage, seizures, tremors, and paralysis.

According to Bowles (2003), dermal application is unlikely to yield problematic blood levels on single doses, though there is a possibility of buildup with repeated daily dosages due to the long half-life of terpenoids in the body (p. 86). Low dilutions in a carrier as well as short periods of usage are considered safe.

Essential oils, such as rue, mugwort, wormwood, thuja, and pennyroyal are considered to be neurotoxins and potential abortifacients and should be avoided in aromatherapy applications. Sage, spike lavender, and camphor have moderate ketone content and are generally considered safe for external application. Other oils, such as cedar, peppermint, rosemary, spearmint, and yarrow have such a low ketone content that concern is minimal. Standard safety practice for the above oils is to avoid internal use, keep away from children, and avoid long-term daily use.

Essential oils rich in camphor should not be used on infants or young children. Camphor is known to easily cross the skin, the mucous membranes, and the placental barrier. In large doses it can cause significant hepatotoxicity and/or neurotoxicity. Ingestion of even small doses of camphor can cause fatal poisoning in children. Remember to keep all essential oils away from children and out of their reach.

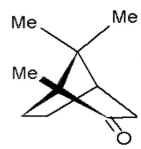

Figure 4-21   Camphor

General therapeutic actions of ketones:

- ▶ strong mucolytics
- ▶ promote skin/tissue regeneration
- ▶ wound healing agents
- ▶ calming to nervous system, sedative

Examples of Ketones Found in Essential Oils

camphor	Rosemary ct camphor, Spike lavender, *Lavendula stoechas*, Camphor oil, Sage (Figure 4-21)
d-carvone	Caraway, Dill
l-carvone	Spearmint
fenchone	Fennel, Lavender, Thuja
menthone	Peppermint oil and other *Mentha* species (Figure 4-22)
nootkatone	Grapefruit
piperitone	Peppermint, *Eucalyptus polybractea*
pulegone	Pennyroyal oils, Peppermint
thujone	Thuja, Sage, Wormwood
verbenone	Rosemary ct verbenone

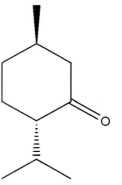

Figure 4-22   Menthone

Essential Oils Rich in Ketones

Dill, *Eucalyptus dives*, Hyssop, Mugwort, Sage (*Salvia officinalis*), Thuja

Oxides

Oxides are organic compounds that have an oxygen molecule situated between two carbon molecules. Oxides are fairly unstable and oxidize rapidly on exposure to air or water. Oxides are also susceptible to heat. The major oxide to be found within essential oils is the chemical 1,8 cineole, which is also known as eucalyptol. **Oxide compounds have names that end in *–ole* or *–oxide*.**

General therapeutic actions of oxides:

- ▶ antiviral
- ▶ expectorant
- ▶ respiratory stimulant

Examples of Oxides

1,8 cineole; Eucalyptol	Eucalyptus, Niaouli, Tea tree (Figure 4-23)
bisabolol oxide	German chamomile
bisabolone oxide	German chamomile

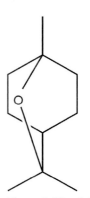

Figure 4-23   1,8 cineole syn eucalyptol

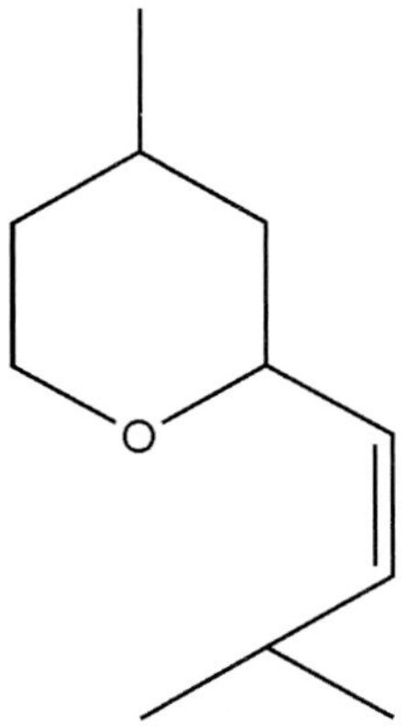

Figure 4-24 Rose oxide

rose oxide	Rose (Figure 4-24)
sclareol oxide	Clary sage

Essential Oils Rich in Oxides

Cajeput, *Eucalyptus globulus* and other eucalyptus species, Niaouli, Tea tree

Sesquiterpene Lactones

Yarnell (2003) describes sesquiterpene lactones as a subcategory of sesquiterpenes with a characteristic lactone ring structure derived ultimately from farnesyl pyrophosphate (p. 47). Sesquiterpenes lactones are uncommon in essential oils but are found as the bitter principle in many of the Asteraceae family, including *Achillea millefolium*, *Arnica montana*, and *Tanacetum annum*. They are only slightly soluble in water, slow to volatize, and do not readily oxidize. According to Schnaubelt (2004), "sesquiterpene lactones are among the pharmacologically most active molecules found in essential oils and are the most effective mucolytics in medical aromatherapy (p. 109)." The essential oil of *Inula graveolens* contains some sesquiterpene lactones and is used for the treatment of asthma and bronchitis. **Lactone compounds have names that end in *–lactone* or *–ine*.**

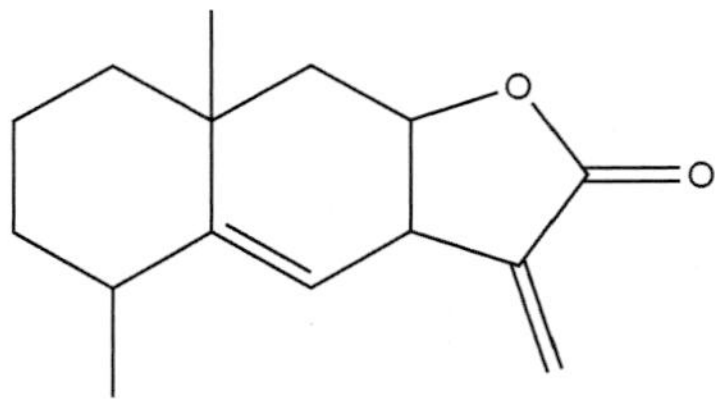

Figure 4-25 Alantolactone

General therapeutic actions of lactones include:

- mucolytic and expectorant
- anti-inflammatory
- smooth muscle relaxant
- antimicrobial

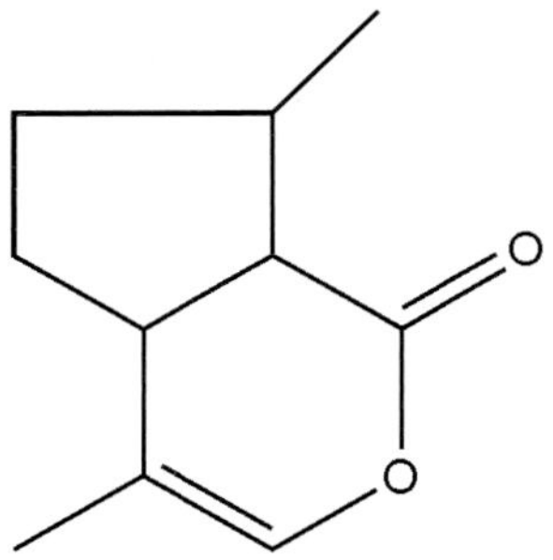

Figure 4-26 Nepetalactone

Examples of Sesquiterpene Lactones

alantolactone	*Inula helenium, Inula graveolens* (Figure 4-25)
isolantolactone	*Inula graveolens*
nepetalactone	Catnip (*Nepeta cataria*) (Figure 4-26)

Essential Oils Rich in Sesquiterpene Lactones

Inula graveolens, Catnip

Furanocoumarins

Coumarins are a type of lactone and **furanocoumarins** are a type of coumarin. The furanocoumarins are most often found within citrus oils and angelica root. Bergaptene is the most common furanocoumarin and is responsible for the photosensitizing action of bergamot essential oil. Furanocoumarins are very slightly soluble in water.

General therapeutic actions of furanocoumarins include:

- photosensitizers
- antifungal, antiviral (Clarke, 2002)

Examples of Furanocoumarins

angellicin   Angelica root
bergaptene   Bergamot (Figure 4-27)

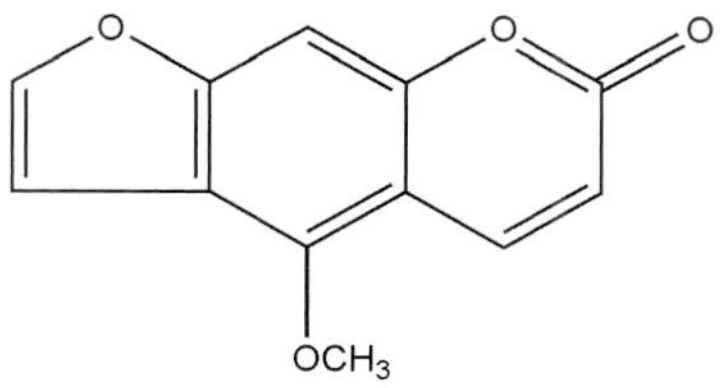

Essential Oils Rich in Furanocoumarins

Angelica root, Bergamot, Expressed citrus oils

Furanocoumarin Toxicity and Safety Information

Essential oils rich in furanocoumarins exhibit phototoxic effects. Phototoxic or photosensitizing compounds are substances that can cause rapid tanning or burns under the influence of ultraviolet light. Furanocoumarins are able to absorb ultraviolet light, thereby producing a burning or tanning effect on the skin.

Figure 4-27   Bergaptene

IN PRACTICE

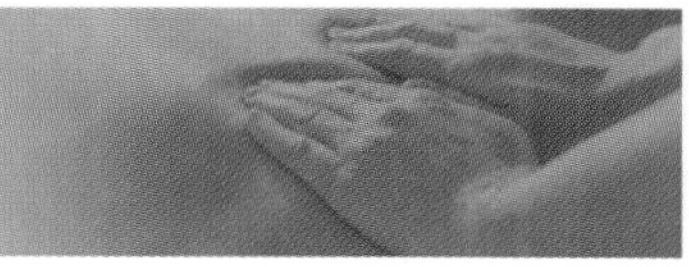

Case Study 4.1

Chemistry Applied

J. is a forty-year-old self-employed woman who is a self-proclaimed type "A" personality. She is under considerable stress (perhaps self-induced) every day and feels she has no time to relax. She suffers with bouts of bronchitis as it is winter and feels that it is caused by her stress and hence lowered immunity. J. also complains about her neck and shoulders being tight and somewhat tender/painful as well as nights of insomnia. J. came to have an aromatherapy massage by referral from a friend.

For the full-body massage blend, I chose the following essential oils:

■ Lavender (*Lavandula angustifolia*)—rich in esters and sedative alcohol, linalol, for their relaxing and balancing effects on the CNS
■ German chamomile (*Matricaria recutita*)—rich in sesquiterpenes, for its ability to calm and soothe the nervous system and musculoskeletal system
■ Ginger (*Zingiber officinale*)—rich in sesquiterpenes, calming and soothing to the nervous system as well as warming and slightly analgesic for muscular aches and pains

Massage Blend: 3% dilution/1oz oil

Lavender   10 drops
German chamomile   3 drops
Ginger   5 drops
100% Apricot kernel oil

Take-Home Diffusor Synergy: This synergy was designed to address lowered immunity as well as her bronchitis.

■ Eucalyptus (*Eucalyptus globulus*)—rich in oxide, 1,8 cineole, for its expectorating action
■ Cinnamon leaf (*Cinnamomum zeylanicum*)—rich in phenols for its immune enhancing capabilities
■ Tea tree (*Melaleuca alternifolia*)—rich in monoterpene alcohols, for its immune enhancing capabilities and supportive to Eucalyptus 1,8 cineole content, for its expectorating action
■ Lemon (*Citrus limon*)—rich in monoterpenes, for its antiseptic action, and to support the other essential oils in blend

Synergy

Eucalyptus   20 drops
Cinnamon leaf   7 drops
Tea tree   12 drops
Lemon   25 drops

Recommended use: In electronic nebulizing diffusor, on timer for 10 to 20 minutes an hour while at home. Also, place 5 to 10 drops in a 1oz spritzer to spray in car or around work space as needed or desired.

The following essential oils are considered to be phototoxic: Bergamot (0.4%), Expressed lime (0.7%), Tagetes (0.05%), and Angelica root (0.78%). The percentages that follow each oil are the maximum level recommended for retail products according to Tisserand and Balacs (1995).

Guidelines have been established for dosage levels considered to be safe for the application of essential oils with phototoxic furanocoumarins. The dilution rate has been indicated above by the inclusion of parenthesis around a percentage. When combining two or more known photosensitizers, it is important to ensure that the total furanocoumarin content is below 0.4% (less than 2 to 3 drops per ounce of carrier). Also, it would be prudent when using photosensitizing oils that the client be asked to avoid direct sun or sun beds for a minimum of twelve to twenty-four hours.

SUMMARY

- Through the study of the basic chemistry of essential oils, you are better equipped to not only interact with individuals in the medical and health professions with regard to the therapeutic benefits of essential oils but also to create safe and effective blends for clients.
- Organic chemistry was once known as the study of living organisms and/or substances that were derived from living organisms; it is now defined as the scientific study of the structure, properties, composition, reactions, and preparation of chemical compounds of carbon and hydrogen.
- Each chemical family has been provided a section on the general therapeutic actions attributed to its family. The system of attributing general properties to each chemical family has been called the structure energy system.
- Essential oils contain simple hydrocarbons in the form of terpenes and oxygenated hydrocarbons, also known as substituted hydrocarbons, in the form of alcohols, phenols, esters, aldehydes, ketones, oxides, lactones, and furanocoumarins.
- Phenol compounds are potential liver toxins when taken internally, skin irritants when applied in high dilutions or undiluted. Phenol compounds are best used diluted in a carrier and in low dilutions.
- Furanocoumarins are most often found within citrus oils and angelica root and are responsible for the photosensitizing action of these essential oils.
- Ketone compounds have a greater toxicity when taken internally and although dermal application seems unlikely to produce negative effects it would be prudent of the practitioner to only apply essential oils rich in ketones in low dilutions and over a short period of time.

NEW TERMINOLOGY

Alcohols	Furanocoumarins
Aldehydes	Hydrocarbons
Biosynthesized	Isoprene unit
Esters	Ketones
Functional group	Monoterpenes

Organic chemistry

Oxides

Phenols

Phenylpropanoids

Sesquiterpenes

Sesquiterpene lactones

Structure energy system

Terpenes

REFERENCES

Bowles, E.J. (2003). *The Chemistry of Aromatherapeutic Oils*. Crows Nest, Australia: Allen & Unwin.

Clarke, S. (2002). *Essential Chemistry for Safe Aromatherapy*. Edinburgh, UK: Churchill Livingstone.

Food and Agriculture Organization of the United Nations. (1995). *Flavors and Fragrances of Plant Origin*, Appendix 1. Retrieved on August 28, 2005, from http://www.fao.org/documents/show_cdr.asp?url_file=/docrep/V5350E/V5350e06.htm.

Merck Pharmaceuticals. *Poisoning*. Retrieved on February 23, 2006, from http://www.merck.com/mrkshared/mmanual/section19/chapter263/263b.jsp.

Mills, S., and Bone, K. (2000). *Principles and Practice of Phytotherapy*. London: Harcourt Publishers.

Schnaubelt, K. (1995). *Advanced Aromatherapy*. Rochester, VT: Healing Arts Press.

Schnaubelt, K. (2004). *Aromatherapy Lifestyle*. San Rafael, CA: Terra Linda Scent.

Theis, N., and Lerdau, M. (2003). The Evolution of Function in Plant Secondary Metabolites. *International Journal of Plant Sciences 164* (3 Suppl.): S93–S102.

Tisserand, R., and Balacs, T. (1995). *Essential Oil Safety*. New York: Churchill Livingstone.

U.S. Environmental Protection Agency (1997). *Methyl Salicylate: Establishment of an Exemption from Requirement of a Tolerance*. Retrieved on February 23, 2006, from http://www.epa.gov/fedrgstr/EPA-PEST/1997/November/Day-19/p30251.htm.

Yarnell, E. (2003). *Phytochemistry and Pharmacy for Practitioners of Botanical Medicine*. Wenatchee, WA: Healing Mountain Publishing.

Further Recommended Reading

Bowles, E.J. (2003). *The Chemistry of Aromatherapeutic Oils*. Crows Nest, Australia: Allen & Unwin.

Clarke, S. (2002). *Essential Chemistry for Safe Aromatherapy*. Edinburgh, UK: Churchill Livingstone.

Schnaubelt, K. (1995). *Advanced Aromatherapy*. Rochester, VT: Healing Arts Press.

WORKSHEET

Chemistry

Based upon the essential oils you have learned about so far in the course, categorize each one based upon the core or main biochemical family (ies). For instance, lavender would be categorized under alcohols, specifically a sedative alcohol (linalol), and esters (linalyl acetate).

▨ **MONOTERPENES**

▨ **ALDEHYDES**

▨ **SESQUITERPENES**

▨ **KETONES**

▨ **ALCOHOLS**

▨ **OXIDES**

▨ **PHENOLS**

▨ **SESQUITERPENE LECTONES**

▨ **PHENYLPROPANOIDS**

▨ **FURANOCOUMARINS**

▨ **ESTERS**

CHAPTER TEST

1. The simplest organic compounds and the basic backbone of essential oils are:

   a. sesquiterpenes

   b. aldehydes

   c. hydrocarbons

   d. oxygenated hydrocarbons

2. Monoterpenes are based upon the joining of two isoprene units so they have _____ carbon atoms.

   a. 5

   b. 20

   c. 35

   d. 10

3. The following is an example of an aldehyde:

   a. citronellol

   b. geranial

   c. patchoulol

   d. limonene

4. An ester is the product of a chemical reaction between an organic acid and _____.

   a. an aldehyde

   b. a hydrocarbon

   c. a ketone

   d. an alcohol

5. Phenols are similar to alcohols since they have an —OH group, however they differ because the —OH group is directly attached to a:

   a. benzene ring

   b. hydrocarbon

   c. carbonyl group

   d. phenolic acid

6. An example of an essential oil rich in aldehydes is:

   a. spearmint

   b. tangerine

   c. cardamom

   d. lemongrass

7. Bergaptene is the most common furanocoumarin to be found in citrus oils and is responsible for the_____ action of oils such as bergamot.

    a. nervous system toxicity

    b. urinary stimulating

    c. photosensitizing

    d. calming

8. 1,8 cineole is also known as:

    a. an aldehyde

    b. eucalyptol

    c. gingerol

    d. bisabolene

9. The following is an example of a phenol compound:

    a. linalol

    b. menthol

    c. thymol

    d. citronellal

10. Furanocoumarins are known to be potent_____ and caution should be used when using them in the presence of the sun.

    a. mucous membrane irritants

    b. photosensitizers

    c. dermal irritants

    d. liver toxins

REVIEW QUESTIONS

1. What is the importance of having an understanding of the chemistry of essential oils?

2. Discuss why the general therapeutic actions provided for each chemical family may be inadequate in understanding the full scope of activity of an individual essential oil.

3. Discuss the issue of safety as it applies to the knowledge of the chemistry and activity of aromatic compounds.

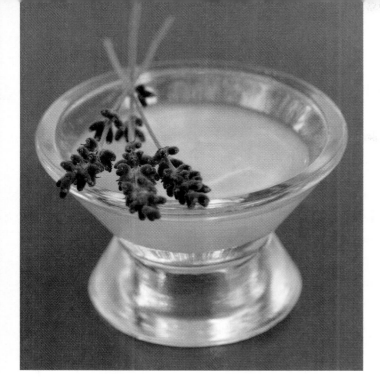

Aromatic Blending

LEARNING OBJECTIVES

After reading this chapter, you will be able to

1. List three core reasons a consultation is performed.
2. Describe two basic communication skills.
3. List, describe, and utilize three approaches to designing a blend.
4. Demonstrate knowledge and application of blending factor.
5. List and describe the three elements in the structure for creating a synergy.
6. Develop an aromatherapy massage blend.
7. Demonstrate knowledge of various dosage considerations and describe potential dilution rates used in aromatherapy applications.

INTRODUCTION

The art and science of blending is one of the most fascinating, dynamic, and creative aspects of aromatherapy. Considered a mystery to some and a science to others, this chapter has been designed to support and enhance skills for effective yet creative and unique blending. Designing a unique blend for each client is the very heart of holistic aromatherapy. In the words of Maury (1989), "To reach the individual we need an individual remedy. Each of us is a unique message. It is only the unique remedy which will suffice. We must, therefore, seek odoriferous substances which present affinities with the human being we intend to treat, those which will compensate for his deficiencies and those which will make his faculties blossom. It was by searching for this remedy that we encountered the individual prescription which on all points represents the identity of the individual" (p. 94).

STAGE ONE: THE CONSULTATION (ASSESSMENT)

Holistic therapies, such as aromatherapy and bodywork, foster a cooperative relationship between client and practitioner with the goal of attaining optimal physical, mental, emotional, social, and spiritual well-being. It emphasizes the need to look at the whole person, including analysis of physical, nutritional, environmental, emotional, social, spiritual, and lifestyle aspects of the individual.

A consultation is designed to collect information or data regarding the client's current state of health; general lifestyle, including diet and exercise; emotional well-being; and current/past medical history. A consultation supports the therapist's understanding of the nature of the condition, how it is affecting the individual client, and what intervention would be most beneficial.

In massage therapy this is often termed an assessment, which Rattray and Ludwig (2000) define as "an educated evaluation of a client's condition and physical basis for his symptoms in order to determine a course of treatment" (p. 107).

A consultation is not designed to diagnose an illness or disorder as these are beyond the scope of practice for massage therapists and bodyworkers. Only physicians are able to diagnose.

Within a holistic framework, the consultation is designed to:

- gather information from the client including the client's current state of health, general lifestyle (including diet and exercise), emotional well-being, and current/past medical history
- evaluate the nature of the condition to be addressed, whether it be physical, emotional/mental, spiritual/energetic, or a combination of all three
- provide the foundation for designing and performing a safe, knowledgeable, and effective treatment based upon the individual's needs

Standard Consultation Form

Many massage therapists and bodyworkers will use a standard consultation or health intake form that was provided to them during their training, or they will utilize forms provided by other therapists or by organizations such as the Associated Bodyworker and Massage Professionals association. These intake forms are suitable for aromatherapy massage and bodywork. When integrating aromatherapy into your bodywork or massage sessions, you may wish to add the following questions:

1. Do you have any known allergies to nuts, seeds, or other vegetable oils?
2. Do you have any known allergies to different scents or aromas?

Standard consultation forms will typically have a disclaimer at the end. It may be prudent to add in a note about the use of aromatherapy. An example of a disclaimer statement for aromatherapy would be: I understand that aromatherapy is provided for the basic purpose of enhancing the massage or bodywork technique and is not designed to diagnose, prescribe, or treat any physical or emotional illness. I understand that the practitioner will be using a variety of herbal and aromatic oils and to my knowledge I have no known allergies to the oils being utilized.

Basic Communication Skills

According to Rattray and Ludwig (2000), one of the strengths of massage therapy lies in the fact that massage therapists spend more time with the client than do most other healthcare practitioners. Basic communication skills are critical at every stage of the healing process and particularly during the consultation phase of the session. Communication skills are the essential tools by which a therapist is able to develop a relationship and means of interaction with the client. Two important aspects of good communication skills involve: attending and active listening.

Attending

Attending refers to the manner in which the therapist is present with the client, both physically and psychologically. Effective attending communicates to the client that the therapist is fully present and actively engaged with them. Effective attending also provides a safe space for the client to open up and explore their life and current "crisis" or illness and to develop a trusting relationship with the therapist.

The basic elements of effective attending include:

■ **Squaring off:** "Squaring off" means positioning one's body so that it is in alignment with the client, indicating to the client that the therapist is actively engaged and involved with the client (e.g., eye to eye, shoulder to shoulder).

■ **Reduce barriers:** Adopt an open, nondefensive posture. This usually takes the form of having uncrossed arms and legs, since crossed arms and legs can be misconstrued as signs of lessened involvement with or availability to your client

■ **Maintain eye contact:** Maintaining good eye contact with the client is another way of saying "I'm with you," "I'm interested in what you have to say." The occasional look away is expected, however one should attempt to maintain eye contact as much as possible.

■ **Be relaxed and comfortable:** Being relaxed and comfortable with your goals, intentions, boundaries, and knowledge as a therapist will allow the client to feel more relaxed, comfortable, and confident in your skills as a practitioner.

■ **Maintain awareness:** Your source of communication as a therapist is your body and your voice. It is helpful during the consultation to maintain a "gentle awareness" of the cues and messages that you may be sending to a client based upon facial or bodily expressions. Both your verbal and nonverbal behavior should indicate a clear-cut willingness to work with the client without judgment.

Active Listening

Morris (1997) says that **active listening** is "demonstrating that we are energetically engaged in the discussion—not just passive listeners, and that we have brought in our intellect and knowledge too." Actively listening to your client, as well as being receptive to the unspoken dialogue being communicated, can offer valuable assistance in the creation of a unique treatment program for the individual.

Active listening involves:

- ▶ listening to and understanding the client's verbal messages
- ▶ observing and reading the client's nonverbal behavior, including their posture, facial expressions, movement, and tone of voice
- ▶ listening to and understanding a client's story within the context of their life, culture, and beliefs
- ▶ listening for hints of disharmony, unhappiness, or stress within a client's life

Attending and active listening during a consultation will allow the therapist to better create an effective aromatherapy massage treatment plan based upon the individual's needs and goals.

Response Skills

Response skills are those skills that enable the therapist to respond appropriately to the client. We will discuss the use of empathy below.

The Use of Empathy

Basic **empathy** involves listening to clients, understanding them and their concerns to the degree that this is possible, and communicating this understanding to them so that they might understand themselves more fully and act on their understanding. Basic empathy is the skill that enables you to communicate your understanding of the client's world and life to the client.

Empathy is different from sympathy, as sympathy is most often an expression of pity, compassion, commiseration, and condolence. Sympathy often denotes agreement of the client's dilemma. Empathic listening, like mindfulness, is helpful in building a relationship of trust with the client. It also shows the client that you respect them and are there to listen to what their concerns are.

"It means entering the private perceptual world of the other and becoming thoroughly at home in it. It involves being sensitive, moment by moment, to the changing felt meanings which flow in this other person, to the fear or rage or tenderness of confusion or whatever that he or she is experiencing. It means temporarily living in the other's life, moving about in it delicately without making judgments." *Karl Rogers*

STAGE TWO: DEVELOPING A TREATMENT FRAMEWORK

Upon completion of the consultation, the following questions could serve as starting points to creating an effective aromatic massage session.

1. What appears to be the overall perception of the core problem/issue?
2. Should I be treating the physical ailment, the mental/emotional element, or the spiritual/energetic element? How can I combine the three?
3. If a physical disorder is present, is it chronic or acute? If there is acute pain, is it contraindicated for massage, or could I attempt to treat it symptomatically with one form of treatment?
4. What is the client's goal in having this treatment and what is my intention? Does the client have a willingness in the healing process?
5. What information do I feel I have intuitively received?
6. How can I utilize essential oils to facilitate the healing process?
7. Which essential oils immediately come to mind for this individual?
8. Do I need to refer this client for diagnosis or other treatments, e.g., chiropractic?

> Holistic therapies focus on healing the patient by addressing the nature of the disease within the context of the whole person. The holistic therapist seeks to understand the potential contributing factors of disharmony as well as the potential pathways for supporting the body in reaching its optimal state of being.

The treatment framework also includes your approach to the blending process. Three possible approaches include:

Physiological Approach

Based upon the consultation, you may decide to blend solely for the physiological condition presented. A physiological approach to blending bases the selection of essential oils upon their chemistry and/or known therapeutic actions. Physiological blends place their emphasis on the activity of the blend rather than the aroma. If one is blending for a physical ailment, there will certainly be times when the aroma is not necessarily "attractive," however it will continue to act effectively on the condition being treated.

Example of a Physiologically Based Synergy

This is a synergy designed for the treatment of adult chronic bronchitis and lowered immune response.

Eucalyptus *(Eucalyptus globulus)*: Rich in the oxide 1,8 cineole. Expectorant and respiratory stimulant.

Rosemary ct. camphor *(Rosmarinus officinalis)*: Rich in camphor and 1,8 cineole. General expectorant and strong mucolytic activity.

Peppermint *(Mentha × piperita)*: Rich in the alcohol, menthol, and ketone, menthone. Opens up airways and enhances immune system.

Thyme ct. thymol *(Thymus vulgaris)*: Rich in the phenol, thymol. Supports and enhances immune system.

Emotional/Mental/Spiritual Approach

On the other hand, you may wish to blend solely based upon the emotional/mental/ spiritual aspects of the client. When blending for emotional/mental/spiritual purposes, the emphasis is placed on the aroma of the blend and its emotional/subtle therapeutic properties.

Example of an Emotional Design

This is a blend designed for an individual who has a high degree of stress, feels ungrounded, is having a difficult time feeling self-worth, and suffers with bouts of anxiety.

> **Vetiver** *(Vetiveria zizanioides)*: To ground and center, reduce anxiety and stress.
>
> **Frankincense** *(Boswellia carterii)*: For all around healing purposes, reduce anxiety and stress.
>
> **Rose** *(Rosa × damascena)*: For self-nurturing and self-love, to calm and soothe.

Holistic (Combination) Approach

Most often an aromatherapy blend is designed to address the whole person and hence includes essential oils for physical, mental/emotional, and spiritual/energetic purposes. For this type of blend, both its therapeutic intent as well as its perceived pleasantness of aroma by the client is important.

Example of a Combination Design

This blend is designed for an individual who is currently experiencing tension, tightness, and general discomfort in the neck and shoulders. Underlying this condition is incredible stress due to time pressures at work and financial concerns. The individual is also feeling anxious, tired, and a bit depressed about her ability to remain calm at home given the circumstances at work and with finances.

> **Black pepper** *(Piper nigrum)*: For its analgesic properties as well as its ability to provide strength and courage.
>
> **Clary sage** *(Salvia sclarea)*: Antidepressant; for its euphoric and calming abilities; it supports and enhances black pepper and peppermint for the relief of muscular aches and pains; soothes anxiety.
>
> **Grapefruit** *(Citrus × paradisi)*: To provide an uplifting element to overall blend; good for stress-related conditions and supports the release of tension/anxiety.
>
> **Peppermint** *(Mentha × piperita)*: To support black pepper as an analgesic; to enhance energy flow to avoid stagnation and fatigue.

↳ STAGE THREE: DEVELOPING AN AROMATIC BLEND

Step 1: Design Synergy

Step 2: Choose Carrier Oil or Other Delivery System

Step 3: Dosage: At What Dilution?

Step 4: The Blending Factor

Step 5: Perform Massage

Step 6: Document

Step 7: Follow-Up Evaluation

Step 1: Design Synergy

A synergy is the combination of three to five essential oils without a carrier oil or other base product, such as a cream or lotion. Creating an effective synergy requires a deep understanding of one's repertoire of essential oils, a solid treatment plan based upon the information gained from the consultation, and a blending approach. Designing an effective synergy or combination of essential oils is the first step toward developing the individualized therapeutic massage oil to be used during a session. The following structure may be used in selecting essential oils.

■ **Core essential oil:** The core essential oil is chosen based upon your primary purpose/goal and is considered the heart of the synergy. For example, if a client comes in with chronic tendinitis, which is causing great stress due to the pain, then your primary purpose could be the relief of pain and inflammation in the subacute phase of tendinitis. The secondary purpose could be to provide relief from stress.

Let's say we choose Lavender (*Lavandula angustifolia*) for its ability to reduce pain and inflammation. Lavender is also beneficial for the relief of stress.

■ **Enhancer essential oil:** The enhancer essential oil strengthens the core essential oil in its purpose and therapeutic action. For instance, above we have chosen an essential oil for its pain-relieving and anti-inflammatory properties.

We could choose German chamomile (*Matricaria recutita*) for its reputation as one of the best anti-inflammatory agents and for its ability to relieve stress. German chamomile will not only enhance the therapeutic activity of the first essential oil but will also add to its psychological benefits as well.

■ **Harmonizing essential oil:** The harmonizing essential oil supports and enhances the vitality and purpose of the overall synergy. The harmonizing essential oil often has a decisive impact on the overall aroma and is chosen for both its aroma and ability to enhance the goals of the synergy.

If you are creating a blend solely for a physical condition, then the essential oil chosen can simply further the goal of the above two essential oils or, if it is possible to address an emotional aspect of the condition, then the harmonizing essential oil can be added for its influence on the emotional state of the individual and hence the aroma of the final blend.

Professional Insight

The Shroud of Secrecy

Blending for aromatherapy purposes often seems as if it is hidden in a shroud of secrecy, which can be intimidating or disempowering to the newcomer and practitioner alike. Sometimes individuals appear to doubt that they have the ability to blend "right," and often individuals will choose to go with an already designed blend from a book rather than venture into the world of blending. The secret behind a good blend is the understanding of each essential oil that creates it. To truly create great blends, one must have a strong knowledge of and experience with each individual essential oil within one's repertoire of oils. If one knows each essential oil intimately, including its aroma, its core therapeutic properties (anti-inflammatory, etc.), its core aromatic applications (sprains, etc.), and its general psychological attributes, then one can, with ease, design an effective aromatic blend. This knowledge base is greatly enhanced with personal and professional experience and observations of the efficacy of the essential oil being used.

Based upon the primary purpose of the above blend, we could add sweet marjoram (*Origanum marjorana*) to support the analgesic and relaxing/soothing properties of lavender and German chamomile.

■ **Additional essential oils:** If it is desired or warranted, you can decide to add one or two additional essential oils. These additions would be either an enhancer or harmonizing essential oil. For instance, continuing on with the client above, you could decide that an additional essential oil would be of benefit for the overall effectiveness of the treatment. Let's say we add helichrysum (*Helichrysum italicum*) for its anti-inflammatory and healing properties. The final synergy would be a combination of lavender, German chamomile, sweet marjoram, and helichrysum.

Do They Smell Good Together?

Once the essential oils have been chosen, the next step is to ensure they smell good together. This is always done *before* blending them together. Remove the caps from all four bottles, place them together in your hands to ensure that all the lids are the same height, and then waft the bottles under your nose. Notice if they complement one another, if they smell good together, and if they appear to merge well as a group. If one essential oil seems to not merge very well with the others, you may decide to replace that one with another of similar therapeutic action. Whether blending for emotional/mental/spiritual or physical benefits, the oils should be complementary to one another in action and aroma.

The next step in blending is to decide on the carrier oil or other base product.

Step 2: Choose Carrier Oil or Other Delivery System

The choice of carrier oils or other delivery systems, such as a cream, gel, or lotion, is an essential aspect of the blending process. Carrier oils can be mixed together to create an additional therapeutic substance that will be further enhanced with the addition of the synergy of essential oils. A variety of carrier oils will be covered in depth in Chapter 6, while other base products will be covered in Chapters 8 and 9.

For the example used above, tendinitis/stress, you could choose to blend the following base oils to fill a one-ounce bottle for the massage session:

    10 percent Arnica herbal oil
    10 percent St. John's wort herbal oil
    80 percent Apricot kernel oil

Step 3: Dosage: At What Dilution?

According to Mills and Bone (2000), "The subject of appropriate dose is probably the most controversial aspect of contemporary Western herbal medicine" (p. 116). This could be said of the practice of aromatherapy as well. The vast majority of traditional aromatherapists adopt a low dilution, between 1 and 3 percent, when blending with essential oils. High dosages and undiluted applications are still considered by many within the aromatherapy industry to be highly controversial, while others believe that these higher dilutions are warranted at certain times and for specific conditions.

Indeed, many research and empirical studies appear to be confirming that sometimes a higher dilution and even an undiluted application is what is called for, particularly if treating a viral, bacterial, or fungal infection. And while it would not be prudent to assume one dosage is necessarily more worthy or more correct or incorrect than another, it is necessary to understand that dosage decisions are truly based upon the practitioner's knowledge and experience with applying essential oils as well as available safety knowledge.

Another aspect to great blending is to have a strong sense of purpose for the blend. *Attempting to accomplish diverse goals in a blend can dilute its overall efficacy.* It would be impossible to create a blend for chronic bronchitis and varicose veins. These two conditions not only require different oils but also different methods of application.

As bodyworkers and massage therapists, you may choose to work with two or three blends with different dilutions. For instance, you may choose to use a 5 percent dilution for localized treatment of acute muscular aches and pains of the neck and back and a 2.5 percent dilution for the rest of the body. Indeed, higher dilutions are often meant to be applied to a smaller, more localized area whereas a lower dilution may be utilized for full-body massage and/or more emotional treatment work.

Perhaps in the future, as aromatherapy develops, more defined or coherent guidelines for dosage will arise. For now, dosage decisions must be made within a framework of reasons.

Dosage depends on:

▶ the condition being treated and whether it is in an acute or chronic state
▶ the method of application and the area of the body to be covered
▶ the safety data of essential oils to be used, established guidelines when applicable
▶ the integrity of the skin that it will be applied to
▶ the age of the individual who will be using the blend/synergy
▶ the specific goal of treatment
▶ the knowledge and confidence of the practitioner
▶ the current commonly or generally accepted dosage

Traditional Dosage Chart

Percentage	Drops per Ounce of Carrier	Indicated For
1 percent or less	2 to 6 drops	Children, infants, pregnancy, face creams
1.5 percent	9 drops	Subtle aromatherapy, emotional and energetic work, pregnancy, frail/elderly, face creams and oils
2.5 percent	15 drops	Holistic aromatherapy, general massage work, general to stronger skin care
5 percent	30 drops	Stronger dilution, treatment massage, localized treatment work, wound healing
10 percent	60 drops	Strong dilution acute physical symptom relief, localized treatment work
10 to 15 percent	60 to 90 drops	Same as 5-10 percent. An uncommon dilution but may increase therapeutic activity depending on purpose and condition for which it is being applied, treatment work on localized area

More Advanced Blending Dilutions

>25% Often used in more advanced treatment blends under qualified and confident practitioners; Used for localized treatment work on small area. Caution is expressed with choice of essential oils.

IN PRACTICE 5.1

The Drop Controversy

The traditional dosage chart reveals percentages and number of drops and has been provided here due to its ease and simplicity of use. Drops and percentages have long been used by aromatherapists as measurements for the dosage of essential oil/ within a given delivery system, carrier, or base product.

According to research by Svoboda, Ruzickova, Allan, and Hampson (2001), however, this system has some serious flaws. First, 20 drops per milliliter appears to be a myth. Based upon their findings, a milliliter of essential oil can be anywhere from 20 to 40 drops depending on the essential oil, the company it comes from, and the dropper size used to dispense it. During the research project, it was also found that each essential oil drop varies in volume, weight, and viscosity.

The researchers believe that this ence may have a potential effect on the therapeutic value of a blend as well as the financial cost (e.g., 20 drops of rose essential oil compared to 20 drops of eucalyptus).

Drops and percentages are still the most commonly used measurements for aromatherapy applications and hence for the purpose of this text we shall use this method.

The aromatherapy industry will continue to change and grow on its own time; for now, the recognition of the inadequacy of drops is observed with an eye toward developing better methods in the future.

>40% Rare to almost unheard of within mainstream aromatherapy. Tiger balm is an example of such high dilution. It is highly effective as an analgesic for muscular aches and pains. Used for localized treatment work on small area. Caution is expressed with choice of essential oils.

100% For most forms of inhalation and for the creation of synergies or undiluted applications; can be useful for insect bites, burns, cuts and scrapes, spot acne treatment, spot muscle ache or spasm treatment, digestive upset treatment, fungal or bacteria infection, headaches or migraines, etc. Used for localized treatment work on small area. Caution is expressed with choice of essential oils.

For the tendinitis/stress blend, we will use a 5 percent dilution, which means 30 drops for the one ounce of carrier oils.

⟶ MEASUREMENT AND DILUTION CHARTS

Measurement Chart				
1ml	20 drops			
5mls	100 drops	1 teaspoon		
10mls	200 drops	2 teaspoons	⅓ ounce	
15mls	300 drops	1 tablespoon	½ ounce	
30mls	600 drops	2 tablespoons	1 ounce	
60mls	1200 drops	4 tablespoons	2 ounces	
120mls	2400 drops	8 tablespoons	4 ounces	1/2 cup
240mls	3600 drops	16 tablespoons	8 ounces	1 cup

Dilution Chart

Carrier Oil in Ounces	.5% Dilution	1%	2.5%	3%	5%	10%
½ ounce	1–2 drops	3 drops	7–8 drops	9 drops	15 drops	30 drops
1 ounce	3 drops	6 drops	15 drops	18 drops	30 drops	60 drops
2 ounces	6 drops	12 drops	30 drops	36 drops	60 drops	120 drops
4 ounces	12 drops	24 drops	60 drops	72 drops	120 drops	240 drops

Step 4: The Blending Factor

Based upon the example provided, we now have the synergy, carrier oils, and dilution decided as follows:

Essential oils: Lavender, German chamomile, Sweet marjoram, and Helichrysum.

Carrier oils: 10 percent Arnica herbal oil

10 percent St. John's wort herbal oil

80 percent Apricot kernel oil

Dilution: 5 percent

The final step in creating the blend is to decide how many drops of each essential oil to use. This can be accomplished by using the blending factor. The blending factor is a concept I learned during my education in aromatherapy at the Raworth Centre of Natural Medicine in England. Over the years, many have found that it is an invaluable tool for creating well-balanced blends. The blending factor can be thought of in terms of an aromatic potency scale and is utilized as a tool for determining the appropriate and specific number of drops for each essential oil within a given blend or synergy.

Blending Factor Scale (1 to 10)

1 = Powerful aroma, use less in blend

10 = Tends to be more volatile, lighter aroma, use more in blend

Perceiving Blending Factor

The following exercise is meant to help support your awareness of what determines an individual essential oil's blending factor.

Step 1: Choose three essential oils out of your repertoire of oils.

Step 2: Remove the lids off all three bottles.

Step 3: Using both your hands, hold the bottles together so that all the tops are at the same height.

Step 4: Swirl the bottles under your nose, slowly, a number of times. Then pause a moment and repeat. Repeat as needed to gain further insight.

Step 5: Decide which of the three is the most potent (which one seems to be standing out the strongest), and then place this one down on the table. Then with the remaining two bottles repeat Steps Three, Four, and Five.

With only three oils, once you have determined the second most potent essential oil, the remaining oil would be considered the least potent. You then have the oils in a line from most potent to less potent, which means the first one will have the least amount of drops, while the third one will have the most and the second a middle number of drops.

You will have a chance to work on an exercise to help support your application of the blending factor at the end of this section.

Setting a Blending Factor

If you find that you are using an essential oil for which no blending factor has been given, you can use the above exercise to figure it out. Often it is best to compare the unknown essential oil to an essential oil from the same botanical family. For instance, the blending factor for fir (*Abies alba*) has not been provided. Fir belongs in the same family as pine (*Pinus sylvestris*) and cedarwood (*Cedrus atlantica*), both of which have known blending factors.

Flexible Blending Factor

The blending factor provides the beginning blender with a way of figuring out how many drops of each essential oil should go into the blend. The blending factor is by no means written in stone, for it is meant to be flexible to the essential oils in your repertoire. This means that we acknowledge that essential oils vary in strength from company to company, from year to year, harvest to harvest, and so forth. So one should feel free to adopt different blending factor numbers based upon a comparison with other oils of stable potency, such as Roman chamomile (*Chamaemelum nobile)* or neroli (*Citrus aurantium*), which would always be more potent (BF: #1), or citrus oils which are always more volatile and lighter.

Potency or Therapeutic Activity

The blending factor is based upon potency of aroma and, to a much smaller degree (if at all), therapeutic potency. I would compare blending factors as follows: Roman chamomile has a blending factor of 1, which means it is very "potent" and only a small amount needs to be used for a blend or synergy in relation to other oils being blended. Lavender (*Lavandula angustifolia*), on the other hand, has a blending factor of 7, which means a medium or higher percentage of lavender can be used than Roman chamomile.

I would also use the concept of blending factor when deciding on how many drops of each essential oil to put in a bath. I would use less of "potent" oils, such as neroli and Roman chamomile (2 to 3 drops per bath), a medium amount of geranium (*Pelargonium graveolens*) or ylang ylang (*Cananga odorata*) (3 to 5 drops per bath), and a higher number of drops for mandarin (*Citrus reticulata*) or lavender (7 to 10 drops per bath).

Blending Factor in Practice

Continuing on with our example for tendinitis/stress, we can decide on drops as follows:

Essential Oil	Blending Factor	Drops
Lavender	7	12
German chamomile	1	3
Sweet marjoram	3	6
Helichrysum	5	9
Total	5% dilution =	30

There are two ways of figuring out the drops: by mathematical equation or by intuitive observation. I have never been fond of mathematical equations, and essential oils do not always fit into precise calculations, so the first number chosen is, in a sense, a bit random while at the same time maintaining its relation to the others. In this example, German chamomile and sweet marjoram are the two most potent essential oils, while helichrysum is a little more potent than lavender. Hence, I chose to work with the most potent oils first by designating 3 drops for German chamomile and 6 drops for sweet marjoram. This added up to 9 drops leaving 21 drops to be divided between the other two oils. I then examined the varying strengths of the helichrysum and lavender in my repertoire of essential oils and decided on 9 drops for helichrysum and 12 drops for lavender.

The mathematical equation method of figuring out exact drops would be performed as follows:

Essential Oil	Blending Factor	Drops
Lavender	7	
German chamomile	1	
Sweet marjoram	3	
Helichrysum	5	

First add up the total blending factors: 7 + 1 + 3 + 5 = 16

Then divide the blending factor number for each essential oil by 16, which would look something like this.

Essential Oil	Blending Factor	
Lavender	7	7 divided by 16 = .4375
German chamomile	1	1 divided by 16 = .0625
Sweet marjoram	3	3 divided by 16 = .1875
Helichrysum	5	5 divided by 16 = .3125

You now have the percentage for each essential oil that will make up the 30 drops for the 5 percent dilution. To obtain the actual number of drops, you would then multiply the percentage for each essential oil by 30.

Essential Oil	Blending Factor	
Lavender	7	.4375 * 30 = 13 drops
German chamomile	1	.0625 * 30 = 2 drops
Sweet marjoram	3	.1875 * 30 = 6 drops
Helichrysum	5	.3125 * 30 = 9 drops

The final blend would then look like this:

Essential Oil	Blending Factor	
Lavender	7	13
German chamomile	1	2
Sweet marjoram	3	6
Helichrysum	5	9
Total	5% dilution =	30

As you can see, the final results using the mathematical formula are pretty close to what I originally got with the more intuitive approach.

Step 5: Perform Massage

With the massage blend prepared, you are now ready to apply it with your chosen massage and bodywork technique.

Blending Factor Chart		
Common Name	**Latin Name**	**Blending Factor**
Angelica	*Angelica archangelica*	2 to 3
Basil	*Ocimum basilicum*	4
Bergamot	*Citrus bergamia*	7
Birch	*Betula lenta*	2
Black pepper	*Piper nigrum*	3 to 4
Cardamon	*Elettaria cardamomum*	4
Cedarwood	*Cedrus atlantica*	5 to 6
Roman chamomile	*Chamaemelum nobile*	1

Blending Factor Chart (*Continued*)

Common Name	Latin Name	Blending Factor
German chamomile	*Matricaria recutita*	1
Clary sage	*Salvia sclarea*	2 to 3
Cypress	*Cupressus sempervirens*	5
Eucalyptus	*Eucalyptus globulus*	4 to 5
Fennel	*Foeniculum vulgare*	3
Frankincense	*Boswellia carterii*	3 to 4
Geranium	*Pelargonium graveolens*	3
Ginger	*Zingiber officinale*	4
Grapefruit	*Citrus paradisi*	6
Helichrysum	*Helichrysum italicum*	5
Jasmine	*Jasminum officinale*	1
Juniper berry	*Juniperus communis*	4
Laurel, bay	*Laurus nobilis*	2
Lavender	*Lavandula angustifolia*	7
Lemon	*Citrus limon*	4 to 5
Lemongrass	*Cymbopogon citratus*	1
Mandarin	*Citrus reticulata*	7
Sweet marjoram	*Origanum marjorana*	3
Melissa	*Melissa officinalis*	1
Myrrh	*Commiphora myrrhanee*	4 to 5
Neroli	*Citrus aurantium*	2
Orange	*Citrus sinensis*	7
Patchouli	*Pogostemom cablin*	5
Peppermint	*Mentha x piperita*	1 to 2
Pine	*Pinus sylvestris*	4 to 5
Ravensara	*Ravensara aromatica*	7
Rose	*Rosa x damascena*	1
Rosemary	*Rosmarinus officinalis*	2 to 3
Sandalwood	*Santalum album*	6
Tea tree	*Melaleuca alternifolia*	3
Thyme	*Thymus vulgaris*	1
Vetiver	*Vetiveria zizanioides*	1
Yarrow	*Achillea millefolium*	3
Ylang ylang	*Cananga odorata*	4

↳ BLENDING OBSERVATIONS

The following are a series of observations about blending. They are listed here to serve as helpful guidance during the blending process.

■ **Blend essential oils first:** When creating an aromatherapy massage oil, cream, gel, or other application, it is best to blend the essential oils together first. The essential oils will merge together more quickly this way. If you add each essential oil separately directly into a base product, it will take longer for them to blend together.

■ **Glass: a valuable tool:** Whether creating a blend or a synergy, it is most beneficial to blend in a glass container rather than plastic. Plastic seems to alter the aroma and dull the therapeutic synergistic blending of the oils themselves. It is also possible that some small quantity of essential oil is naturally drawn into the plastic as well. For these reasons, avoid using plastic for blending essential oils. One can always add the synergy into a base product and then into a plastic bottle for immediate use, when needed or desired. Glass, on the other hand, appears to support the successful integration of the essential oils and should be used as the first vehicle for blending.

■ **Shake-down:** Once you have placed 3 to 5 essential oils inside a glass bottle, it is important to swirl and shake the oils around. This can be accomplished by placing the lid securely on the bottle and then gently shaking. This will allow the oils to move around, interact, and merge together. One should shake the bottle for at least 2 to 3 minutes. Once you have done this, open the bottle and see how the blend is merging together.

IN PRACTICE 5.2

Glass or Plastic: An Essential Controversy

The best medium to blend essential oils is glass, particularly amber or blue cobalt glass. However, in the real world, we understand that this is not always possible nor is it always desirable.

When opting for plastic, only use a dark-colored PET (Polyethylene Terephthalate) plastic, as it is least likely to leach out the valuable essential oils or affect the chemical composition of your blends. PET bottles are lightweight, tough, and highly resistant to dilute acids, oils, and alcohols. They are available in different colors and are recyclable; they can be recognized by the triangular recycle symbol with the number 1 in the center. PET plastics can be recycled into a variety of other products, including ski coat fibers, fleece vests, and sleeping bag linings. Never store undiluted essential oils in PET bottles; always use glass for essential oil synergies.

When using plastic, fill the container halfway with your base material first, then add your selected essential oils or synergy. Finish filling with base material, cap or cover, and shake well to blend.

IN PRACTICE 5.3

To Shake or Not To Shake

There appears to be some differences of opinion within the aromatherapy community as to whether one should shake their blends or not. This appears to be a matter of opinion rather than of scientific fact, so it is truly up to the individual to decide what feels right to them.

Many subtle/energetic aromatherapy practitioners believe that a blend/synergy should be gently rolled in the hand. It should be noted that homeopathic remedies use shaking as an important aspect of potentizing the remedy. According to the National Center for Complementary and Alternative Medicine, "A concept that became 'potentization,' which holds that systematically diluting a substance, with vigorous shaking at each step of dilution, makes the remedy more, not less, effective by extracting the vital essence of the substance" (http://nccam.nih.gov/health/homeopathy/).

Other aromatherapists believe that a blend should be shaken to ensure the oils have been properly blended together. In the authors' experience, shaking a blend is most beneficial. Either way appears to be fine as both methods have been employed for years with great success.

Sometimes one of the essential oils is still taking over the aroma; this can mean one of two things: either the synergy needs to be shaken more or more drops of the other essential oils in the blend need to be added. It is wise, before adding additional drops, to repeat the shaking of the bottle a few more times. This can sometimes have the effect of merging the essential oils more closely together. If after this exercise one of the essential oils is still showing up more than it should, you can add a drop or two of the other oils in the blend. This can often have an immediate balancing effect on the whole blend. (See In Practice 5.3 To Shake or Not To Shake.)

■ **Synergizing time:** If you have ever blended before, you will have noticed how a blend or synergy can change over time. Like all relationships, the interaction of one essential oil with another, as well as the interaction of a large number of chemical constituents, is bound to create an ongoing dialogue as they figure out ways to merge, enhance, or dull the other. Basically, when essential oils are blended together, it takes time for them to merge. Synergizing time takes into account that a blend or synergy will continue to change and evolve over time.

SUMMARY

■ An aromatherapy consultation is designed to gather information about the client, evaluate the condition(s) to be addressed, and to provide a framework for designing an individualized aromatic program.

■ Attending and active listening are basic communication skills that enable the therapist to develop a therapeutic relationship with the client and to enhance the therapist's ability to design an effective treatment approach.

■ Three possible approaches to blending include a physiological approach, an emotional/mental/spiritual approach, and a holistic (combination) approach.

■ The three elements in structuring an effective synergy include a core essential oil that addresses the primary purpose of the blend; an enhancer essential oil that strengthens the core essential oil in its purpose and therapeutic action; and a harmonizing essential oil that supports and enhances the vitality and overall purpose of the synergy.

■ Vegetable and herbal carrier oils can be blended together to create an additional therapeutic substance, which enhances the overall activity of the essential oils.

■ The dosage/dilution of essential oils ranges from 1 percent or less to 100 percent. The choice of what dilution to use depends on a number of factors including condition being treated, method of application, safety of essential oils being used, integrity of skin, age of individual, currently accepted dilution levels, and the confidence and experience of the practitioner.

■ The standard aromatherapy massage dilution is 2.5 percent or 15 drops of essential oil for every one ounce of carrier.

■ The blending factor is an aromatic potency scale that may be utilized as a tool for determining the number of drops for each essential oil within a synergy or blend.

■ Essential oils will merge together more quickly when blended together first without a base (e.g., cream, vegetable oil).

■ It is best to utilize glass for blending essential oils, but if it is necessary to use plastic, it is important to utilize PET plastic.

NEW TERMINOLOGY

Active listening	Empathy
Attending	Enhancer essential oil
Blending factor	Harmonizing essential oil
Core essential oil	Synergy
Dosage/dilution	

REFERENCES

Maury, M. (1989). *Marguerite Maury's Guide to Aromatherapy: The Secret of Life and Youth*. Essex, England: C.W. Daniel Company.

Mills, S., and Bone, K. (2000). *Principles and Practice of Phytotherapy*. London: Churchill Livingstone.

Morris, L. (1997). Focused Listening. *International Journal of Aromatherapy 8* (1), 16–17.

Rattray, F., and Ludwig, L. (2000). *Clinical Massage Therapy*. Toronto, Ontario: Talus Incorporated.

Svoboda, K.P., Ruzickova, G., Allan, R., and Hampson, J.B. (2001). An investigation into drop sizes of essential oils using different dropper types. *International Journal of Aromatherapy 10* (3/4), 99–103.

WORKSHEET

Blending Practicum

With your partner, perform a standard massage consultation, adding any questions you would like to in order to create an effective aromatherapy massage blend. Select essential oils which have been covered in the course so far.

Name:_____   Date:_____

Primary purpose:_____

Secondary purpose: _____

Discuss your blending approach:_____

_____

_____

Essential oils selected

Essential Oil – Common Name	Essential Oil – *Latin Name*	Why Chosen?

You will be blending a 1-ounce bottle of oil with a 2.5 percent dilution rate. Using the blending factor, figure out how many drops of each essential oil will go into the blend:

Essential Oils	Blending Factor	Drops

Dilution 2.5 percent in 1 ounce   Total drops: 15

Blend massage oil and give to partner to use at home.

CHAPTER TEST

1. List four types of information a consultation is designed to collect.

   a.

   b.

   c.

   d.

2. Effective attending communicates to the client that the therapist is fully present and actively engaged with them.

   _____True   _____False

3. The blending factor reveals the _____ of an essential oil.

   a. aromatic potency

   b. note

   c. core purpose

   d. harmonizing action

4. Designate the number of drops for each essential oil based upon the blending factor. The total number of drops to be used is 60.

   Cypress   BF: 5   Drops: _____

   Eucalyptus   BF: 4 to 5   Drops: _____

   Rosemary   BF: 2 to 3   Drops: _____

5. It appears that essential oils merge more quickly together when blended _____.

   a. into water first

   b. directly into the base oil

   c. together in a glass container first

   d. as a perfume

6. A physiological approach to blending bases the selection of essential oils upon the _____ and/or _____. (select two from below)

   a. emotional aspects

   b. chemistry

   c. known therapeutic actions

   d. energetic properties

7. If you are blending for an emotional reason, it is important that the client finds the blend _____.

    a. therapeutic

    b. pleasant

    c. chemical-based

    d. unappealing

8. An essential oil with a blending factor of 10 means:

    a. less potent

    b. not potent at all

    c. more potent

    d. equally potent

9. The standard synergy or blend typically has _____ essential oils.

    a. 0 to 1

    b. 8 to 12

    c. 3 to 5

    d. 5 to 25

10. The holistic aromatherapy massage oil dilution is most commonly:

    a. 1 percent

    b. 5 percent

    c. .5 percent

    d. 2.5 percent

REVIEW QUESTIONS

1. Discuss the idea of dosage in aromatherapy.

2. Complete the following chart.

Create a blend for muscular aches and pains: 2.5 percent dilution in a 60 mls base

Essential Oils	Blending Factor	Drops
Peppermint	1 to 2	
Rosemary	2 to 3	
Black pepper	3 to 4	
Total		30

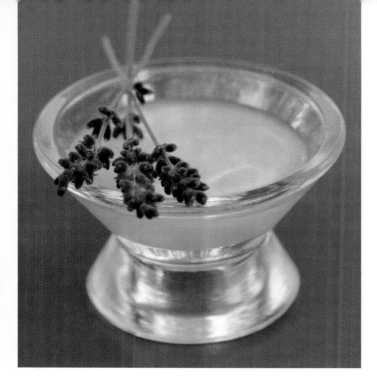

Aromatherapy and the Skin

➔ LEARNING OBJECTIVES

After reading this chapter, you will be able to

1. Describe the basic structure and list five functions of the skin.
2. Discuss the ability of essential oils to penetrate the skin and list six factors that influence their ability to be absorbed dermally.
3. List seven potential therapeutic benefits of applying essential oils to the skin.
4. Describe eight therapeutic actions essential oils have on the skin and provide at least three samples of essential oils with each therapeutic action.
5. Describe and list therapeutic benefits of a range of vegetable carrier oils, herbal oils, and other raw material.
6. List and describe important fat-soluble vitamins and nutrients found in vegetable carrier oils.
7. Create effective aromatherapy blends for a variety of skin types and conditions.

INTRODUCTION

Werner and Benjamin (1998) best summarize the interaction between the bodyworker and the skin by saying "Massage practitioners speak in a language of touch. The messages practitioners give are invitations to a number of different possibilities: to enjoy a state of well-being; to heal and repair what is broken; to reacquaint a client with his or her own body. All this happens through the skin, a medium equipped like no other tissue in the body to take in information and respond to it, mostly on a subconscious level" (p. 1).

⤳ ANATOMY AND PHYSIOLOGY OF THE SKIN

The skin consists of three main layers:

> the epidermis—the outermost layer
> the dermis—the middle layer
> the subcutanea—the innermost layer

The Epidermis

The epidermis consists of five layers, in which the transformation from living cells to dead cells occurs (Figure 6-1). These five layers, beginning with the outermost layer, include:

A. **The stratum corneum.** This is the layer of the epidermis that is exposed to the environment and *consists of nonliving skin cells composed of keratin protein*. These cells are constantly being shed as cells move upward from the lower layers of the epidermis to the surface.

On the surface of the stratum corneum is a light layer of oil from the sebaceous glands and water from the sudoriferous glands, which create what is known as the **acid mantle**. This is a slightly acidic layer on our skin that protects the skin from infection. The acidity of an adult skin is around 5pH to 6pH.

THE SKIN

- covers an average of eighteen square feet and weighs about seven pounds
- contains one hundred sweat glands, twelve feet of blood vessels, and hundreds of sensory receptors for touch, heat, and cold in each square centimeter of skin
- serves as a protective barrier, when unbroken
- serves as our first line of defense against disease and bacterial invasion
- regulates body temperatures by constricting blood vessels in cold temperatures to preserve body heat and producing sweat in warm temperatures to cool the body by water evaporation
- detoxifies the body by excreting wastes
- breathes (takes in oxygen and releases carbon dioxide)
- absorbs nutrients and manufactures vitamin D
- protects the body from ultraviolet damage from the sun by producing melanin, a tan
- is also our largest sensory organ

Kusmirek (2002) points out that the skin's acid mantle is vital to the skin's health as it is our first line of defense against germs and contains elements that maintain crucial moisture. According to Kusmirek, vegetable oils support this crucial system.

B. **The stratum lucidum.** This is known as the barrier and clear layer. It is thin and poorly defined, varying in thickness from one cell to noticeable thickness on the palms of the hands and the soles of the feet. It is composed of hardened skin cells (nonliving) made of keratin, similar to the stratum corneum.

C. **The stratum granulosm.** This is known as the transitional layer because the cells are changing. They are beginning to die, harden, or become keratinized, and have lost significant oil and water content. It is one to four cellular layers thick.

D. **The stratum spinosum.** It is five to eight layers thick and has lost some of its oil and water content. The cells flatten as they rise from the lower part of these layers to the upper part, becoming almost tilelike.

E. **The stratum germinativum.** This is the deepest layer of the epidermis. You may notice that cells in this layer are cube-shaped. *It is the only layer of the epidermis that undergoes cell reproduction* (**mitosis**). Skin rejuvenation begins with this layer; many factors, such as age, diet, circulation, exposure to heat, cold, light, drugs, and smoking, will influence the rate of cell regeneration. The average life cycle of each new cell is about five to six weeks. Any skin care treatment aimed at improving the skin will need at least six weeks to two months before any real improvement can be expected.

Langerhans' Cells

Immune cells in the epidermis Langerhans' cells are **phagocytic cells** (cells that ingest and destroy foreign matter, such as microorganisms or debris) that play a role in immunity. They are found mainly in the stratum spinosum and stratum germinativum layers of the epidermis, though they can also be found in other organs

Figure 6-1 The three layers of the skin

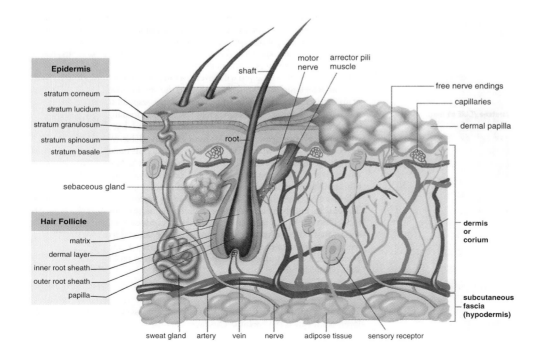

Epidermis
- stratum corneum
- stratum lucidum
- stratum granulosum
- stratum spinosum
- stratum basale

sebaceous gland

Hair Follicle
- matrix
- dermal layer
- inner root sheath
- outer root sheath
- papilla

shaft
root
motor nerve
arrector pili muscle
free nerve endings
capillaries
dermal papilla
dermis or corium
subcutaneous fascia (hypodermis)

sweat gland   artery   vein   nerve   adipose tissue   sensory receptor throughout the body. Langerhans' cells seem to be present in lymphatic nodes as well. According to Funnel (nd), "These cells participate in the cutaneous immune response and migrate from skin to lymph nodes."

These immune system cells send dendrites to the very surface layer of the stratum corneum. They are exposed to everything happening at the surface, and they come into contact with everything applied to the skin. Langerhans' cells are involved with the skin's reaction, such as in dermatitis or sensitization. Materials aimed at activating the skin's natural defense system can have truly far-reaching effects. And these are capabilities that have long been claimed for aromatherapy.

The Dermis

The thicker layer beneath the epidermis is the dermis, also called the "true skin" because most vital functions of the skin are carried out there. The dermis is made up of the following structures:

■ **Connective tissue:** **Connective tissue** gives the skin strength, resiliency, and flexibility. There are two main types of fibers that make up the connective tissue (fibrous material) in the dermis: elastin and collagen. **Elastin** is a protein component of the fibers that give the skin its elasticity—the ability to stretch and return to its original shape. **Collagen** is a complex, long-chained protein that is tough and does not stretch easily. It gives the skin strength and makes up about 75 percent of the fibrous material. The connective tissue fibers are supported in a gel-like substance composed mostly of mucopolysaccharides, particularly hyaluronic acid. **Hyaluronic acid** attracts and retains water to maintain moisture and flexibility in the skin.

■ **Blood and lymph vessels:** The dermis is well supplied with blood vessels, both arterioles and capillaries that originate from arteries and veins in the subcutaneous layer. Capillary loops arise vertically from fine vessels and supply the papillary structures with nutrients while carrying away waste products. Lymph vessels take up fluid from the capillaries that has been diffused but not reabsorbed by them. This helps prevent swelling. They also help remove waste products.

■ **Hair follicles:** Extending from deep in the dermis to the surface of the skin, the hair follicle is a tubular structure that is lined with epithelial tissue and houses the growing hair. The only muscle in the skin is the erector pili muscle, which is attached to each hair follicle. It causes the hair to stand on end, reacting to cold or emotion. The hair follicle is considered to be a site of entrance into the dermal layer of the skin, and hence the bloodstream, for essential oils.

■ **Glands:** The **sebaceous glands** are attached to the hair follicle and produce oil called sebum (See Figure 6-2) that is secreted onto the surface of the skin. Sebum lubricates the hair follicle and hair shaft and acts as an emollient for the skin, protecting it from moisture loss. It also acts as an antibacterial agent. Some researchers believe that sebum's primary function may be as a pheromone, a hormone whose scent attracts the opposite sex. Sebaceous glands are most concentrated on the face, scalp, neck, upper back, and chest.

Figure 6-2   The sebaceous gland

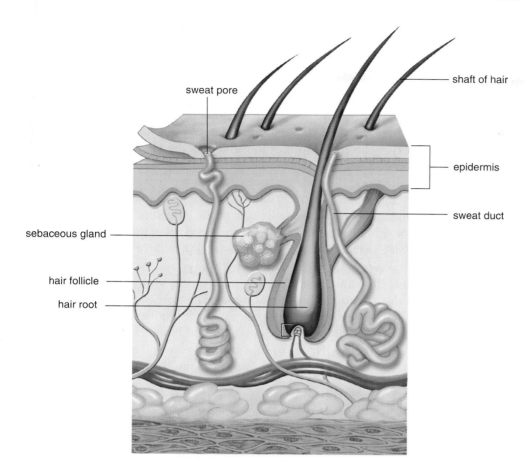

The **sudoriferous glands**, also known as the sweat glands, help to maintain body temperature by secreting perspiration. The hypothalamus is the key regulator of body temperature and responds to the temperature of circulating blood. Sympathetic nerves, in response to raised body temperature, stimulate sweat glands. The evaporation of perspiration from the skin's surface cools the body. There are two types of sudoriferous glands: the apocrine (the larger) and eccrine (the smaller).

◼ **Sensory nerves (and the importance of touch):** The skin is our largest sense organ, containing a large number of nerve endings, and is the first sense to develop. According to Field (2003), touch is critical for growth and human development, communication and learning, comfort and reassurance, and to build emotional bonds. She comments that alternative treatments, such as massage therapy and acupuncture, are helping to bring touch therapy back to medicine, where, since prerecorded time, it legitimately reigned as the primary form of therapy.

The Subcutanea

Below the dermis is the third layer called the subcutaneous layer. It varies in thickness and is made of a fatty tissue that gives the body smoothness and contour. It serves as a shock absorber and cushion for the vital organs, stores energy, and is an effective insulator. It also houses a network of arteries that form capillaries that branch into the dermis layer.

⤷ THE SKIN: A PATHWAY ONTO AND INTO THE BODY

The popular application of essential oils to the skin has been contributed to the seminal work of Marguerite Maury entitled *Marguerite Maury's Guide to Aromatherapy: The Secret of Life and Youth*, published in France in 1961. In her book, Maury (1989) quotes Dr. Badmadjeff as saying: "If it is possible to influence an individual from the outside to the point of modifying his philosophy, it must be done by means of aromatherapy substance—and through the skin." During her career Maury sought and found, via dermal application, a method of application for essential oils that was capable both of "influencing the muscular tonus, the quality and aspect of the skin and the tissues, and to obtain a better functioning and a normalization of the individual's rhythm" (Maury, 1989, p. 108). Maury was able to successfully merge aromatherapy with massage.

In 1992, Tony Balacs wrote: "Aromatherapists tend to believe that the recipients of aromatherapy massage will gain benefit in three ways: from absorbing the essential oil through the skin, from inhaling the vapor, and from the massage itself." And indeed, this statement holds true today. The skin is a pathway onto the body whereby essential oils exert their influence on the skin itself as well as a pathway into the body where essential oils may enter general blood circulation, possibly influencing the whole body. See Figure 6-3 for the Pathways Chart.

Figure 6-3   The skin: a pathway into the body

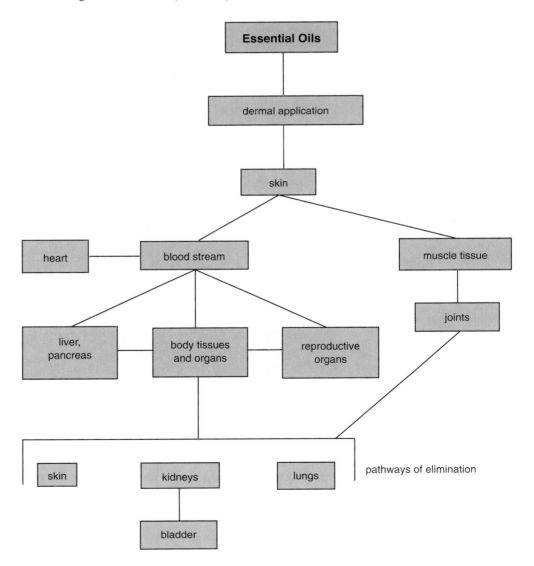

According to Balacs (1992), "the skin is highly efficient at transporting small, relatively fat-soluble molecules like essential oils into the body's interior, especially when aided by a circulation-stimulating massage." Factors that affect the degree to which essential oils are absorbed into the skin include:

■ **Temperature of the skin:** Skin that has been warmed through bathing or the application of a compress tends to be more permeable than cold skin.

■ **Hydration of the skin:** Skin exhibiting good hydration tends to be more permeable than dehydrated skin.

■ **Lipophilic nature and molecular structure:** Essential oils are known to be highly lipophilic, which means they are attracted to fat. Essential oils are also known to have a small molecular structure that enables them to permeate through the stratum corneum into the dermal layer and on into systemic blood circulation.

■ **Skin integrity:** The condition of the skin has an affect on the permeability of essential oils. Damaged or compromised skin is often more permeable than healthy skin. Caution should be used in dosage and choice of essential oils for treatment of damaged or compromised skin conditions.

■ **Hair follicles and thickness of skin:** It has long been assumed that one of the entrance pathways for essential oils is through the hair follicles. Areas with a greater number of hair follicles may allow increased essential oil penetration, whereas areas of the skin that are thick, such as the feet and hands, may reduce or slow down the penetration of essential oils.

■ **Occlusion:** Occlusion refers to the process of applying essential oils and then covering the area with something like a bodywrap or compress. This occlusion will allow for greater penetration of essential oils.

Once essential oils have been absorbed through the skin, they are able to affect the muscles and joints as well as body tissue and organs. Bowles (2003) writes: "It is not known to what extent essential oil constituents penetrate to the adipose layer from a dermal application, though dermally applied oils do appear to have anti-inflammatory and analgesic effects on muscles and joints without having to enter the systemic circulation" (p. 121).

Essential oils are then excreted in the urine, feces, perspiration, and breath. According to Cooksley (1996), essential oils take fifteen minutes to twelve hours to be fully absorbed and about three to six hours to be expelled in a normal healthy body. Absorption and excretion times increase for individuals with obesity or who have poor circulation or thickened skin. With regard to absorption, not all components of an essential oil are absorbed equally; rather, some constituents penetrate more quickly than others. As Buckle (2003) points out, in the case of lavender, most of the two main constituents, linalol and linalyl-acetate, were absorbed within twenty minutes and eliminated within ninety minutes.

Buckle (2003) further comments that the study of where essential oils go when they are absorbed and how they are absorbed and eliminated by the body is still not fully understood. What is known is that essential oils exert a profound influence on overall well-being when used correctly.

For massage therapists and bodyworkers, the application of essential oils to the skin can offer the following therapeutic benefits:

▶ relax and soothe muscles and joints
▶ reduce muscle spasms
▶ relieve nerve pain
▶ reduce inflammation
▶ provide a cooling or warming effect
▶ provide antibacterial, antifungal, or antiviral activity and support
▶ relax and soothe the nervous system
▶ provide specific therapeutic benefits for common skin conditions
▶ aid in the treatment of sprains, strains, and repetitive movement injuries

The remainder of this chapter will focus on the application of essential oils, vegetable oils, herbal oils, and other raw material that may be applied to the skin for massage and bodywork purposes. Table 6.1 lists the therapeutic benefits essential oils have for the skin. In the next chapter we will explore two other pathways into the body: inhalation and olfaction.

TABLE 6.1

Essential Oil Therapeutics for the Skin

Therapeutic Action	Essential Oils
Anti-inflammatory—a substance that soothes and reduces inflammation	German chamomile, Frankincense, Helichrysum, Lavender, Myrrh, Patchouli, Sandalwood, Yarrow
Antibacterial—a substance that destroys bacteria	Basil ct. linalol, Cinnamon leaf, Eucalyptus, Lemongrass, Niaouli, Palmarosa, Sage, Tea tree, Thyme, Yarrow
Antifungal—a substance that destroys or inhibits fungal growth	Cinnamon leaf, Clove bud, Lemongrass, Myrrh, Niaouli, Palmarosa, Patchouli, Tea tree, Thyme
Antiseptic—a substance that destroys or prevents the growth of microbes	Bergamot, Roman chamomile, Cypress, Frankincense, Grapefruit, Lavender, Lemon, Lemongrass, Sweet marjoram, Scots pine, Tea tree
Astringent—a substance that causes cells to shrink; contracts, tightens, and binds tissues	Cedarwood, Cypress, Geranium, Lemon, Patchouli, Rose
Circulatory Stimulant/Tonic—a substance that enhances or increases blood circulation	Carrot seed, Black pepper, Juniper, Laurel, Lemon, Lemongrass, Pine, Rosemary ct. camphor or cineole
Cellular Rejuvenation—a substance that enhances cellular reproduction	Carrot seed, German chamomile, Helichrysum, Lavender, Palmarosa
Detoxifier—a substance that enhances the removal of toxic substances from the body	Carrot seed, Cypress, Fennel, Grapefruit, Juniper berry, Lemon
Nervine/Relaxant—a substance that relaxes the nervous system; can reduce or soothe nervous disorders	Angelica root, Bergamot, German chamomile, Roman chamomile, Frankincense, Lavender, Mandarin, Sweet marjoram, Melissa, Neroli, Sweet orange, Petitgrain, Rose, Sandalwood, Vetiver, Ylang ylang
Vulnerary—a substance that promotes wound healing	Carrot seed, German chamomile, Roman chamomile, Frankincense, Helichrysum, Lavender, Myrrh, Neroli, Patchouli, Rosemary ct. verbenon, Sage, Yarrow

↪ VEGETABLE OILS IN PRACTICE

Vegetable oils are an intrinsic part of the *materia medica* or repertoire of an aromatherapist as carrier oils and as therapeutic substances with astounding benefits for holistic bodywork and massage (Kusmirek, 2002). As **carrier oils**, vegetable, nut, or seed oils are used *to dilute essential oils and carry them onto the skin and into the body*. As therapeutic substances, vegetable oils are a good source of oil-soluble vitamins, such as A, D, and E, as well as essential fatty acids, all of which are needed by the skin to maintain its health, tone, and elasticity.

Expeller pressed organic unrefined vegetable oils are the best oils for the skin as these are extracted at low temperatures and do not go through a refining process, thus preserving the valuable nutrients of the oil. Refined oils have generally been extracted through the use of high temperatures and have undergone subsequent processing, including deodorizing the oil to remove the taste and smell, bleaching, and other refining. In doing so, the vitamin content of the oil is reduced and the essential fatty acid content largely destroyed rendering an oil with little to no therapeutic value.

According to Erasmus (1993), "the oils available in supermarkets, corner groceries, and convenience stores, whether from safflower, walnut, sunflower, corn, grape seed, soybean, sesame, rice bran, canola, almond, peanut, avocado, other seed or nut sources, or oil blends, are fully refined and deodorized, and are either solvent-extracted or a mixture of expeller-pressed and solvent-extracted oils. Fully processed oils are the equivalent of refined sugars, and can therefore be called 'white' oils (p.98)."

The application of high-quality, unrefined organic vegetable oils offers an array of valuable nutrients to support, nourish, and enhance the functions of the skin. These nutrients include:

Fat-Soluble Vitamins and Nutrients Found in Vegetable Oils

■ **Vitamin E:** The vitamin E family is referred to as "tocopherals" that includes alpha, beta, gamma, and delta tocopherals. Alpha-tocopheral is considered by some to be the most biologically active. Vitamin E is one of the most important **antioxidants**, which means that it is able to prevent cell damage from the destructive elements of free radicals. Free radicals, when in excess, can damage healthy tissue, destroy the collagen and elastin fibers that support the skin, and interfere with the formation of fresh, healthy skin cells, making our complexions blotchy and dull.

Vitamin E helps to protect the skin against environmental pollutants. It is used topically to reduce scar formation and to treat burns, including radiation burns. Vitamin E assists wound healing and has great repairing and regenerating properties. In conjunction with beta-carotene, vitamin E may decrease the harmful effects of the sun. Research studies are showing that vitamin E could be an important component of a healthy immune system. Oils with vitamin E could therefore be used to support the Langerhans' cells in the skin with their immune function.

■ **Vitamin A:** Vitamin A is an essential vitamin for cellular growth and repair of body tissues. It plays a crucial role in preserving the integrity of red blood cell membranes as well as the skin. Vitamin A is particularly important for the mucous cells lining the respiratory, digestive, urinary, and reproductive tracts as well as the membranes of the eyes and the ducts of secretory glands. Some symptoms of deficiency include rough, dry, scaly skin; lack of tearing; problems with gums and teeth; loss of smell and appetite; and night blindness.

■ **Beta-carotene:** Beta-carotene is one of over five hundred carotenes that occur in nature. Beta-carotene, a precursor to vitamin A, is considered to be one of the most active of the carotenes. "It is a potent scavenger of toxic oxygen radicals, especially those produced by chemicals in the air and those generated by our own metabolism. It has stronger immune-stimulating and thymic supportive activity than vitamin A" (Golen, 1995, p. 132). Oils rich in beta-carotene tend to be a rich orange color.

Beta-carotene is found in carrot phytol, palm oil, and algae. Palm oil also contains the carotene lycopene, which appears to have more anticancer abilities then beta-carotene. According to Pizzorno and Murray (2000), "beta-carotene may play a role in protecting the skin from the damaging effects of the sun, beta-carotene functions as a cellular screen against sunlight-induced free radical change" (p. 607).

■ **Vitamin D:** This works with calcium to build bones, teeth, and healthy skin. It promotes healing and is good for burns and abrasions. According to Kusmirek (2002), avocado oil is the only vegetable oil that contains vitamin D.

■ **Lecithin:** This is an important component of cellular membranes, particularly those of the brain and nerves. It is a powerful emulsifying agent and helps to remove fats and cholesterol from the blood.

Essential Fatty Acids Found in Vegetable Oils

Essential fatty acids (EFAs) are called "essential" because our bodies cannot manufacture them, therefore we must consume them in our diets and apply them to our skin. Essential fatty acids are an important part of the membranes of every cell in our body. According to Murray and Beutler (1996), without a healthy membrane, cells lose their ability to hold water, vital nutrients, and electrolytes. They also lose their ability to communicate with other cells and be controlled by regulating hormones.

Unrefined polyunsaturated oils, such as flax seed, evening primrose, borage, passionflower, and rosehip seed oil, are rich in EFAs. Fatty oils rich in EFAs are extremely reactive and are easily damaged by light, heat, and oxygen exposure. Keep oils rich in EFAs refrigerated. The following are essential fatty acids found in oils used for aromatherapy and massage purposes.

■ **Linoleic acid:** Linoleic acid is an essential fatty acid that is important in building the membranes that surround every skin cell. It helps to strengthen the protective lipid barrier that lies beneath the surface of the skin and guards against moisture loss. Lack of linoleic acid can lead to serious skin problems, premature aging, and can reduce the strength of the skin's supporting collagen fibers, which may slow wound healing and can trigger hair loss. Linoleic acid is converted into gamma linoleic acid in the body.

■ **Oleic acid:** Oleic acid is a monounsaturated fatty acid. Vegetable oils with a high content of oleic acid are more resistant to the damaging affects of heat and light.

■ **Gamma linoleic acid (GLA):** This is a very important fatty acid that helps in the formation of prostaglandins. Prostaglandins play an important role in the inflammatory process, blood clotting, stimulating smooth muscle in the uterus, inhibit the secretion of gastrointestinal acid, and increase the secretion of a protective mucous layer in the stomach. Oils rich in gamma linoleic acid can play an important role in treating inflammatory conditions including eczema, psoriasis, and rheumatoid arthritis. Apart from breast milk, evening primrose oil, black currant, and borage seed oil are the main sources.

⟶ COMMON CARRIER OILS

■ **Almond, Sweet** *Prunus amygdalus* var. *dulcis*

Sensory info: Pale yellow, light to no aroma.

Shelf life: Medium to long (6 to 12 months). Best to refrigerate to prolong shelf life.

Dosage: Can be used 100 percent or in a blend of other oils.

Nutrient profile: Monounsaturated oil contains valuable trace minerals. High in oleic acid, which helps to keep it stable.

Therapeutic applications: A good emollient, it protects and nourishes the skin. Helps relieve itching, soreness, dryness, and inflammation of the skin, e.g., eczema. Good for all skin types, particularly dry skin.

■ **Apricot** *Prunus armeniaca*

Sensory info: Pale yellow. Light texture, easily absorbed.

Shelf life: Medium to long (6 to 12 months). Can keep refrigerated to prolong shelf life.

Dosage: Can be used 100 percent or in a blend of other oils.

Nutrient profile: Contains vitamins, especially A and E, and trace minerals. High in oleic acid, which helps to keep it stable.

Therapeutic applications: All skin types, especially mature, dry, sensitive, or inflamed skin. Good facial oil as it encourages the skin to secrete its own natural oils. Good moisturizer for scalp. A great combination for massage is 50 percent apricot kernel and 50 percent sunflower oil.

■ **Avocado** *Persea americana*

Sensory info: Dark green to light green to almost clear. Thick, heavy oil, but very penetrating, easily absorbed. Green color is due to large amounts of chlorophyll (Earle, 1992).

Shelf life: Short life (3 to 6 months), degrades quickly unless preserved.

Dosage: Can be used 10 percent in a blend of other oils, depending on purpose.

Nutrient profile: Contains vitamins, especially A, B, and D, proteins, lecithin, and sterol (up to 10 percent).

Therapeutic applications: Revitalizing and regenerating. A wonderful emollient for the skin. Promotes cellular regeneration. Can be used as a natural sunscreen. According to Kusmirek (2002): "repeated massage applications with avocado and sesame reveal an increase in hydration of the upper layers of the skin and an improvement in the skin's elastic properties" (p. 98). Can be used for all skin types, especially dry, dehydrated, fragile, or mature skin; also for dry eczema or psoriasis.

▣ Grape seed   *Vitis vinifera*

Sensory info: A very popular oil as it has a light texture, is nongreasy, easily absorbed, and has very little smell. Almost colorless to pale green. Most grape seed oil on the market is solvent extraction although some expeller pressed oils are available. Expeller pressed is preferred.

Shelf life: Medium to long (6 to 12 months). Can keep refrigerated to prolong shelf life.

Dosage: Can be used 100 percent or in a blend of other oils.

Nutrient profile: Low cholesterol content. Contains vitamins, minerals, and proteins, but not as nourishing as other oils.

Therapeutic applications: All skin types.

▣ Hazelnut   *Corylus avellana*

Sensory info: Light to dark yellow oil.

Shelf life: Stable and long lasting.

Dosage: Medium to long (6 to 12 months). Can keep refrigerated to prolong shelf life.

Nutrient profile: Contains vitamins A and B. Rich in vitamin E.

Therapeutic applications: This oil is highly recommended as a carrier oil because of its ability to penetrate the epidermis without leaving the skin greasy (Kusmirek, 2002). Indicated for dry, dehydrated, or sensitive skin types. Great emollient.

▣ Jojoba   *Simmondsia chinensis*

Sensory info: Liquid wax from desert plant. Golden to light yellow. Light, fine texture; very penetrating; odorless.

Shelf life: Stable and long lasting.

Dosage: Can be used 100 percent or in a blend of other oils.

Nutrient profile: Contains proteins, vitamins, especially E, minerals, and a waxy substance that mimics collagen.

Therapeutic applications: Jojoba has been used for acne to dissolve clogged pores and support the skin's natural pH balance. It has natural anti-inflammatory properties, making it helpful for eczema, psoriasis, and inflamed skin. Wonderful all around skin care oil. Hair care: dry scalp, dandruff. Smoothes cuticles. Can reduce wrinkles by increasing hydration. Can prevent or reduce stretch marks. Indicated for oily, combination, or acne skin types although all skin types will benefit.

▪ Olive *Olea europaea*

Sensory info: Greeny yellow to yellow. Rich and sticky, strong smell.

Shelf life: Stable. Medium to long. Do not refrigerate but keep in cool location.

Dosage: Can be used 100 percent or in a blend of other oils.

Nutrient profile: Moderately saturated oil. Contains vitamins, especially E, minerals, and proteins.

Therapeutic applications: Has disinfecting and wound-healing properties, which makes it helpful for infected skin, itchy, sore, inflamed, chapped, and scaly skin. Useful in treating eczema and psoriasis. Softening and soothing. Indicated for sensitive skin.

▪ Palm oil *Elaeis guineensis*

Sensory info: Yellow to reddish, solid mass like coconut oil.

Shelf life: Stable. This oil can be solvent extracted or cold pressed. Cold pressed is recommended.

Dosage: Can be used 100 percent or in a blend of other oils.

Nutrient profile: 51 percent saturated fat. Palm oil is similar in composition as coconut oil.

Therapeutic applications: According to Pizzorno and Murray (2000), "Palm oil carotenes appear to give much better antioxidant protection than other sources" (p. 606). Due to its high content of carotenes, palm oil would be beneficial in regenerative skin care, including postsurgical wounds as well as aging or premature aging skin. Palm oil may be beneficial for enhancing the immune system via the Langerhans' cells in the skin and for photosensitivity disorders. Palm oil serves as a good emollient for the skin.

▪ Rose Hip *Rosa rubiginosa*

Sensory info: Very pleasant aroma, pinkish red color, emollient to the touch.

Shelf life: Low to medium stability. Must be kept refrigerated.

Dosage: Can be used 10 to 20 percent in a blend of other oils.

Nutrient profile: A complex system of unsaturated essential fatty acids, contains high amounts of linoleic acid and vitamin C, as well as smaller amounts of trans-retinoic acid.

Therapeutic applications: One of the best tissue regenerators for scars, skin burns, and premature aging (not oily or acne skin as it blocks the pores). Rosehip seed oil is high in essential fatty acids. It is believed to be a powerful tissue regenerator and has been used to help heal burns and sunburns, improve the appearance and texture of scars, and reduce wrinkles. It is indigenous to the Andes and is commonly sold as Rosa Mosquet or Muscat oil.

▪ Shea butter *Butyrospermum parkii*

Sensory info: A yellow butter, soft yet thick; becomes liquid at body temperature.

Shelf life: Medium to long. (6 to 12 months). Keep cool or in refrigerator.

Dosage: Can be used 100 percent or in a blend of other oils.

Nutrient profile: Has a high content of non-saponfiable fats, including Kariten, Allantoin, and vitamins F, E, and A.

Therapeutic applications: Shea butter is a heavenly butter/oil that has been traditionally used by natives of Africa for its softening, emollient qualities for the skin. Shea butter increases microcirculation in the skin and hence is beneficial in wound healing, scar tissue formation, and cellular rejuvenation. Shea butter is perfect for keeping the skin soft, supple, and healthy. Prevents chapping and irritation, softens rough skin, and protects against sunburn. It is also a beautiful addition to skin care creams and salves.

■ Sunflower   *Helianthus annuus*

Sensory info: Pale yellow, light in texture.

Shelf life: Rich oleic acid makes it more stable, although not as stable as jojoba. Medium shelf life (6 to 12 months).

Dosage: Can be used 100 percent or in a blend of other oils.

Nutrient profile: Unsaturated oil. Contains vitamins and minerals and some lecithin.

Therapeutic applications: It is good for all skin types. Great texture for massage and skin care preparations.

■ Walnut   *Juglans regia*

Sensory info: Pale yellow to golden; medium texture.

Shelf life: Medium shelf life (6 to 12 months).

Dosage: Can be used 100 percent or in a blend of other oils.

Nutrient profile: Rich, unsaturated fatty acid oil. Rich in linoleic acid and good content of GLA.

Therapeutic applications: Great emollient and helps the skin to retain moisture. Indicated for mature, inflamed, or sensitive skin types. Has regenerative activity.

↪ HERBAL OILS

Herbal oils are infusions of medicinal herbs most commonly in an olive oil or sunflower oil base. Typically, fresh (which has been dried to some extent to remove all moisture) or dried plant material is placed in a jar and then covered with the chosen vegetable oil. This mixture is then placed in the sun for two to four weeks or longer and then strained. These herbal infusions are then applied to the skin for a variety of therapeutic benefits, depending on the medicinal plant used. To learn more about infusing herbal oils, we recommend James Green's book, *The Herbal Medicine Makers Handbook,* or Rosemary Gladstar's *Herbal Healing for Women*.

The three most common herbal infusions utilized by massage therapists and bodyworkers will be discussed below; however, it is important to remember that a wide range of medicinal plants may be used to create therapeutic herbal oils for application to the skin.

▦ Calendula *(Calendula officinalis)*

Calendula is an annual herbaceous plant, 1 to 2 feet high, with medium-green leaves and a much branching fragrant stem. The daisylike flowers can be a delightful variety of light orange, yellow, and even golden to dark yellow flowers. It will flower all summer long and well into autumn. It is one of the easiest plants to grow and one that provides great joy.

Therapeutic benefits: Calendula has been shown to be an effective antimicrobial (both antiviral and antibacterial), anti-inflammatory, antifungal, and vulnerary herbal oil. Clinical trials have shown that calendula increases cell proliferation and encourages the granulation process of wound healing.

Calendula is indicated for:

- wound healing/tissue repair
- inflamed skin conditions
- poorly healing wounds
- cracked skin conditions
- burns
- insect bites
- cracked nipples due to breastfeeding (nontoxic to baby)
- damaged tissue, ulcers

▦ Arnica *(Arnica montana)*

Arnica is a perennial herb and a member of the Asteraceae (compositae) family. It grows 30 to 60 cm tall and has yellow-orange flowers. *Arnica montana* occurs naturally in Central and Northern Europe. Other species of arnica that exhibit the same therapeutic benefits include *Arnica cordifolia* and *Arnica latifolia*. These species are found predominantly in the western United States.

Therapeutic benefits: Arnica has been shown to provide antimicrobial, anti-inflammatory, wound healing and analgesic effects. According to Moore (1993), "arnica works by stimulating and dilating blood vessels, particularly the specialized capillaries that control whether blood is piped into the small peripheral capillary beds or is shunted over to small veins, bypassing more widespread blood dispersal. Good, diffused blood transport and circulation into injured, bruised, or inflamed tissues helps speed up resolution and removal of waste products" (p. 49).

Safety data: Only apply arnica on unbroken skin. Arnica is considered to be toxic internally. Avoid use if client has allergies to other species within the Asteraceae family, e.g., ragweed, German chamomile. Extended use may cause eczema (Mills and Bone, 2000).

Arnica is indicated for:

- bruises
- sprains and strains
- counterirritant to treat rheumatism
- burns, including sunburns
- hyperextensions
- arthritis, bursitis, or myalgia
- joint stiffness

■ St. John's Wort (*Hypericum perforatum*)

St. John's wort is a perennial herb with small bright-yellow flowers. It is native to Europe and Asia and naturalized in the United States and Australia. It grows abundantly in the Pacific Northwest and Canada. St. John's wort flowers in early summer. The infused oil is made from the flower buds just before they open.

Therapeutic benefits: St. John's wort is known for a wide range of therapeutic activity. As an herbal oil, it has been shown to be an effective antimicrobial, anti-inflammatory, analgesic, and vulnerary agent.

St. John's wort is indicated for:
- insect bites
- burns, including sunburns
- damaged tissue, slow healing wounds or ulcers
- bruises
- herpes lesions
- myalgia (muscle pain)
- dermal inflammation
- sprains and bruises (not as potent as arnica)

⤳ OTHER RAW MATERIAL

■ Coconut oil

For hundreds of years, Philippine and Hawaiian women have been utilizing coconut oil to protect the skin and soften the hair.

Coconut oil can be used to:

soften rough, dry skin

reduce chronic skin inflammation

soothe skin rashes

limit the damage to the skin from excessive sun exposure

Coconut oil also serves as an excellent ingredient for salves and creams as a thickening and emulsifying substance. Coconut is a solid oil that can occlude the skin when used alone; however, the use of coconut with other vegetable oils or in creams reduces the occluding action of coconut by itself.

■ Cocoa butter

Cocoa butter is the ivory-colored natural fat of the cocoa bean extracted during the manufacturing process of producing chocolate and cocoa powder. Cocoa butter is solid at room temperature but it has a low melting point (just below body temperature), and it does change from a solid to a liquid quickly. Besides smelling like chocolate, cocoa butter is a wonderful emollient butter for the skin. It can be added into a homemade cream or gently (low heat, indirect heat) melted down with other carrier oils.

■ Beeswax and honey

Beeswax comes from the honeycomb of the honey bee. Beeswax will have a dark to light yellow color and will have a unique sweet honeylike aroma. It is used as an

IN PRACTICE 6.1

Use of Honey

Salt Scrub and Honey Foot Treatment
Make Salt Scrub by combining the following ingredients:

4 tbsp. of sea salt

1 tbsp. apricot kernel oil

3 drops tangerine (*Citrus reticulata*) essential oil

1 teaspoon warmed honey

Mix the ingredients well. Prior to massage, scrub the feet with the salts and place feet in hot/warm water foot bath. Leave for 5 to 10 minutes; remove feet from foot bath and dry them; send client into massage room and ask them to prepare for the massage treatment.

emulsifier and thickening agent in the creation of homemade creams, lotions, and salves. The best beeswax is local unprocessed beeswax, rich in color and vibrant with aroma.

Honey is used in spa and bodywork treatments for its ability as a natural humectant. Honey helps attract and retain moisture in the skin, making the skin soft and supple. Honey is being used for back and bodycare treatments, foot spa treatments, and for the face and neck. Research studies are showing that honey has a natural ability to protect the skin from free radicals, and it may be employed as an antioxidant agent in skin care products. Honey has been historically used for its antimicrobial properties, and in many countries honey is still considered a medicine and not just a sweetener for teas and cereals.

AROMATIC APPLICATIONS FOR THE SKIN

Skin Types

Although everyone's skin is basically the same physiologically, characteristic differences result from heredity, lifestyle, or age, and the skin is classified as a certain "type." As a massage therapist or bodyworker, it is important to be able to understand skin types so as to select the most beneficial essential oils, base oils, and methods of application for each client. Although it is outside the scope of practice for therapists to "diagnose" skin type, you may certainly educate your clients as to the characteristics of various skin textures and ask them which best describes their skin type. In this way you can further customize your massage and body care blends by using base vegetable oils and/or herbal oils along with specific essential oils that will work best with each client's skin type and goals.

Normal Skin

For our purposes in "skin typing," normal skin indicates that the water and oil glands on the face are producing just the right amount to hydrate (add moisture) and protect the skin (prevent moisture loss). Normal skin's appearance is moist, plump, and dewy. The pores are small to medium in size. There are few or no blemishes and minimal sun damage. The skin is of medium thickness and has good tone. Normal skin is soft, smooth, and firm. It may have some oiliness in the "T zone" (the forehead, nose, and chin), but unless the oil is excessive, the skin is still considered normal.

ESSENTIAL OILS: Any essential oil, particularly Carrot seed, Clary sage, Frankincense, Geranium, Lavender, Neroli, Rose, Sandalwood, Vetiver

VEGETABLE OILS: Grapeseed, Jojoba, Sweet almond, Apricot kernel, Shea butter, Sunflower

Oily Skin/Acne Prone

Oily skin has sebaceous glands that are too active. The pores are visibly more noticeable than in other skin types and are medium-to-large in size. Oily skin has a shiny appearance and is usually thicker, firmer, and less sensitive than the other types. Oily skin appears most often among those aged twelve to twenty-two, but some people may have oily skin all their lives, although it should gradually become less oily with age. While there is a tendency for clogged pores, blackheads, and blemishes, the good news for oily skin is that it usually has a youthful appearance and does not show the signs of aging as quickly as the other skin types.

ESSENTIAL OILS: Cedarwood, Clary sage, Cypress, Frankincense, Geranium, Helichrysum, Juniper berry, Lavender, Lemon, Lemongrass, Melissa, Niaouli, Palmarosa, Patchouli, Petitgrain, Rose, Tea tree, Ylang ylang

VEGETABLE OILS: Grapeseed, Jojoba, Hazelnut, Sunflower

Dry Skin

Dry skin has a lack of oil, a lack of water, or both. Skin that is lacking in oil is called simple dry skin. Skin that is lacking in water is called dehydrated skin. If the skin is thin and the pores are barely visible, it is probably lacking in oil (and possibly water as well). If the skin is thick with visible pores but has the characteristics of dry skin, it is probably only lacking water.

Dry skin can be seen in people of all ages. Women tend to have drier skin than men do, and fair-skinned people have dry skin more often than dark-skinned people do. Dry skin can feel tight and may have visible flaking. It is often delicate, easily irritated, and usually sensitive to cold weather. Dry skin has a matte finish with no sheen and can have a rough feel to it.

ESSENTIAL OILS: German chamomile, Roman chamomile, Clary sage, Fennel, Lavender, Myrrh, Sandalwood, Vetiver, Ylang ylang

VEGETABLE OILS: Apricot kernel, Sweet almond, Avocado, Hazelnut, Jojoba, Olive, Shea butter, Sunflower, Walnut

Sensitive Skin

Sensitive skin is characterized by overreaction to external influences. Certain cosmetics, handling, and environmental factors (such as sun, wind, and temperature extremes) easily irritate it. Exposure can result in redness, a rash, itching, stinging, or burning. Sensitive skin has a tendency to develop distended or broken capillaries as well as allergies, and it usually sunburns easily.

Sensitivity can be present in normal, dry, and oily skins and at any age. However, it is most common among people of Celtic descent, particularly redheads and people with blond hair and blue eyes. Sensitive skin is thinner than other skin types; the nerve endings and blood vessels tend to be closer to the surface, which is thought to be one of the causes of the oversensitivity.

Sensitive skin needs to be treated gently. The cause of irritation can vary with each individual, so a sensitive skin care program can also vary. Generally, however, products that contain alcohol, artificial colors, and artificial fragrances should be avoided. Highly active ingredients, such as alpha hydroxy acids, may also need to be avoided. Essential oils may or may not be able to be used. If used, it should be in a low dilution with soothing and gentle oils. Preservatives have also been known to cause problems for some people.

ESSENTIAL OILS: German chamomile, Roman chamomile, Frankincense, Helichrysum, Lavender, Neroli, Rose, Sandalwood

VEGETABLE OILS: Apricot kernel, Grapeseed, Hazelnut, Jojoba, Olive, Shea butter, Sunflower, Walnut

Aging/Mature Skin

"Aging" is a characteristic that may be combined with any of the other skin types, for example, aging/sensitive skin or aging/blemished skin, or it can simply mean mature skin. When the aging condition is present, it may be appropriate for the individual, or it may be "premature." Appropriate aging occurs naturally from the passage of time and the slowing down of the glandular functions in the skin, lessening its ability to rejuvenate. Premature aging is the result of overexposure to the sun (the number one cause), smoking, improper skin care, mistreatment, poor lifestyle habits, or health problems. In these cases, the skin looks older than it should.

ESSENTIAL OILS: Carrot seed, German chamomile, Roman chamomile, Frankincense, Geranium, Helichrysum, Lavender, Lemon, Myrrh, Neroli, Palmarosa, Rose, Sandalwood, Vetiver

VEGETABLE OILS: Apricot kernel, Avocado, Grapeseed, Jojoba, Palm, Rosehip seed, Shea butter, Sunflower, Walnut

Common Skin Conditions

Most skin disorders, for example, boils, acne, impetigo, and herpes simplex, commonly contraindicate massage, at least locally. The following conditions often benefit from massage. (**NOTE:** Cellulite will be covered in Chapter Ten under Lymph and Immune Health.)

◾ **Psoriasis: Psoriasis** is noted when the skin has well-demarcated raised red patches or thickening of the skin caused by rapid cell division (up to 1000 times faster than normal skin cell division). The skin has the appearance of being scaly and dry, and it may itch and bleed. Psoriasis is thought to be caused by chemical or mechanical irritations, change of climate, genetic disposition or stress-related reactions. Psoriasis most often occurs around the elbows, knees, scalp, and back, although it can occur anywhere on the body. Stress tends to aggravate conditions of psoriasis.

According to Bensouilah (2003), psoriasis is a particularly difficult condition to treat and, not surprisingly, the more severe the symptoms, the more difficult it is to provide effective treatment. However, she goes on to say that aromatherapists should not be deterred from attempting to address the distressing symptoms of psoriasis. Aromatherapy is used to provide relief of symptoms, reduce stress, and provide a supportive role to other natural therapies such as naturopathy or homeopathy.

THERAPEUTIC GOALS

- Reduce itching and/or inflammation
- Aid in healing the skin, avoiding scar formation
- Reduce stress

ESSENTIAL OILS: German chamomile, Roman chamomile, Cypress, Frankincense, Helichrysum, Lavender, Myrrh, Neroli, Patchouli, Rose, Sandalwood, Vetiver, Ylang ylang

BASE MATERIAL: Shea butter, Calendula, Aloe vera gel with hydrosols of Lavender and German chamomile

▓ **Scars:** Scars are marks left on the skin after healing from an injury, trauma, or surgery. When the skin has been wounded, fibroblast cells repair the tissue. Sometimes fewer collagen and elastic cells are present during the healing process, and the result is skin that is firmer and less elastic. Old scars are difficult to change but can be improved with a diligent program. Using essential oils while the skin is healing can minimize or prevent scarring. The application of essential oils on old scar tissue can also lead to a healthier and loving relationship to the scar and its possible painful memory. According to Werner and Benjamin (1998), massage is locally contraindicated during the acute state of any injury in which the skin has been damaged, however, in the subacute state, massage may improve the quality of the healing process.

Types of Scars

▓ **Keloid:** Keloid scar is actually a thick, puckered, itchy cluster of scar tissue that grows beyond the edges of a wound or incision. Keloid scars can be very nodular in nature. You may notice a somewhat darker color of the keloid scar tissue compared to the rest of the skin. Keloids occur when the body continues to produce tough, fibrous protein (known as collagen) after a wound has healed, causing a raised mass of scar tissue that goes outside the edges of the initial wound or incision.

▓ **Hypertrophic:** Scars are thick and raised and often darker in color than surrounding skin. They differ from keloid scars in that they are usually confined to the original area of damage. Hypertrophic scar formation is not a part of normal wound healing and can develop over time. These kinds of scars are a problem in patients with a genetic predisposition (tendency) to scarring and in deep wounds that require a long time to heal.

THERAPEUTIC GOALS

- reduce inflammation
- aid in healing the skin
- reduce scar formation
- keep skin supple
- address emotional issues

ESSENTIAL OILS: Carrot seed, German chamomile, Frankincense, Helichrysum, Lavender, Lavendin, Myrrh, Neroli, Palmarosa, Patchouli, Rose, Rosemary ct. camphor or ct. verbenon, Sage, Sandalwood, Tea tree, Ylang ylang

BASE MATERIAL: Jojoba, Rosehip seed oil, Calendula oil, St. John's wort, Shea butter

AROMATHERAPY APPLICATIONS: Massage blend, 2.5 to 5 percent dilution

gel

cream or lotion

Sample scar formulation:

25 to 30 percent rosehip seed oil

25 percent calendula herbal oil

50 percent jojoba

essential oils (in order of quantity): helichrysum, carrot seed, rosemary ct. verbenon, lavendin (*Lavandula × intermedia*).

■ **Eczema/Dermatitis: Eczema/dermatitis** is an inflammatory skin disorder usually brought on by an outside agent. Dermatitis can be accompanied by eruptions, redness in the skin, dry or scaly skin, and/or swelling. Eczema is a more superficial form of dermatitis, affecting the epidermal layer. With eczema the skin is red, dry patchy skin, with a rash that can be either dry or weeping. Inflammation occurs and the eczema can be raw, painful and sometimes bleeding.

There are different types of eczema, including **contact eczema** caused by an allergic reaction to irritating substances, for example, chemicals, rubber, metals, soaps, and washing powders; **varicose eczema**, which is commonly present in people with varicose veins and the elderly; **atopic eczema**, which is often found in people with a family history of allergic reactions to, for example, hay fever or asthma; and **discoid eczema**, which can be seen as scaly, itchy, round-shaped patches found on the limbs.

According to Rattray and Ludwig (2000), "Massage is not completely contraindicated for dermatitis and eczema. If the lesions are open and oozing, they are avoided. If open lesions are not observed, and with the agreement of the client, gentle massage using essential oils over the lesions may be helpful. Care is taken to ensure that the client does not react to the carrier, lotion, or essential oil" (p. 1147).

THERAPEUTIC GOALS

- reduce itching and/or inflammation
- aid in healing the skin, avoiding scar formation
- reduce stress

ESSENTIAL OILS: Carrot seed, German chamomile, Roman chamomile, Cypress, Frankincense, Geranium, Helichrysum, Lavender, Melissa, Myrrh, Palmarosa, Rose, Tea tree, Sandalwood, Vetiver, Ylang ylang

BASE MATERIAL: Jojoba, Sunflower, Apricot kernel, Shea butter, Calendula, Aloe vera gel with hydrosols of lavender and German chamomile

IN PRACTICE

Case Study 6.1

Chronic Eczema and Stress

B. is a thirty-six-year-old woman who has been suffering with chronic eczema for several years. She has small-to-medium patches on her neck, hands, and arms. The skin is inflamed and itchy. She feels that stress is a major contributing factor to the current episode. B. is currently in the midst of a divorce and is under considerable pressure at work. B. is hoping that massage and aromatherapy can help relieve her stress as well as relieve the inflammation and itchiness caused by the eczema.

Massage Oil Blend: Soothe Stress/Eczema

20% Calendula herbal oil

20% Jojoba oil

60% Apricot kernel

■ German chamomile (*Matricaria recutita*): anti-inflammatory, stress-relieving, soothes itching, 5 drops

■ Helichrysum (*Helichrysum italicum*): anti-inflammatory, soothes the skin and emotions, 7 drops
■ Lavender (*Lavandula angustifolia*): anti-inflammatory, reduces itching and stress, 12 drops
■ Geranium (*Pelargonium graveolens*): balancing, soothing to emotions, 6 drops

2 oz. glass bottle/ 2.5% dilution

A full-body relaxation massage was provided. The remaining massage oil blend was given to the client for home use. She would apply the oil to specific areas affected by the eczema twice a day and as needed or desired. She could also rub on neck to help with stress relief. After the session the client reported feeling very relaxed. On a two-week follow–up, B. reported a significant improvement in the eczema that she said had almost completely disappeared. She also reported feeling much more relaxed and was enjoying using the blend.

SUMMARY

■ The skin is comprised of three layers: the epidermis, the dermis, and the subcutanea. The skin functions as a protective covering and is our first line of defense. The skin helps regulate body temperature, absorbs valuable nutrients, detoxifies, breathes, plays a role in immunity via the Langerhans' cells, and is our largest sensory organ.
■ Factors that affect the degree to which essential oils are absorbed into the skin include temperature and hydration of the skin, the skin's integrity, the lipophilic nature of the essential oils, the number of hair follicles, thickness of the skin, as well as occlusion of the area to which they are applied.

- Essential oils applied to the skin have the ability to affect the muscles and joints, and they may exert an anti-inflammatory or analgesic effect, relieve nerve pain, provide a cooling or warming effect, reduce muscle spasms, and assist in the treatment of a variety of musculoskeletal conditions.
- Essential oils exhibit a wide range of activity on the skin, from anti-inflammatory actions of such oils as German chamomile to vulnerary actions of such oils as helichrysum.
- Vegetable oils are called carrier or base oils and are utilized to dilute essential oils for application to the skin. Vegetable oils also provide valuable nutrients for the skin and help to maintain the skin's health, tone, and elasticity. The best vegetable oils to use for massage are those that are organic, unrefined, or minimally processed.
- The application of high-quality, unrefined organic vegetable oils offers an array of valuable nutrients to support, nourish, and enhance the functions of the skin, including such nutrients as vitamins A, D, and E, beta-carotene, lecithin, and essential fatty acids (EFAs).
- Herbal oils are sunflower or olive oil infusions with medicinal plants. The three most common herbal oils used in massage therapy include arnica, calendula, and St. John's wort. Herbal oils can be used at a 20 percent dilution with other vegetable carrier oils.
- The five basic skin types are normal, oily or acne prone, dry, sensitive, and aging/mature. Each skin type has numerous essential oils and vegetable oils that may support and improve the skin's overall health and appearance.

NEW TERMINOLOGY

Acid mantle

Antioxidants

Atopic eczema

Carrier oils

Collagen

Connective tissue

Contact eczema

Discoid eczema

Eczema/dermatitis

Elastin

Herbal oils

Hyaluronic acid

Langerhans' cells

Mitosis

Phagocytic cells

Psoriasis

Sebaceous glands

Sudoriferous glands

Varicose eczema

REFERENCES

Balacs, T. (1992). Dermal Crossing. *International Journal of Aromatherapy 4* (2), 23–25.

Bensouilah, J. (2003). Psoriasis and Aromatherapy. *International Journal of Aromatherapy 13* (1), 2–7.

Bowles, E.J. (2003). *The Chemistry of Aromatherapeutic Oils*. Crows Nest, Australia: Allen & Unwin.

Buckle, J. (2003). *Clinical Aromatherapy*. Philadelphia, PA: Elsevier Science.

Cooksley, V. (1996). *Aromatherapy—A Lifetime Guide to Healing with Essential Oils.* Englewood Cliffs, New Jersey: Prentice Hall.

Earle, L. (1992). *Vital Oils.* London: Ebury Press, Random House.

Erasmus, U. (1993). *Fats that Heal, Fats that Kill.* Burnaby, Canada: Alive Books.

Field, T. (2003). *Touch.* Boston, MA: Massachusetts Institute of Technology.

Funnel, R. (nd). *What Is a Dendritic Cell?* Retrieved October 2, 2005, from: http://cmmg.biosci.wayne.edu/asg/dendritic.html

Golan, R. (1995). *Optimal Wellness.* New York: Ballantine Books.

Kusmirek, J. (2002). *Liquid Sunshine.* Glastonbury, England: Foramicus.

Maury, M. (1989). *Marguerite Maury's Guide to Aromatherapy: The Secret of Life and Youth.* Essex, England: C.W. Daniel Company.

Mills, S., and Bone, K. (2000). *Principles and Practice of Phytotherapy.* London: Churchill Livingstone.

Moore, M. (1993). *Medicinal Plants of the Pacific Northwest.* Sante Fe, New Mexico: Red Crane Books.

Murray M., and Beutler, J. (1996). *Understanding Fats and Oils.* Encinitas, CA: Progressive Health Publishing.

Pizzorno, J.E., and Murray, T. (2000). *Textbook of Natural Medicine.* London: Churchill Livingstone.

Rattray, F., and Ludwig, L. (2000). *Clinical Massage Therapy.* Toronto, Ontario: Talus Incorporated.

Werner, J., and Benjamin, B. (1998). *A Massage Therapist's Guide to Pathology.* Baltimore, MD: Williams & Wilkins.

WORKSHEET

Aromatherapy and the Skin (Part I)

Name:_____ Date:_____

Exploring Carrier Oils

1) Compare the texture and viscosity of three different vegetable base oils as well as at least one commercially prepared massage lubricant. Note your observations below; discuss with the group.

Name of Oil/Texture	Viscosity			Use with Skin Type:	Notes
	Light	Med	Heavy		
	☐	☐	☐		
	☐	☐	☐		
	☐	☐	☐		
	☐	☐	☐		
	☐	☐	☐		

Base Oils and Skin Types

2) Read the client profiles below. Based on the information given, determine which carrier oils you would choose when creating a base blend for massage. List at least two essential oils you would use.

a) Jill is a secretary at a busy law firm. She is twenty-two years old and lives alone with her two cats. In her teenage years she battled regular breakouts, which seem to have recently returned to her back and shoulders. Lately she has been under a great deal more stress at work than usual. Jill says she has normal-to-oily skin. She tries to avoid foods with peanuts and milk due to sensitivities. She is here for a massage, hoping to reduce stress and improve sleep.

Base Oil/Material	Percentage	Why Chosen?

Essential Oils: _____, _____,
_____

b) Mary is a forty-five-year-old stay-at-home mom. She has three children ranging in age from seven to seventeen. Mary reports having dry skin, and lately she has been feeling depressed because her mother is ill. Mary has no known allergies but is very sensitive to soaps and perfumes and will often get red patches on her skin when using store-bought products. She is here to receive massage or bodywork to help her feel better again.

Base Oil/Material	Percentage	Why Chosen?

Essential Oils: _____, _____,
_____

Aromatherapy and the Skin (Part II)

Your Skin Type

3) Determine your body's skin type from the list below. Select base oils suitable for your skin type and mix in a 1 ounce bottle. Do not add essential oils! Label and keep for next class. List at least two essential oils that you think would be beneficial to your current skin type.

Classify your skin type *(more than one may apply!)*

❑ Mature: slightly older, thinner skin, some fine lines or wrinkles, less elasticity, and possibly sun or age spots

❑ Normal: soft and supple, has firm texture and good color. Doesn't usually suffer from blemishes or dry patches

❑ Normal to Oily: an overproduction of sebum (or oil) in at least the T-zone area, shiny nose, prone to breakouts

❑ Normal to Dry: generally soft skin with some tightness; dry or flaky patches, usually around the mouth and on cheeks or under eyes

❑ Sensitive: skin often turns red or blotchy after washing or applying certain products, reacts to hot and/or cold, chemicals, and environment

❑ Acne Prone: frequent breakouts and blemishes; pores clog easily, causing pimples and blackheads; may be due to hormones, diet, or stress

Select Your Base Oils

Base Oil/Material	Percentage	Why Chosen?

Essential Oils: _____, _____,
_____

CHAPTER TEST

1. The outermost layer of the epidermis is called the:

   a. stratum germinativum

   b. stratum corneum

   c. stratum spinosum

   d. stratum lucidum

2. Langerhans' cells play an important role in:

   a. fatty metabolism

   b. sensory perception

   c. immunity

   d. sweat production

3. List five factors that affect the degree to which essential oils may be absorbed into the skin.

   a.

   b.

   c.

   d.

   e.

4. The application of essential oils to the skin has been contributed to the work of:

   a. Gattefosse

   b. Wildwood

   c. Valnet

   d. Maury

5. Which of the following essential oils would be considered an astringent?

   a. lavender

   b. cypress

   c. ginger

   d. German chamomile

6. Which of the following essential oils would be considered a vulnerary?

   a. spearmint

   b. tangerine

   c. lavender

   d. lemongrass

7. Which of the following fat-soluble vitamins is essential for cellular growth and repair of body tissues?

   a. beta-carotene

   b. vitamin E

   c. lecithin

   d. vitamin A

8. A vegetable rich in _____ is considered to be more stable and more resistant to the damaging effects of heat and light.

   a. linoleic acid

   b. oleic acid

   c. gamma linoleic acid

   d. vitamin D

9. An example of an herbal oil is:

   a. apricot kernel

   b. shea butter

   c. calendula

   d. sunflower

10. Honey has a natural ability to protect the skin from:

   a. excess subcutanea

   b. sunlight

   c. heat

   d. free radicals

REVIEW QUESTIONS

1. Describe the three layers of the skin and discuss the skin's main functions.

2. Discuss the therapeutic benefits of purchasing specialty oils instead of bulk vegetable oils from grocery stores or other large chain stores.

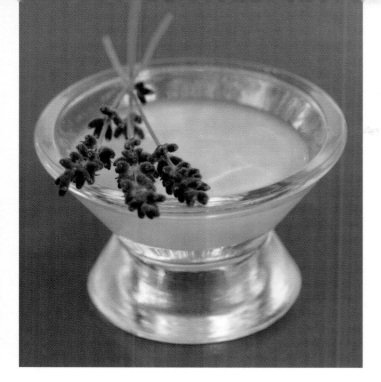

The Nature of Olfaction

 LEARNING OBJECTIVES

After reading this chapter, you will be able to

1. List five potential benefits of olfactory aromatherapy.
2. Describe the basic anatomy and physiology of olfaction.
3. Identify, list, and describe important structures of the limbic system.
4. Define the term stress, discuss its impact on the body/mind, and design a therapeutic blend for stress relief.
5. Describe factors that determine our emotional reactions to an essential oil.
6. Discuss the potential benefits of the memory-based association for aromatherapy massage.
7. List and describe methods of inhalation and diffusion.

INTRODUCTION

Merging touch with aroma can have a profound effect on the emotional, mental, spiritual, and physiological well-being of the client. Traditional aromatherapy practices in many countries utilize massage as the primary method of application. Tisserand (1988) defines traditional aromatherapy practice as "a caring, hands-on therapy which seeks to induce relaxation, to increase energy, to reduce the effects of stress and to restore lost balance to mind, body, and spirit" (p. 1). This chapter is dedicated to exploring the sense of smell and its potential therapeutic applications when combined with massage. The subject of olfaction is vast, but attempts have been made to provide you with information relevant to the integration of aromas with massage and bodywork.

OLFACTION: THE SENSE OF SMELL

Of the five primary senses—touch, taste, smell, sight, and hearing—smell is considered to be the most neglected, overlooked, and least understood or appreciated. According to Gibbons (1986), aromas reach into our emotional life, drawing from the deepest caves in our minds whereby they suggest, stimulate association, evoke, frighten, and arouse us. Maury (1989) comments that the use of odoriferous matter induces a true sentimental and mental liberation, and essential oils free us from encumbering emotions while leaving our faculties unimpaired. Jean Jacques Rousseau is known to have remarked that the sense of smell is the sense of imagination and that scent has always excited the strongest emotions in man.

Our sense of smell is indeed an extraordinary sense capable of altering the landscape of our perceptions and emotions. The integration of natural aromas, in the form of genuine essential oils from plants, with massage can have profound effects on healing mind, body, and spirit.

Potential Benefits of Olfactory Aromatherapy

Olfactory aromatherapy implies the therapeutic use of the sense of smell and the aromas of essential oils to enhance mind/body/spirit well-being. Olfactory research and empirical studies have been able to show that aromas can produce a wide range of effects and can be of great benefit to emotional/psychological conditions and physical health, particularly with stress-related conditions.

To summarize some of the research findings, aromas can:

- ▶ reduce or alleviate stress and anxiety
- ▶ relieve pain
- ▶ induce sleep or relaxation
- ▶ increase alertness and overall performance
- ▶ be used for weight control or loss
- ▶ balance and adjust sleep patterns
- ▶ alleviate nausea
- ▶ affect and improve mood and increase overall emotional well-being
- ▶ useful stress management tool due to impact on autonomic nervous system
- ▶ ease physical ailments, particularly stress-related disorders
- ▶ help shape our impressions of self and others

OUR SENSE OF SMELL

- The sense of smell is very underestimated. Smell is our first primary defense mechanism. Our reaction to smell is quicker at 0.5 seconds than to pain at 0.9 seconds, although we react more quickly to auditory stimuli at 0.15 seconds (Genders).
- The average healthy person can distinguish between ten and forty thousand odors (ad infinitum), many on a subliminal level.

- Smell relays messages from our outer world directly to the brain, influencing the physical body, mind, and emotions.
- Olfactory nerve cells regenerate every thirty to sixty days, clearly underlining their importance.
- Smell is a chemical sense; the receptors respond to chemical stimuli. To arouse sensation, a substance must first be in a gaseous state before going into a mucous solution (olfactory epithelium).

ANATOMY AND PHYSIOLOGY OF OLFACTION

Olfaction is a pathway into the body whereby aromas exert an influence on the body and mind. Figure 7.1 outlines the path of an aroma once it is inhaled or smelled. To understand this pathway, let us explore the anatomy and physiology of olfaction. An odor, smell, or aroma is created by minute gaseous like particles released by various objects or substances. When we smell lavender, for instance, its purple, sweet aroma enters our nasal cavity.

The main functions of the nasal cavity include:

▶ warming, moistening, and cleansing the air we breathe in through the nose
▶ filtering the air of small particles through the nasal hairs
▶ playing a role in voice phonetics, acting as a resonating chamber
▶ containing the olfactory epithelium, located in the upper portion of the nasal cavity

Inside each nasal cavity are two parts: the olfactory part and the respiratory part. The olfactory part is made up of the upper (superior) area and a portion of the central area of the nasal cavity, while the remaining tissue closer to the projection of the nose and a portion of the central area make up the respiratory part. Sniffing increases the airflow through to the upper sinuses and can enhance olfactory perception and the impact of an aroma. Once inside the nose, the aromatic molecules of lavender reach the olfactory epithelium.

Many factors play a role in the rate and magnitude at which an odorant is absorbed into the olfactory epithelium. These factors include:

■ **Solubility of the aroma itself:** **Lipophilic** (fat-loving) substances will dissolve very easily in olfactory epithelium. Essential oils are considered to be lipophilic substances.

■ **Molecular weight of the odorant:** The heavier the molecular weight the more difficult the molecule will have in moving in the air current, and hence absorption is reduced. Essential oils have a low molecular weight and are easily absorbed by olfactory epithelium.

■ **Thickness of mucus layer:** Thickness and viscosity of the olfactory epithelium is variable in each person and can be affected by hormones, diet, and

Figure 7-1 Olfactory pathway into the body

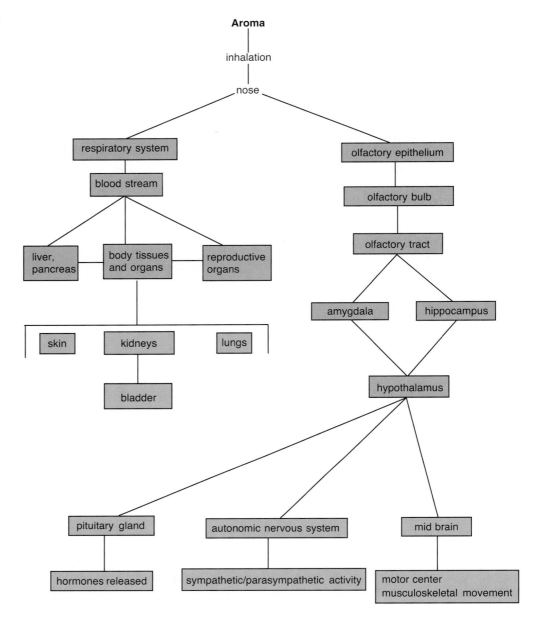

health. A thickened mucus layer slows down the speed of reaction to an odorant and at times can create partial anosmia, reduced sense of smell (e.g., such as during the common cold).

Olfactory Epithelium

Vroon (1994) considers olfactory epithelium to be the actual organ of smell since without it one would be unable to smell. Olfactory epithelium tissue is located at the top and on both sides of the superior nasal cavity and is about the size of a small postage stamp. The tissue is made of three types of cells: the **olfactory receptor neurons**, which transduce the odor to electrical signals; the **supporting cells**, which protect the receptor neurons, secrete mucus, and remove mucus and dead sensory cells; and the **basal cells**, which are found on the underside of the epithelium.

Olfactory basal cells are capable of **neurogenesis**, which means they are capable of creating new nerve tissue to replace the old. Because olfactory cilia are exposed directly to the air and everything the air contains, their lives are short. Olfactory epithelium regenerates every thirty to sixty days. This incredible ability of the olfactory tissue to reproduce nerve tissue illustrates its importance to human survival and the experience of living.

The olfactory epithelium in each nostril contains between three to five million **receptor cells** (for a total of six to ten million), also known as olfactory receptor neurons. These **olfactory receptor neurons** function as **chemoreceptors**, which means they register chemical sensory input, such as volatile, gaseous substances like essential oils. The dendrites (that part of the nerve cell that receives nerve impulses and sends impulses to the cell body) of olfactory receptor neurons project directly onto the surface of the nasal mucus membrane, with each dendrite ending in several fine hairlike projections known as **cilia**. These cilia extend beyond the epithelium surface into the mucosa and are considered to be naked neurons, meaning they are in direct contact with the outside world. Tisserand (1988) notes that "smell is the only sense in which the receptor nerve endings are in direct contact with the outside world" (p. 116). Receptors for the sense of smell are found in the cilia.

Receptors and Odor Identification

On October 4, 2004, Dr. Linda Buck of the Basic Sciences Division at the Fred Hutchinson Cancer Research Center in Seattle, WA and Dr. Richard Axel of Columbia University in New York were awarded the Nobel Prize in Physiology or Medicine. According to the Nobel Assembly at Karolinska Institute, the two researchers were being recognized for their discoveries of odorant receptors and the organization of the olfactory system (Nobelprize.org). The two researchers were among many who were attempting to understand what has been called the most enigmatic of our five senses: the sense of smell.

It was 1991 when Buck and Axel published their seminal paper entitled "*A novel multigene family may encode odorant receptors: A molecular basis for odor recognition.*" During their research, Axel and Buck successfully identified approximately 350 different odor receptors. Axel and Buck also found that the receptors don't act alone, but rather each odorant interacts with a number of receptors. As each odorant contains different odor molecules, these individual molecules seem to fit into a number of different receptors that work together in identifying the aroma or odorant. According to the *Seattle Times*' (2004) "Sweet Whiff of Success" article, Axel and Buck found that one receptor can recognize different odorants, but different odorants are recognized by different combinations of receptors.

In the same article, Buck commented that a good analogy for understanding how olfactory receptors work is to consider the letters of the alphabet. You can put together an endless array of words with only twenty-six letters. The same is true of different olfactory receptors acting together with each arrangement providing you with a different smell.

Axel and Buck, working independently of each other, also discovered that when information about a smell goes from receptors in the nose to the olfactory bulb in the brain and then to the olfactory cortex in the brain, there is a different organization or "map" at each level. Each odor is "deconstructed" into tiny parts, going to numerous different receptors, and it (the odor) is eventually brought together into single neurons in the olfactory cortex (the limbic system). From the olfactory cortex, information continues up to the higher levels of the cerebral cortex.

Nerve Transmission of Odors

Once an odorant or aroma has been received by the olfactory epithelium, a nerve impulse is initiated into the olfactory bulb. The **olfactory bulb** sits on top of the cribiform plate of the ethmoid bone and is continuous with the olfactory tract. The axons of olfactory neurons synapse with the dendrites of the mitral cells in the olfactory bulb. The cranial nerve is made up of the axons of the olfactory neurons. The olfactory bulb serves as the first site of odor recognition before it is passed along the olfactory tract.

The **olfactory tract** is a band of white matter that moves slightly upward and divides into two roots, the outer root that projects directly into the limbic system, specifically the amygdala and septum; and the inner root that projects into the olfactory cortex, which then connects to the temporal and frontal cerebral lobes. The temporal and frontal lobes then interpret and perceive the odor. Thus, olfactory nerve projection encompasses some higher olfactory areas of the brain and the entire limbic region along with associated pathways.

↳ THE LIMBIC SYSTEM

The **limbic system**, also known as the emotional brain, is considered to be one of the oldest parts of the human brain and is referred to as the Paleomammalian or Rhinencephalon brain (the smell brain). Our ancestors utilized the sense of smell to a much greater degree than we do today. With the growing evolutionary emphasis in Western culture on sight (and a corresponding growth in the size of the cerebral cortex), the sense of smell has fallen into decline, even though the system itself remains intact. The limbic region persists, with profound effects on our body chemistry and emotional well-being.

The limbic system's main functions are in the realm of emotions, instinctive behavior and responses, motivational drives, learning, and memory. Nerve impulses, such as those received by aromatic molecules, that reach the limbic system activate smell-related emotions and behaviors. They play a major role in many emotions such as pain, pleasure, anger, rage, fear, sorrow, sexual feelings, docility, and affection. According to Dr. Michael Shipley (1986), a neurobiologist at the University of Cincinnati College of Medicine, the amount of human brain tissue devoted to smell is still very great. Although we don't seem to be very aware of smells, they have a very privileged and intimate access to those parts of the brain where we really live.

The limbic system includes the amygdala, the anterior thalamus, the nucleus accumbens, the hypothalamus, the septum, and the hippocampus including the cingulate gyrus and parahippocampal gyrus. Additional parts of the brain associated with the processing of the sense of smell include the cortex, the frontal lobes, and the temporal lobes. For the purpose of brevity, we shall focus our attention on the amygdala, the hypothalamus and the hippocampus.

The Amygdala

The **amygdala** is an almond-shaped mass located deep within the temporal lobes, close to the hypothalamus and adjacent to the hippocampus. The amygdala receives stimuli from the five senses, but none so directly as the sense of smell. Unlike other sensory perceptions, olfactory stimuli reach directly to the amygdala without first going through the thalamus for relaying. The amygdala is hard-wired to respond to

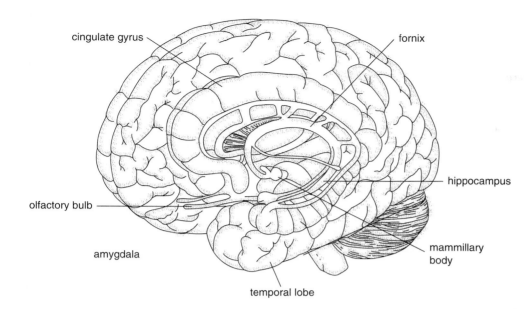

Figure 7-2 Structures of the limbic system are shaded in this partially transparent view of the brain

fear by initiating the "flight or fight" response that activates the sympathetic nervous system. For instance, the smell of fire alerts the amygdala, which then initiates the "flight or fight" response. It is thought that this is an innate response designed to perform a survival function.

Alexander (2000) comments: "the amygdala houses the main circuits that color our experience with emotion" (p. 110). It is responsible for assigning emotional significance to sensory information, including intensity (e.g., from mildly interesting to incredibly interesting).

The amygdala, along with the hippocampus, is crucial for the formation of memories. The amygdala couples a learned sensory stimulus (lavender = relaxing) to an adaptive response (soothes and reduces activity in the sympathetic nervous system). "Once the amygdala attaches emotional significance to sensory information, its emotional evaluation is passed on to the hippocampus, which organizes the information and integrates it with previous memories of similar sensory details. The greater the emotional significance assigned by the amygdala, the more intently the memory is permanently recorded by the hippocampus" (Ratey, 2001, p. 211).

According to Molavi (1997), the main outputs of the amygdala are to the hypothalamus and the brain stem autonomic centers. This means that what affects the amygdala has far reaching effects on the autonomic nervous systems as well as the endocrine system.

Aroma → Amygdala → Hypothalamus → Brain stem → Controls various autonomic functions such as respiration and the regulation of heart rhythms.

The Hypothalamus

The **hypothalamus** lies below the thalamus and above the pituitary gland in the heart of the brain. The main functions of the hypothalamus include:

■ **Control center for autonomic nervous system activity:** The hypothalamus controls and integrates autonomic nervous system activity (sympathetic and parasympathetic divisions) that stimulates smooth muscle, regulates the rate of the contraction of cardiac muscle, and controls the secretion of many glands. It is the main regulator of visceral activities (e.g., heart rate, digestion, sweating, vasoconstriction, eye blinking).

■ **Expression of emotions:** The hypothalamus integrates autonomic and visceral responses with the individual's emotional or physical state of being. For instance, if an individual is feeling anxious, then the hypothalamus could trigger the sympathetic nervous system into activity. The hypothalamus plays a role in emotional responses such as anger, fear, pain, and pleasure.

■ **Regulates body temperature.**

■ **Controls endocrine system/functions:** In response to information from internal and external stimuli, the hypothalamus is able to control the entire endocrine system via its connections with the pituitary gland.

■ **Regulates hunger sensations, metabolism, and thirst sensations.**

■ **Works with other parts of the brain in the regulation of sleeping and waking states.**

■ **Involved in the control and expression of sexual behavior:** A "specialized sexual center nuclei within the posterior portion of the hypothalamus responds to sexual stimulation of the tactile receptors within the genital organs. The experience of orgasm involves neural activity with the sexual center of the hypothalamus" (DeGraaff and Fox, 1985, p. 391).

Information from olfaction and the limbic system is one source of input for the hypothalamus. In response to olfactory information, the hypothalamus will send neuronal signals to the autonomic nervous system, the brain stem, or the pituitary gland. "Through control of the hypothalamus, the limbic region influences the entire endocrine system of hormones thus exerting an affect on nerves, hormones, body temperature, insulin production, appetite, thirst, caloric levels, digestion, stress, repulsion, and sexual arousal" (Gibbons, 1986).

Outgoing messages from the hypothalamus can be sent via various paths as diagramed below:

hypothalamus → autonomic nervous system → symp/para response
→ brain stem motor centers → skeletal muscles
→ pituitary gland → hormones

The Hippocampus (Parahippocampal gyrus)

The **hippocampus** is a curved band of gray matter located inside the temporal lobe (humans have two hippocampi, one in each side of the brain). It forms a part of the limbic system and plays a part in learning and memory. The hippocampus is vital for short-term memory as well as for the consolidation of that memory into a long-term form. Research has shown that the hippocampus is crucial for the development and formation of new memories about experienced events (episodic or autobiographical memory).

The hippocampus, like the olfactory epithelium, is capable of neurogenesis, which means the hippocampus is capable of producing new neurons. According to Sapolsky (2004), the rate of neurogenesis can be regulated. For instance, an enriched learning environment and exercise can increase the rate of neurogenesis, while stress actually inhibits neurogenesis. It has been shown that the hippocampus shrinks in size when an individual is under stress. Alexander (2000) states that people that pour out the stress hormones (glucocorticoids) have a diminished hippocampus and hence a reduced ability to make new memories or draw on older memories (p. 112).

Bodyworkers and massage therapists are able to utilize the intimate connection of smell with memory for enhancing the therapeutic benefit of their treatments. By providing the client with a small bottle of the aromatherapy blend used during the session to take home, one may activate the aromatic memory-based association, thereby allowing the client to feel as if they were back in the massage room, emotionally, physically, and spiritually. How does this work?

AROMATIC MEMORY-BASED RESPONSE

According to Kirk-Smith (n/d), a neutral odor can be easily paired with an emotional state, in a single session, so that it will evoke the same emotional state in another circumstance at a later time. I call this an aromatic memory-based response.

Phase One: Initial Experience

A client arrives for their aromatic massage or bodywork session. The client has specifically requested aromatherapy for their session. The client feels comfortable speaking to the therapist, and the therapist learns about her client, enhancing the therapist's abilities to customize a blend to meet the needs of the client. The client is then given a full-body massage with the blend created for her. The massage is relaxing, nourishing, and refreshing. The client is relaxed and feels taken care of. All the while a waft of aroma lingers around the room, mesmerizing the client, adding to the relaxation.

On a physiological level, this experience could trigger a lowering of blood pressure, a relaxed stomach or colon, breathing slows down and becomes more relaxed, and muscle spasms relax. On a psychological level, this experience could bring about feelings of peace, joy, happiness, and the feeling of nourishment. On an energetic level, this experience could release energy blockages and release toxic energy particles. All these levels will get locked into the memory frame and will be stored in the limbic system.

Phase Two: Lock-and-Key Mechanism

After the session, the therapist provides the remaining blend for the client to take home. Hours or days later the client will be able to smell the blend her therapist made for her, and the client will respond as if she were with the practitioner; she will experience relaxation or excitation as dictated by the initial experience. The potential benefits of this memory-based association is far-reaching as it will allow the client to access the state of relaxation and comfort that were originally felt during a massage session.

How this happens is by the means of the lock-and-key mechanism. It is based upon the long-term memory of a specific aroma or combination thereof. The aroma is the key which unlocks the memory of the experience and emotion.

Experience + Emotion + Aroma (key) = Memory (= Experience + Emotion) (lock)

IN PRACTICE 7.1

Aromatic Memories

Aromas can stir up lost memories and emotions. In fact, memories attached to a particular aroma/smell are considered to be some of the longest lasting forms of memory. For example, the smell of apple pie baking may remind you of being at home with your family, and you may feel comforted by this aroma. On the other hand, the smell of an antiseptic-type aroma may remind you of being in a hospital when you or someone in your family was sick. Memories can have both positive and negative connotations. Take a moment to reflect on memories and emotions you have that are related to a specific aroma or smell.

Creating a Therapeutic Memory-Based Association for Your Clients or Self

The aroma used to "condition" should be a scent that does not have memories already attached to it, a neutral or novel aroma is the best. Use aromas that the client perceives as pleasant. A pleasant aroma + a pleasant experience = aroma is perceived as more pleasant and hence more therapeutic.

Have the client smell the blend you have made for them prior to beginning the massage session or place a few drops of the blend on a tissue and place it under the face cradle or directly on the floor beneath the face cradle. You can also have a short stool to place the tissue a bit higher up yet still just below the face cradle. This will enhance the client's association between the aroma and the experience of the massage.

Since repeated exposure to a specific aroma can increase the connection and memory, and hence the response the client experiences, it is vital for you to provide the same synergy or blend to the client for home use.

EMOTIONS AND AROMA

Although it is beyond dispute that aromas have a direct influence on behavior, the question of which aroma triggers which emotion or behavior is not. This is largely due to the "great individual differences in the perception of a smell and the appreciation of the smell, and thus in any ensuing action" (Vroon, 1994, p. 122) or emotional state. The appreciation of a particular aroma appears to be largely an acquired one rather than an innate response. The exceptions are aromas that clearly signal danger, as these aromas are able to trigger the innate "fight or flight" response.

Therefore, one must recognize that aromatherapy books that attempt to attribute specific emotional states do so out of generalized characteristics of that essential oil, either via morphological considerations or therapeutic emotional representations; for example, lavender is a sedative and hence will be emotionally calming. Essential oils are known to exhibit both psychological and physiological effects. These effects are summarized below.

■ **Psychological/emotional level:** Pleasant vs. Unpleasant vs. No specific effect
The psychological impact of an aroma will depend greatly on the individual's ability to smell the aroma being presented. The individual will quickly categorize the aroma as either pleasant, unpleasant, or no effect. If the aroma is pleasant, a number of emotional

ESSENTIAL OIL THERAPEUTICS

Sedative and/or relaxing essential oils include:

Angelica root, Bergamot, Cardamon, Roman chamomile, German chamomile, Clary sage, Cypress, Frankincense, Geranium, Jasmine, Lavender, Melissa, Myrrh, Neroli, Patchouli, Petitgrain, Rose, Sandalwood, Tangerine, Vetiver, and Ylang ylang.

Stimulating and/or uplifting and invigorating essential oils include:

Birch, Black pepper, Carrot seed, Eucalyptus, Fennel, Ginger, Grapefruit, Juniper, Laurel, Lemon, Lemongrass, Orange, Palmarosa, Peppermint, Pine, Ravensara, Rosemary, Spearmint, Tea tree, Ylang ylang (has a harmonizing effect).

responses may occur, depending on certain factors. Emotional responses to aromas range from uplifting to calming and from energizing to soothing.

■ **Pharmacological/biochemical level:** Stimulant vs. Sedative vs. No specific effect Tisserand (1988) reported on the studies of two Italian doctors, Giovanni Gatti and Renato Cayola, regarding the action of essential oils on the nervous system. The doctors gave subjects cotton balls impregnated with one of several essential oils. Essential oils identified as sedatives were found to be useful for states of anxiety whereas oils found to be stimulants were found to be useful for depression. Tisserand also reports on another Italian, Rovesti, who found that mixtures of essential oils are more pleasant than single oils for individuals suffering with nervous tension. Although the idea of utilizing stimulating oils for depression and sedative oils for anxiety is a useful tool, ultimately the choice of essential oils will have to do with the individual and their own perceptions of the effects of a given aroma.

What Determines Our General Reaction to a Particular Aroma?

Aromas do not by definition have a positive or negative influence nor does a specific aroma by definition elicit a specific mood. Smell-evoked emotions or behavior evolve out of experiences that occur in the presence of those aromas. To have meaning, an individual must develop a relationship with the aroma based upon associations and actual experiences.

Some factors that determine our general reaction to a particular aroma or smell include:

▶ previous experience of that aroma or one of similar aroma
▶ our current emotional state when exposed to the odor/aroma
▶ whether the aroma is perceived as pleasant or unpleasant
▶ any auto-suggested relations (e.g., this oil is known to be relaxing or anxiety relieving) and most importantly
▶ the environment in which the aroma is introduced (e.g., is your office busy with the phone ringing and people coming in [this type of environment may be perceived as stressful], or is your space soothing, comforting, and nurturing to be in?).

AROMATHERAPY RESEARCH

Aromatherapy Massage and Emotional Well-Being

Harris (2004) reported that a small pilot study conducted in a U.K. day hospital found that aromatherapy massage, performed with customized blends for each client, improved mood, increased relaxation, and lessened depression in the short term (p. 6).

Wilkinson et al. (1999) found that massage with or without essential oils appears to reduce levels of anxiety; however, the addition of essential oils seems to enhance the effect of massage and to improve physical and psychological symptoms, as well as overall quality of life.

Inhalation Effects of Aromas

Barker et al. (n/d) found that the aroma of peppermint may promote a general arousal of attention so participants stay focused on their task and increase performance.

Saeki (2000) found that a lavender footbath is associated with small but significant changes in autonomic activity.

Kim et al. (n/d) found that the inhalation of lavender, marjoram, eucalyptus, rosemary, and peppermint had a major effect on decreasing pain and depression levels for patients suffering with arthritis.

AROMATHERAPY AND STRESS

Having covered some of the basic anatomy and physiology of olfaction, it should come as no surprise that essential oils and their aromas can play a role in reducing not only stress but stress-related disorders. According to Sapolsky (2004), "the diseases of modern times are ones of slow accumulation of damage, such as heart disease, cancer, cerebrovascular disorders. We have also come to recognize the vastly complex intertwining of our biology and our emotions, the endless ways in which our personality, feelings, and thoughts both reflect and influence the events in our bodies. We have come to appreciate that stress can make us sick, and a critical shift in medicine has been the recognition that many of the damaging diseases of slow accumulation can be either caused or made far worse by stress" (p. 3).

The 2005 Massage Therapy Industry Fact Sheet from the American Massage Therapy Association (AMTA) reports that "Americans most often choose to get a massage for medical reasons, relaxation and stress relief. 32% of adult Americans who received massage in the past 5 years did so for medical purposes, such as for muscle soreness and spasm, injury recovery and rehabilitation, and pain relief. 26% of consumers who had a massage in the past 5 years cited relaxation and stress relief as the main reason for getting a massage."

So, what is stress? Stress, or the stress response, can be defined as the body's response to any demand made upon it. A stressor is anything that can trigger the stress response. Each stressor may initiate a differing reaction depending on the type of stressor, the duration it persists, the abilities of the individual to cope, and the amount of social support the individual has in his/her life.

The two types of stressors include external stressors and internal stressors. According to the University of Maryland Medical Center (2004): **external stressors** include adverse physical conditions (such as pain or hot or cold temperatures) or stressful psychological environments (such as poor working conditions or abusive relationships). **Internal stressors** can be physical (infections, inflammation) or psychological. An example of an internal psychological stressor is intense worry about a harmful event that may or may not occur. Sapolksy (2004) elucidates on this further by saying "sustained psychological stress is a recent invention, mostly limited to humans and other social primates. We can experience wildly strong emotions (provoking our bodies into a stress response) linked to mere thoughts" (p. 5).

Duration of Stressors

Not all stress is bad stress. Stress is to the human condition what tension is to the violin string—too little and the music is dull and raspy; too much and the music is shrill or the string snaps. Understanding the types of stressors as well as their possible duration can be beneficial in creating techniques that can support one's ability to cope with stress. According to the American Psychological Association (n/d), stress can be acute (short-lived), episodic, or chronic (longer time frame).

Acute stress is the most common form of stress we all experience on a day-to-day basis. Acute stress is short-term and can be thrilling and exciting in small doses, but too much can be exhausting and overwhelming. An example of acute stress is when you are on a time schedule and you're running late.

Acute stress doesn't have time to do extensive damage to your health because it is short-term stress. The most common symptoms of acute stress include emotional distress, a combination of anger, irritability, or anxiety and depression; tension headaches; muscular aches and pains; upset digestive system, including heartburn, flatulence, diarrhea, constipation, or irritable bowel syndrome; rapid heartbeat; sweaty palms; migraines; shortness of breath; or chest pain. All forms of acute stress tend to be manageable.

Episodic acute stress is similar to what has been commonly called type A personality. Episodic acute stress is when an individual is always in a rush; they take on too much, have too many irons in the fire, and seem to always be doing something or going somewhere. If something can go wrong, it often does. Episodic acute stress is similar to acute stress, however episodic stress has acute stressors daily or even hourly.

In some instances the individual has made it a way of life. Individuals who live with acute episodic stress are often overaroused, short-tempered, irritable, anxious, and tense. They seem to live off their own nervous energy. Symptoms of episodic stress include persistent tension headaches, migraines, hypertension, chest pain, and heart disease.

Chronic stress is when acute stress becomes long-term. This is the grinding form of stress that can wear people down over time. Chronic stress can be caused by many different life events, including poverty, dysfunctional families, long-term relationship problems, persistent financial worries, loneliness, challenging marriages, or a despised job or career.

The Stress Response

The autonomic nervous system works to maintain a state of balance in relation to external and internal conditions through the involuntary regulation of the internal organs, blood vessels, and glands. The autonomic nervous system is responsible for our responses to stress and relaxation. The sympathetic and parasympathetic nervous systems make up the two opposites of the autonomic nervous system. Ideally, there should be a balance between these two systems. A long-term imbalance prevents healing and leads to disease.

The sympathetic nervous system controls functions that include those associated with action: fight or flight. Stress is the most common cause of sympathetic system activation. The parasympathetic system, on the other hand, is responsible for mediating calm and relaxation. It functions to create a state of rest and repair. The stress response, in varying degrees, may result in:

■ **A rapid mobilization of energy from storage sites and the inhibition of further storage:** In chronic stress the body is unable to store extra energy and hence fatigue becomes more common. Glucose and the simplest forms of proteins and fats come to the rescue. These substances are secreted by fat cells, the liver, and muscles.

■ **An increase in heart rate, blood pressure, and breathing rate:** Chronic stress may lead to cardiovascular disease.

■ **Inhibited digestion:** Chronic stress may lead to peptic ulcers and other digestive disorders.

■ **Inhibited growth and reproduction:** Chronic stress may lead to low sperm count and low testosterone levels. Sexual behavior and interest may decline.

■ **Curtailed growth and tissue repair:** Chronic stress may lead to slow healing wounds.

■ **Decrease in sexual drive:** During chronic stress, females are less likely to carry pregnancy to full term and are less likely to ovulate. Males have trouble with erections and secrete less testosterone.

■ **Inhibited immunity:** Chronic stress may lead to increased vulnerability to infectious diseases, e.g., bacteria, fungi.

■ **Blunted pain perception:** Acute stress analgesia is common.

■ **Loss of cognitive and sensory skills:** Chronic stress may result in increasing the rate of loss of brain cells during aging, and hence memory loss increases. When individuals are under stress, the hippocampus shrinks in size, which means memory and new learning may be impaired to varying degrees. Stress affecting the hippocampus include emotional stressors, such as chronic or recurring depression and post-traumatic stress disorder.

Based upon the impact of stress as outlined above, it is understandable that episodic, chronic, and acute stress can either lead to or exacerbate a variety of health problems including those listed in Table 7.1.

The stress response requires that the body spend more time dealing with the stressor and hence less time on other activities necessary to maintaining health. Finding ways to reduce and cope with the stress response would be highly useful for each of us.

Activating the Relaxation Response

Rattray and Ludwig (2000) believe that "the stress reduction massage is the basis of every massage treatment performed, regardless of the condition being treated." It is now widely known that massage therapy is an effective technique for stress reduction and can be used to address many of the conditions considered to be stress-related as listed above. In 1988 Tisserand observed that the power of aromatherapy

	TABLE 7.1
Conditions Commonly Caused By or Made Worse By Stress	

Angina	Diabetes – Type II Adult Onset	Reduced feelings of pleasure
Anxiety	Depression	Rheumatoid arthritis
Asthma	Headaches/Migraines	Skin disorders: hives, psoriasis, rosacea, eczema
Autoimmune disorders	Immune suppression	Sleep disturbances: insomnia
Cancer	Irritable bowel syndrome	Slow wound healing
Cardiovascular disease	Lack of sexual drive	Substance abuse
Common cold	Menstrual irregularities	Susceptibility to infections
Constipation	Muscle tension	Ulcers
Depression	Muscular and joint pain	Ulcerative colitis
Eating disorders	Premenstrual syndrome	
Hypertension		

in counteracting stress lies in the combination of essential oils and massage, both of which are capable of relaxing and reducing stress, reducing pain, lowering blood pressure, stimulating/enhancing the immune system, and relieving muscular tension. The integration of genuine essential oils with massage offers a profound approach to potentially reduce the damaging effects of stress on the body, mind, and spirit.

Therapeutic goals:

- ▶ reduce pain and muscular tension
- ▶ facilitate immune system function
- ▶ enhance a healing and calm emotional state
- ▶ decrease sympathetic nervous system firing
- ▶ encourage stress-reducing activities and coping skills

Aromatherapy applications:

- ▶ massage oil, 2.5 to 5 percent dilution
- ▶ gel for sore neck and shoulders or for headache
- ▶ hydrotherapy: home baths
- ▶ self-massage
- ▶ diffusion

Blending for Stress

The choice of essential oils for stress relief can be based upon either the physical manifestations of stress (e.g., tight neck and shoulders or constipation) or for the emotional manifestations (e.g., anxiety, worry, or depression). When blending for relaxation and emotional purposes, it is crucial that the client find the aroma blend pleasant.

This can be accomplished by preselecting essential oils that you believe would be most beneficial for the client and then holding the bottles together and allowing the client to provide feedback on their perception and reaction to the aroma. Once the client has confirmed that the aroma is pleasant, then you can feel confident that the blend will be of benefit during the massage.

Table 7.2 has been designed to support the application of essential oils for a variety of emotional states. The essential oils provided under each emotional state are given based upon their general physiological action, nature, and potential inherent messages (e.g., relax, sedate, ground).

TABLE 7.2

Essential Oils for Emotional Support and Healing

Emotional State	Essential Oils
Anger, Irritability	Angelica root, Bergamot, Cardamom, Cedarwood, Roman chamomile, German chamomile, Clary sage, Frankincense, Jasmine, Laurel, Lavender, Myrrh, Neroli, Palmarosa, Petitgrain, Rose, Sandalwood, Tangerine, Ylang ylang
Anxiety	Angelica root, Bergamot, Cedarwood, Roman or German chamomile, Clary sage, Geranium, Jasmine, Lavender, Sweet marjoram, Melissa, Myrrh, Neroli, Palmarosa, Patchouli, Petitgrain, Rose, Sandalwood, Tangerine, Vetiver, Ylang ylang
Aphrodisiac, Frigidity	Cardamom, Cinnamon leaf, Clary sage, Fennel, Ginger, Helichrysum, Jasmine, Neroli, Patchouli, Rose, Sandalwood, Ylang ylang
Burnout, Exhaustion	Basil ct. linalol, Roman or German chamomile, Cinnamon leaf, Cypress, Frankincense, Geranium, Helichrysum, Lavender, Lemon, Orange, Peppermint, Rose, Rosemary, and Tangerine
Calming/Soothing	Bergamot, Roman chamomile, German chamomile, Clary sage, Lavender, Melissa, Myrrh, Neroli, Petitgrain, Vetiver
Clarity	Birch, Eucalyptus, Grapefruit, Juniper, Laurel, Lemon, Lemongrass, Palmarosa, Peppermint, Pine, Rosemary, Sage, Spearmint
Cleansing	Carrot seed, Cedarwood, Eucalyptus, Grapefruit, Juniper, Laurel, Lemon, Lemongrass, Orange, Peppermint, Rosemary, Sage
Confusion, Indecision	Angelica root, Black pepper, Cypress, Ginger, Laurel, Lemongrass, Palmarosa, Pine, Rosemary, Sage, Vetiver
Confidence, Insecurity	Angelica root, Black pepper, Cardamom, Eucalyptus, Jasmine, Juniper, Lavender, Pine
Courage	Angelica root, Black pepper, Laurel, Myrrh, Peppermint, Rosemary, Sage, Yarrow
Depression	Bergamot, Cardamom, Clary sage, Frankincense, Geranium, Ginger, Grapefruit, Jasmine, Juniper, Neroli, Orange, Palmarosa, Rose, Tangerine, Ylang ylang
Emotional Turmoil	Angelica root, Cardamom, Roman chamomile, Clary sage, Cypress, Frankincense, Jasmine, Laurel, Lavender, Sweet marjoram, Myrrh, Neroli, Palmarosa, Patchouli, Pine, Rose, Tangerine, Vetiver, Ylang ylang

TABLE 7.2   (*Continued*)

Emotional State	Essential Oils
Fears	Angelica root, Black pepper, Cypress, Geranium, Ginger, Laurel, Lavender, Peppermint, Rosemary, Thyme
Grounding	Angelica root, Ginger, Myrrh, Vetiver
Grieving, Loss	Bergamot, Neroli, Patchouli, Rose, Tangerine, Ylang ylang
Heartache	Cardamom, Clary sage, Frankincense, Jasmine, Lavender, Neroli, Rose, Tangerine
Inspiration, Creativity	Bergamot, Cardamom, Clary sage, Fennel, Grapefruit, Jasmine, Juniper, Laurel, Lemon, Neroli, Orange, Palmarosa, Pine, Rosemary
Letting go	Eucalyptus, Grapefruit, Juniper, Laurel, Lemon, Neroli, Orange, Pine
Mood swings	Bergamot, Roman or German chamomile, Clary sage, Cypress, Fennel, Geranium, Lavender, Neroli, Patchouli, Rose, Sage, Tangerine, Vetiver, Ylang ylang
Nervousness	Angelica root, Bergamot, Black pepper, Cardamom, Cedarwood, Clary sage, Frankincense, Lavender, Myrrh, Neroli, Patchouli, Tangerine, Ylang ylang
Nightmares	Bergamot, Roman chamomile, Clary sage, Frankincense, Geranium, Helichrysum, Laurel, Lavender, Sweet marjoram, Neroli, Orange, Rose, Tangerine, Ylang ylang
Panic, Shock	Angelica root, Roman chamomile, Frankincense, Lavender, Neroli, Orange, Palmarosa, Petitgrain, Pine, Rose, Tangerine, Vetiver, Ylang ylang
Spiritual, Protection	Angelica root, Cedarwood, Frankincense, Laurel, Lemongrass, Myrrh, Patchouli, Pine, Rose, Sage
Uplifting	Bergamot, Cardamom, Clary sage, Geranium, Juniper, Laurel, Lemon, Lemongrass, Neroli, Orange, Peppermint, Petitgrain, Pine, Rosemary, Tangerine, Ylang ylang

⟶ DISORDERS OF OLFACTION

Smell is a powerful influence in our lives and affects us in our physical, psychological, and social life. Imagine life without smell! According to extensive research done on anosmia, it appears that life without smell can lead to a lack of drive and motivation, depression, and suppressed appetite with a lack of interest in foods. The following is a list of olfactory disorders that are currently known.

▪ **Anosmia:** Total inability to smell any aromatic substance. Individuals suffering from this condition have an inclination toward depression and reduced libido. The condition can be congenital or the result of a head injury sustained in a car accident or the like. Anosmia can also be caused by long-term exposure to toxic chemicals or surgery.

▪ **Hyposmia:** Partial loss of smell.

▪ **Hyperosmia:** Extreme sensitivity to aromas.

IN PRACTICE 7.2

Exercise Your Sense of Smell

The sense of smell, like muscles and the brain, needs exercise to become stronger. Often when someone thinks they don't have a good sense of smell it is because they don't consciously use it. Also, some individuals don't like the smell of essential oils at first, and often this is because they have been brought up on synthetic odors and are used to the way synthetics smell.

More often than not, however, when that same individual begins to exercise their sense of smell and become more familiar with the natural aromas of essential oils, they begin to experience the vast differences between synthetics and natural aromas.

To exercise the sense of smell, begin by simply observing different aromas/smells within your environment. Then move on to smelling plants when they are in bloom or natural, authentic essential oils. Take time to truly experience the nuances of an aroma. You could even keep a journal of all the different aromas you observe. Share your experiences with others.

■ **Parosmia:** A distortion of imagined odors.

■ **Cacosmia:** Smelling a continuous foul odor.

Causes of Olfactory Disorders

According to Vroon (1994), some diseases that have been found to cause a loss of smell include nasal obstruction, vitamin A deficiency, acute viral hepatitis, disorders of the endocrine system, Turners syndrome, temporal lobe lesions, Parkinson's, Alzheimer's, and changes in estrogen receptors and breast cancer theorized to be secondary to hypothalamic lesions in the brain.

■ **Viral diseases:** Viral diseases such as the flu, common cold, and acute viral hepatitis tend to cause anosmia, which is more often than not a temporary state.

■ **The common cold or smoking:** Inflammation of the nasal mucosa prevents odorous substances from reaching the olfactory area of the nose, causing a temporary loss of smell. This is usual for the common cold or smoking.

■ **Olfactory fading and fatigue:** **Olfactory fading** occurs when our olfactory system adapts to a smell and ceases to register the aroma. An example of olfactory fading would be the smell of our own home that we grow accustomed to and therefore cease to register how it actually smells. **Olfactory fatigue**, on the other hand, is what happens when our olfactory system is exposed to numerous odors within a short span of time. During fatigue we are no longer able to distinguish between one odor and another. This is when it is time to get a good whiff of coffee beans as they help to clear the nasal palate, so to speak.

■ **Pathological processes:** This occurs in the nasal cavities, such as inflammation of mucus membranes, jaw, or sinuses.

■ **Injuries, trauma, or a blow to the head.**

■ **Certain pharmaceutical drugs:** According to Hirsch (2005), "Most patients—and even some doctors—don't realize that many medications can inhibit one's sense of smell. *Most common offenders:* The cholesterol-lowering drug *rosuvastatin* (Crestor). . . the antipsychotics *haloperidol* (Haldol) and *chlorpromazine* (Thorazine). . . the antidepressant *nortriptyline* (Pamelor). . . and the stimulant *methylphenidate* (Ritalin), taken for attention-deficit hyperactivity disorder and mild depression in older adults."

METHODS OF APPLICATION

Throughout this text we will be covering a wide range of methods of application from massage oils, gels, lotions, creams, and salves in chapter 8 to baths, steam inhalations, compresses, hot towels, and aromatic spritzers in chapter 9. Although all methods of application have olfactory benefits, in this chapter we will only be covering direct inhalation and diffusion.

Inhalation

Inhalation refers to the act of breathing in or drawing in a substance such as air or essential oils. Aromatic inhalations are most commonly employed for their effect on the respiratory system and for a variety of emotional states. They are most effective for treating nasal or chest congestion where there is an excess or deficiency of mucus or infection. The inhalation of aromatic substances for respiratory ailments has a long history of use. In some cultures, aromatic plant material is smoked for its expectorating effect. Vicks VapoRub® would be an example of a modern aromatic inhalation substance, although it would not be considered a whole product nor a true aromatherapy product as it utilizes isolated compounds rather than whole essential oils.

Inhalations are also utilized for their ability to relieve emotional distress. Buckle (2003) has reported the use of aromatic inhalations in hospitals to help reduce anxiety, speed transition, and reduce nausea in labor units. Inhaled peppermint appears to relieve postsurgical nausea while inhaled clary sage can help speed delivery. According to Buckle (2003), "In the emergency room we use essential oils such as *Origanum marjorana* (Marjoram) or *Lavandula angustifolia* (Lavender) to help patients calm down so they can tell us what has happened to them more coherently. We also use *Mentha* ✕ *piperita* (Peppermint), *Mentha spicata* (Spearmint) and *Zingiber officinale* (Ginger) to reduce nausea and we offer *Angelica archangelica* (Angelica root or seed) or *Rosa damascena* (Rose) for acute distress" (p. 46).

In general, aromatherapy inhalations are useful for:

- ▶ respiratory issues
- ▶ headaches/migraines
- ▶ insomnia or other sleep disorders
- ▶ motion sickness/nausea
- ▶ anxiety/stress/distress
- ▶ mood altering

Possible techniques to employ for inhalation include:

■ **Direct inhalation:** Direct inhalation refers to the technique of sniffing or inhaling an essential oil directly from a bottle, a handkerchief or a cotton ball. Direct inhalations are most commonly employed for the relief of emotional distress and as supportive therapy for the relief of respiratory congestion or other respiratory ailments. Direct inhalations are also used for their effect on the nervous system.

■ **Direct from bottle:** Create a synergy (undiluted essential oils) utilizing three to five essential oils and place in a small bottle (approx. 5ml). Have client waft bottle under their nose while taking deep inhalations. This can be done three or four times a day or as needed.

■ **Smelling salts:** Create a synergy with a total of twenty to thirty drops utilizing three to five essential oils and place in a 10ml (⅓ ounce) bottle. Once the synergy is in the bottle, fill the remainder of the bottle with either fine or coarse sea salts. Have client waft the bottle under their nose while taking deep inhalations. This can be done three or four times a day or as needed.

■ **Handkerchief or cotton ball:** Place two to four drops of essential oil or synergy on the tissue or cloth. Hold the cloth in the palms of your hand and take two or three deep inhalations through the nose. If using a cotton ball, gently waft the cotton ball under the client's nose. This technique can be used two or three times a day or as needed.

Diffusion

Diffusion refers to a method of transmitting essential oils into the air within a specified area. Three key goals in diffusing essential oils into the environment are to effectively reduce microbes in the air, to alter mood/motivation and emotion, and to support respiratory health. Extensive research has been performed showing the efficacy of essential oils in eliminating or destroying airborne pathogens. Harris (2002) reported that the essential oils of cinnamon (*Cinnamomum zeylanicum*), rosemary (*Rosmarinus officinalis*), eucalyptus (*Eucalyptus globulus*), and lemon (*Citrus limon*) had been found to prevent the transmission of airborne bacterial infections when diffused into the air.

Electric Micro-Diffuser

The electric micro-diffusor differs greatly from the candle diffusor and is considered to be a more appropriate tool to disperse essential oils into traditional and nontraditional health care environments. It does not use candle flames or heat. The electric micro-diffusor consists of two parts: an air pump and a handblown glass expansion chamber (nebulizer) with special internal tubes and baffles. As air is pushed from the pump into the glass chamber, the essential oil "breaks" against the baffles, whereby the essential oil is discharged into the atmosphere in a fine mist of micro droplets.

Aerial dispersion via electric diffuser can be used for:

▶ environmental ambiance
▶ stress/anxiety reduction
▶ insomnia or sleep disorders

DOES HEAT AFFECT THE THERAPEUTIC ACTIVITY OF ESSENTIAL OILS?

According to Harris (2003), a few studies have revealed that there are "no structural chemical changes or alterations when using heat generating diffusers" (p. 33).

However, when an essential oil is exposed to heat, different constituents will evaporate at different times based upon their individual volatility.

- ▶ mood or motivation enhancement
- ▶ increase alertness
- ▶ purify and improve air quality
- ▶ reduce airborne pathogens

Recommended usage: Place two or four milliliters (40 to 80 drops) of essential oil into the glass basin or other holding area. Turn the diffusor on. The standard recommended time to run a nebulizing diffuser is fifteen minutes on and sixty to eighty minutes off. The reason for this is twofold: first, the ionized micro droplets of essential oils will stay suspended in the air during the time the diffuser is off and second, when a nebulizer is run continuously one may experience the reverse of therapeutic benefits due to oversaturation of the essential oils into the air. Therefore, it seems wise to purchase an electric diffuser with a timer.

Clay Candles or Electric Pottery Diffusers

Clay candles and electronic pottery diffusers have a simple design and come in one or two pieces. They typically have an area at the top to place water and essential oil drops and an area beneath that holds a tea candle or electric heating system. They are widely available from aromatherapy and other specialty suppliers. This type of diffuser provides a very simple and affordable method of environmental fragrancing that can be employed for home or office use. Most hospitals, hospices, and other health care facilities do not allow the use of candles in patient rooms.

In general, aromatherapy pottery diffusers are useful for:

- ▶ environmental ambiance
- ▶ stress/anxiety reduction
- ▶ insomnia
- ▶ mood or motivation enhancement
- ▶ increased alertness
- ▶ reduce offensive or negative odors

Recommended usage: Fill the bowl with water (top of diffusor) and add five to ten drops of essential oil. Light candle or plug in diffuser. Do not place essential oils in the cup without water as this will lead to the essential oils being burned by the heat instead of diffused. Also, one may want to avoid placing viscous essential oils, such as benzoin, sandalwood, and vetiver, in the diffuser as these oils will create a resinous substance on the clay that can be difficult to clean or remove.

SUMMARY

- Olfactory aromatherapy refers to the use of the sense of smell and the unique aromas of the different essential oils and their impact on the endocrine, autonomic nervous system, and brain stem. By using the sense of smell, essential oils can exert an effect on the mind/emotions as well as the body/physiological well-being.

- When an aroma is inhaled or smelled, it is received by the olfactory epithelium where it is converted to a nerve impulse that travels to the olfactory bulb and then along the olfactory tract to the limbic region of the brain.

- The limbic system, also referred to as the emotional brain, is made up of the amygdala, the anterior thalamus, the nucleus accumbens, the hypothalamus, the septum, and the hippocampus, including the cingulate gyrus and parahippocampal gyrus. Three important aspects of the limbic system discussed in this chapter include the amygdala, the hypothalamus, and the hippocampus.

- The amygdala is responsible for assigning emotional significance to an aroma, and it plays a role along with the hippocampus in the formation of memory. The hypothalamus has a number of core functions that include a control center for autonomic nervous system activity, expression of emotions, regulation of body temperature, control of endocrine functions, and regulation of sleep/waking states, hunger/thirst sensations, and the expression of sexual behavior. The hippocampus plays a role in learning and memory.

- Our emotional responses to a specific aroma appear to be learned rather than innate. Factors that may determine our general reactions to a particular aroma include previous experience of that aroma or a similar aroma, our emotional state when exposed to the aroma, whether the aroma is perceived as pleasant or unpleasant, and the environment in which the aroma is introduced.

- Stress, or the stress response, can be defined as the body's response to any demand made upon it. Stressors can be external or internal and can be acute (short-term), episodic acute stress (acute stressors daily), or chronic stress. Regardless of the type of stress, it can have a negative impact on the body and can either cause or make worse a number of health conditions.

- Due to the impact of aromas on the limbic region, specifically the hypothalamus, aromatherapy is a useful tool in reducing stress and alleviating stress-related disorders.

- The aromatic memory-based association has a possible role to play in providing continued support for the client's healing when the same remedy used in the massage is provided for home care.

- Inhalations refer to the act of breathing in or drawing in of essential oils for their effects on the respiratory and limbic system. All methods of application from massage oils to diffusion offer this dual effect.

NEW TERMINOLOGY

Acute stress

Amygdala

Anosmia

Basal cells

Cacosmia

Chemoreceptors

Chronic stress

Cilia

Episodic acute stress

External stressors

Hippocampus

Hyperosmia

Hyposmia

Hypothalamus

Internal stressors

Limbic system

Lipophilic

Memory-based response

Neurogenesis

Olfaction

Olfactory bulb

Olfactory epithelium

Olfactory fading

Olfactory fatigue

Olfactory receptor neurons

Olfactory tract

Parosmia

Supporting cells

REFERENCES

Alexander, M. (2000). *How Aromatherapy Works*. Odessa, FL: Spectrum Arts and Publications.

American Psychological Association. (n/d). *The Different Kinds of Stress*. Retrieved March 30, 2006, from http://www.apahelpcenter.org/articles/article.php?id=21.

AMTA (2005). 2005 *Massage Therapy Industry Fact Sheet*. Evanston, IL: American Massage Therapy Association. Retrieved on April 30, 2006, from www.amtamassage.org.

Barker S, Grayhem P, Koon J, Perkins J, Whalen A, and Raudenbush B. Improved performance on clerical tasks associated with administration of peppermint odor. *Perceptual and Motor Skills*, (2003) 97, 1007-10; PubMed ID# 14738372

Buckle, J. (2003). Aromatherapy in the USA. *International Journal of Aromatherapy*, *13* (1), 42–46.

De Graaff, K., and Fox, S. (1985). *Concepts of Human Anatomy and Physiology*, 4th edition. Dubuque, IA: Wm. C. Brown Publishers.

Genders, R. (1972). *Perfumes through the Ages*. New York: G.P. Putnam's Sons.

Gibbons, B. (1986). The Intimate Sense of Smell. *National Geographic*, September 1986.

Harris, B. (2002). Aromatherapy Today Research Notes: Deadly Diffusion. *Aromatherapy Today* 21, pg. 8–9.

Harris, B. (2003). Aromatic Teaser. *Aromatherapy Today* 28, p. 33.

Harris, B. (2004). Research Notes. *Aromatherapy Today*. *30*, 6–7.

Hirsch, A. (2005). *Are You Losing Your Sense of Smell? Bottom Line Secrets*. Retrieved July 25, 2006, from http://www.bottomlinesecrets.com/blpnet/article.html?article_id=35445.

Kim, M.J., Nam, E.S., and Paik, S.I. (n/d). The effects of aromatherapy on pain, depression, and life satisfaction of arthritis patients. College of Nursing, Catholic University of Korea, Korea. Retrieved June 17, 2006 from http://www.kan.or.kr/nurse/nurse_01.php?start=view&year=2005&issue=1&volume=35&spage=186

Kirk-Smith, M. (n/d). Therapeutic Uses of Olfaction. University of Ulster, Newtownabbey, BT37 00QB, Northern Ireland.

Maury, M. (1989). *Marguerite Maury's Guide to Aromatherapy: The Secret of Life and Youth*. Essex, England: C.W. Daniel Company.

Molavi, D.W. (1997). *Neuroscience Tutorial*. Washington University Program in Neuroscience. Retrieved October 10, 2005, from http://thalamus.wustl.edu/course/limbic.html.

Ratey, J. (2001). *A User's Guide to the Brain*. New York: NY: First Vintage Books.

Rattray, F., and Ludwig, L. (2000). *Clinical Massage Therapy*. Toronto, Ontario: Talus Incorporated.

Richardson, S. (1995). The Smell Files. *Discover Magazine, 16* (8), August 1995. Retrieved November 12, 2006, from http://www.discover.com/issues/aug-95/departments/thesmellfiles553/

Saeki, Y. (2000). The effect of foot-bath with or without the essential oil of lavender on the autonomic nervous system: a randomized trial. *International Journal of Aromatherapy, 10* (1/2), 57–61.

Sapolsky, R. (2004). *Why Zebras Don't Get Ulcers*. New York: Henry Holt and Company, LLC.

Seattle Times. (2004). The Sweet Whiff of Success. October 5, 2004, pg. A1, A8.

Shipley, M. (1986). The Intimate Sense of Smell. *National Geographic*, September 1986, p. 333.

Tisserand, R. (1988). *Aromatherapy, To Heal and Tend the Body*. Wilmot, WI: Lotus Press.

University of Maryland. (2004). *What is Stress?* Retrieved July 25, 2006, from http://www.umm.edu/patiented/doc31full.html.

Vroon, P. (1994). *Smell, The Secret Seducer*. New York: Farrar, Straus, and Giroux.

Wilkinson, S., Aldridge, J., Salmon, I., Cain, E., and Wilson, B. (1999). An evaluation of aromatherapy massage in palliative care. Palliative Medicine. *13* (5), 409–17. PubMedID10659113.

WORKSHEET

Aromatherapy and Olfaction (Part I)

Name:_____   Date:_____

Olfactory Exercise

1) Choose one category from which you would like your personal blend created today:

❏ Sedative or Relaxing

❏ Stimulating or Uplifting

❏ Scent Memory of: _____

2) Working with a partner, trade papers. Have a brief conversation about your selection and needs.

Notes: _____

3) Using your partners individualized base oil blend from the previous class (Chapter 7: Aromatherapy and the Skin), create a simple massage oil—1 oz./2.5% dilution for your partner based on the information above.

Total Essential Oil Blend: _____ *drops*

Essential Oil—Common Name	Essential Oil—*Latin Name*	Drops	Why Chosen?

4) Each therapist should now exchange short scalp and shoulder massages with their partner, using an *unscented* oil. Then repeat the process for each partner using their individual aromatherapy blend. Return your partner's worksheet page with their blending information.

5) How did the aromatic massage differ from the unscented?

_____

Did the aromatic massage accomplish your initial blending goal/category?

_____

As the therapist, what did you notice if anything while giving the two massages?

_____

WORKSHEET

Aromatherapy and Olfaction (Part II)

Stress and You

6) Complete the following exercise, then discuss the results with your partner.

My stress level is currently:

❏ very low   ❏ very high

❏ low   ❏ high

❏ medium

What happens for me emotionally when I am stressed is:

_____

What I notice physically when I am stressed is:

_____

How I tend to deal with stress is:

_____

7) Trade papers and create a 3% dilution aromatherapy massage blend for your partner based upon the information provided. Use the blending factor to figure out drops for each essential oil used.

Total Base Blend: _____ *oz. cups lbs.*

Base Oil/Material	Percentage	Why Chosen?

Total Essential Oil Blend: _____ *drops*

Essential Oil—Common Name	Essential Oil—*Latin Name*	Drops	Why Chosen?

8) Exchange full-body relaxation massages with your partner using their stress reduction blend.

9) Following the massage, how do you feel? What kind of emotional or physical responses did you experience?

_____

CHAPTER TEST

1. The sense of smell is also called:

   a. hyperosmia

   b. hyposmia

   c. olfaction

   d. olfactory epithelium

2. List five potential olfactory benefits of aromatherapy.

   a.

   b.

   c.

   d.

   e.

3. The nose contains an olfactory and a respiratory portion.

   _____True   _____False

4. When an individual becomes stressed due to an exam that will happen in a few days, the stressor is termed an _____ stressor.

   a. internal

   b. acute

   c. external

   d. stimulating

5. The sense of smell is a chemical sense, therefore the olfactory neurons function as:

   a. chemoreceptors

   b. bipolar neurons

   c. olfactory epithelium

   d. lipophilic substances

6. The limbic system is considered one of the newest parts of the human brain.

   _____True   _____False

7. Basal cells in the olfactory epithelium are capable of:

   a. lipophilic activity

   b. olfactory perceptions

   c. stimulating the limbic system

   d. neurogenesis

8. The limbic system has also been called:

   a. the hypothalamus

   b. the olfactory epithelium

   c. the emotional brain

   d. a fear system

9. The amygdala houses the main circuits that color our experience with emotion.

   _____True   _____False

10. The nerve tissue within the hippocampus is capable of neurogenesis.

    _____True   _____False

REVIEW QUESTIONS

1. Discuss the potential therapeutic benefits of olfactory aromatherapy.

2. Discuss why it can be challenging to determine the emotional responses to a specific essential oil.

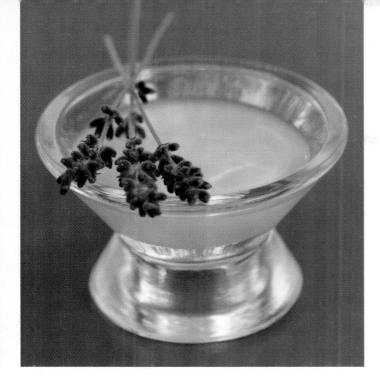

Aromatic Applications and Techniques

LEARNING OBJECTIVES

After reading this chapter, you will be able to

1. Discuss how the integration of aromatherapy can enhance the body/mind/spirit benefits of massage and bodywork.

2. Explain the difference between individualized and generalized aromatherapy blends.

3. Explain the difference between an aromatherapy blend and a synergy.

4. Describe how to make a variety of massage delivery systems, including oils, gels, salves, lotions, and creams.

5. Describe ways of integrating aromatherapy with a variety of massage techniques.

6. List essential oils that may enhance the different massage techniques covered in this chapter.

7. Perform an aromatic facial massage.

INTRODUCTION

The beauty of aromatherapy may lay in its incredible ability to be utilized in just about any massage or bodywork technique and for its ability to address the body, mind, and spirit simultaneously. Aromatherapy is dynamic in its ability to be integrated in a wide range of base products as well as massage techniques. The first half of this chapter focuses on the methods of application for aromatherapy specific to the practice of massage. The second half addresses how to integrate aromatherapy with diverse massage techniques, from relaxation and treatment massage to reflex zone therapy and facial massage.

↪ BODYWORK AND AROMATHERAPY

There are many reasons why people seek massage therapy and other forms of bodywork. Some are stressed out and simply need to relax, while others suffer from injuries or chronic pain. Athletes often use bodywork to maintain flexibility and prevent injury. Some seek bodywork as an adjunct to other complementary therapies, such as chiropractic, biofeedback, or acupuncture. There are those individuals who understand the many health benefits of massage and make it a point to receive regular bodywork, while still others simply "treat" themselves to the perceived luxury only on a birthday or special occasion.

Massage therapy combines the skilled manipulation of soft tissue with movement, technique, and focused intent to help bring about optimal health and wellness. Massage and bodywork can be viewed from either a treatment-based theory, where manual therapies are being employed to address specific signs and symptoms affecting an individual or specific body part; or a wellness-based theory that utilizes various massage and manual therapies to address the whole individual, thus helping to relieve discomforts, improve physical and emotional states, balance energy, increase body awareness, and finally to educate and therefore empower the recipient in establishing and maintaining their own state of well-being.

Integrating aromatherapy into a massage or bodywork practice allows the practitioner to enhance the treatment approach regardless of whether it is treatment-based or wellness-based. Aromatherapy by its very nature will have an impact on the body, mind, and spirit.

Body

The application of aromatherapy blends via massage oils, lotions, gels, or salves are methods of introducing essential oils onto and into the skin. The beneficial healing properties of essential oils and their chemical constituents are then absorbed into the bloodstream through small capillaries and likewise get picked up by the lymphatic system through interstitial fluid. Essential oils are then able to affect the muscles and joints as well as body tissue and organs. Because massage as a therapy shares similar actions on the body as various essential oils, the combination of massage and aromatherapy becomes a natural, well-rehearsed duo for successful bodywork, with each one enhancing the effects of the other.

Mind

Beyond the very physical nature of massage and essential oils as therapeutic agents for the body lies the added benefit of the aroma wafting through the treatment room, relaxing or stimulating the client and quite possibly contributing to a future scent memory that will conjure up memories of the massage and feelings of well-ness when the scent is replayed at a future time. One is able to address the emotional well-being of the client by utilizing specific essential oils for their psychological benefit. One potential approach to address both body and mind is to create a simple, secondary blend specifically created for emotions and use it only locally on the scalp, feet, hands, heart (or where the problem is held emotionally in the body) as a "layer" to the massage session.

Spirit

When we consider the very name "essential oil," we can tune into the fact that this refers to the very essence or life of the plant. This is the utmost pure, innate energy of a plant. Within the essential oil we find not only the chemicals or aromas for healing the body and/or mind, but also the subtle energy or vibration of the plant itself; suitable for healing body, mind, *and* spirit. We should be aware that these substances are most likely affecting the energy body as well as the emotional and physical bodies. Schnaubelt (1999) observes that "very often conditions respond to the use of essential oils regardless of which oils are being used. It appears to be the implementation of aromatherapy alone which brings improvement" (p. 121). It is possible that essential oils, "being representatives of the plant world," are able to communicate with all planes of human consciousness and existence (Schnaubelt, 1999, p. 123).

INDIVIDUALIZED OR GENERALIZED AROMATHERAPY

Holistic aromatherapy, as developed by Marguerite Maury (see Chapter One), lays its emphasis on creating a therapeutic blend for each individual client. In practice, however, this may not always be possible or desirable, particularly in busy clinics and spas. Therefore, it is up to you, the individual practitioner, to decide how you wish to practice aromatherapy.

Individualized Aromatherapy

Individualized aromatherapy blending requires that a skilled and knowledgeable practitioner select and blend essential oils and carrier materials based on the *current* needs and assessment of the client. Such **blends** (a combination of essential oils in a base or carrier) take into account the body/mind/spirit connection and are designed specifically *per individual, per bodywork session.* This way of practicing can be slightly more time-consuming, however with the knowledge and understanding of a specific set of essential oils and blending techniques, you can reduce the time needed to create an individualized blend.

Generalized Aromatherapy

Generalized aromatherapy is the use of pre-blended **synergies** (a combination of essential oils without a base carrier) or **blends** (a combination of essential oils in base or carrier) that address common conditions. Though they are created for specific common concerns or goals, they are not created specifically for the individual client to address their *individual* needs at a given point in time. Utilizing pre-blended aromatics can be very time-efficient and cost-effective, especially in a busy practice or spa. As long as such blends contain only therapeutic-grade essential oils, clients can still enjoy the many health benefits of incorporating aromatherapy into your work. A way to individualize pre-blended synergies is to add one or two essential oils based upon individual needs. See Table 8.1 for samples of generalized synergies and possible additions based upon individual needs.

Whenever customizing a blend, be it an individualized blend or making an addition to a generalized blend, always consider not just the complaint presented, but the "*why*" behind it. For instance, if you are starting with a basic synergy for muscular aches and pains, ask your client *why* they're experiencing so much soreness. If it's because they are unable to sleep at night, then perhaps you would add a couple drops of Roman chamomile and lavender. But if they're sore because they were a weekend warrior and engaged in more physical activity than usual, you might add a few drops of lemon and ginger to the basic synergy instead.

Whether you choose to customize blends for each individual client or utilize pre-blended aromatic products, be sure to explain to clients or potential clients about how you practice aromatherapy. One idea is to design a generalized aromatic treatment for a promotion or your regular menu of services, while offering customized aromatherapy sessions as an option for those who seek it.

IN PRACTICE 8.1

Avoid the Use of Scented or Fragrance Products

Scented or fragrance products are most likely commercially prepared and contain undesirable chemicals and/or synthetic fragrances. Though these can often smell "pretty," they not only negate holistic aromatherapy but they can also elicit allergic or uncomfortable reactions in your clients. Synthetic fragrances do not contain any of the healing qualities of pure, genuine, high-quality essential oils; therefore they do not have the same action on the body. Usually when clients confide that they are "allergic to smells" or "super sensitive," it is because they have been exposed to synthetically fragranced products or massage oils in the past. Once you explain the difference between fragrances or synthetically scented massage oils and those made with pure essential oils, many are willing to at least try the essential oils. In this case a low dilution is recommended.

TABLE 8.1

Generalized Blends with Possible Additions Based Upon Individual Needs

Synergy	Add In:
Muscular Aches and Pains Rosemary (*Rosmarinus officinalis*) Peppermint (*Mentha* x *piperita*) Eucalyptus (*Eucalyptus globulus*)	– Ginger (*Zingiber officinale*) for warming – Lavender (*Lavandula angustifolia*) for relaxing – Lemon (*Citrus limon*) for detoxing
Relaxation Lavender (*Lavandula angustifolia*) Tangerine (*Citrus reticulata*)	– Clary sage (*Salvia sclarea*) for PMS, muscle spasms, cramps – Frankincense (*Boswellia carterii*) for emotional healing, self-reflection – Roman chamomile (*Chamaemelum nobile*) for insomnia or high stress
Uplifting Grapefruit (*Citrus paradisi*) Sweet orange (*Citrus sinensis*)	– Lavender (*Lavandula angustifolia*) for stress relief or anxiety – Ylang ylang (*Cananga odorata*) for stress relief and comfort – Vetiver (*Vetiveria zizanioides*) for grounding

↪ AROMATIC APPLICATIONS FOR MASSAGE

Massage delivery systems are substances that carry essential oils onto the skin and include vegetable oils, gels, lotions, and creams. All types of massage delivery systems can be therapeutically enhanced by adding specific essential oils, tailored to the individual and the goals of the treatment (Figure 8-1).

Preparing Massage Oils

Prepare your base oil by combining various high-quality vegetable oils, such as sweet almond, sunflower, or apricot kernel, along with any desired macerations or herbal-infused oils. Select these base oil ingredients in accordance with your treatment goals and the properties/benefits of each as discussed in Chapter 6. Add approximately 10 drops of all-natural d-alpha tocopherol (vitamin E) per 8 oz. of oil. Store in an airtight jar or bottle, in a cool location, and away from heat or sunlight.

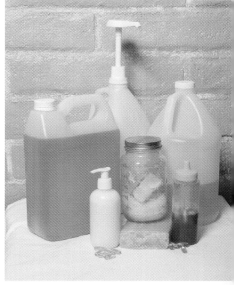

Figure 8-1 Bulk ingredients
Source: © Dennis Gallaher

Select three to five essential oils or a pre-blended synergy to work with based upon client consultation and goals for the bodywork session. Fill a 1 oz. glass or **PET bottle** (polyethylene terephthalate plastic; it is least likely to leach out the valuable essential oils or affect the chemical composition of your blends. See Chapter 5 for further information.) half full with your base oil blend. Add the appropriate number of drops for each essential oil. Add more base oil to fill 1 oz. Cap and shake vigorously for several minutes. The blend is now ready to use.

Massage Lotions, Gels, and Creams

Unscented massage lotions, gels, and creams differ from regular lotions, gels, and creams in that they are designed specifically to be used for massage. They are available from several massage and aromatherapy supply companies. Be sure to check the ingredient list to ensure the product has ingredients you find acceptable. Most commercially prepared base products will contain at least a small amount of preservative to guard against contamination. Look for natural preservatives, such as vitamin E, grapefruit seed extract, or rosemary extract, or the minimal amount of food-grade preservatives necessary to protect the product.

IN PRACTICE 8.2

Time Saving Hints

Carrier Oils

Mix enough base oil to create multiple blends and to supply your facility for several weeks. Herbal oils that should be used at a lower percentage (10%), such as rose hip, evening primrose, or calendula, should be added to smaller, individual bottles just before using.

Blends

Create two or three basic aromatic synergies consisting of fewer essential oils (only two or three) for common complaints such as stress reduction or improving energy. Then to individualize your blend, simply listen to your client and add a few drops more of one or two carefully selected essential oils for their specific needs. These synergies can then be added to your carrier of choice as needed.

Another option is to create your own massage lotion/gel with the sample recipe provided below.

Preparing Massage Lotions, Gels, and Creams

Select three to five essential oils to work with based upon client consultation or comments and goals for the bodywork session. For massage lotions and gels, it is usually most convenient to use a 1 or 2 oz. PET bottle with squeeze or flip top lid. Fill the PET bottle half full with your base lotion or gel. Add the appropriate number of drops for each essential oil. Add more lotion or gel to fill the remaining 1 or 2 oz. Cap and shake vigorously for several minutes. The blend is now ready to use. For massage cream, use a glass bowl or measuring cup and glass or wood stirring rod to mix the essential oils into the cream; then spoon into a glass jar for storing.

Dilution/Dosage Recommendations

For blending into a carrier oil, lotion, or oil-based gel, a dosage of 2.5 to 5 percent is recommended. However, there is an occasional justification for increasing dosage as high as 10 percent for local acute inflammations, chronic pain, and when using specific local techniques. See Chapter 5 for more detailed blending dilutions.

MAKE YOUR OWN MASSAGE LOTION

Creating your own homemade massage lotions and gels can be both fun and economical, not to mention providing you and your clients with a high-quality, all-natural therapeutic treat.

Supplies

16 oz. glass/pyrex measuring cup

Large pot (to fit measuring cup)

Burner or stove

8 oz. bottle with flip top or pump

5 oz. vegetable oil (sweet almond, apricot kernel, sunflower, herbal infused, etc.)

3 oz. distilled water

1 tsp. beeswax

2 vitamin E capsules (100% d-alpha tocopherol, 500 iu)
Essential oils of choice

To Make

Place measuring cup in pot and fill pot with warm water to reach ⅔ up the sides of the measuring cup. Put vegetable oil and beeswax inside the measuring cup. Place pot with measuring cup on burner and heat to medium-high, stirring continuously until the beeswax is completely melted. Remove measuring cup from heat; set aside. Pour distilled water into the lotion bottle. When slightly cooled, pour oil/wax mixture into lotion bottle. Immediately cap and shake vigorously for several minutes. Puncture two vitamin E capsules and squeeze the liquid into the lotion bottle; discard gel caps. Add chosen essential oils, recap, and continue to shake for several more minutes.

Variation

To create a massage lubricant that is more gel-like in consistency, simply change your ratios of oil, water, and wax slightly. Try 6 oz. oils with 2 oz. distilled water and increase wax to 1½ tsp. Follow the same process and remember to shake extremely well, or put the water in a blender and slowly add the melted wax/oil mixture until emulsified and then pour into bottle.

Note

It is best to use new bottles for each batch to help guard against contamination. Make certain all of your tools and containers are clean and sterilized before working. Make smaller amounts of massage lotions/gels that can be used up in a timely manner. Although you can store extra in the fridge for a period of time, beneficial properties of some vegetable and essential oils are better off simply in a cool, dark place. Always shake your lotion/gel before using, especially if some separation has occurred. If your lotion turns lumpy, spotted, or has a foul odor, be sure to toss it out and start fresh with a new batch.

↪ GELS, SALVES, FACIAL CREAMS/OILS

Gels

Aloe vera gel is different from massage gel and deserves a separate mention. Concentrated aloe vera gel is increasingly being employed for aromatic applications for the skin and muscular system, due to its cooling and hydrating effects and for localized applications for muscular aches and pains, varicose veins, burns, and wound healing. Aloe vera gel is one of the best gels, since it adds its own healing attributes. Aloe vera is used for wound healing, burns, and other tissue damage. Aloe vera is also considered an immune-enhancer and exhibits antifungal activity (Pizzorno and Murray, 2000, p. 582). A concentrated aloe vera gel is available in most health food stores.

Aloe vera is a succulent perennial plant belonging to the lily family that grows wild in Madagascar and large portions of the African continent. Because of its many therapeutic uses, it is now commercially cultivated in the United States, Japan, and countries in the Caribbean and Mediterranean. Aloe vera is a common houseplant. The aloe plant is best known for its healing aloe vera gel, a thin, clear, jellylike substance that can be squeezed or scraped from the inner part of the fleshy leaf. A soothing juice is also made from this gel (Figure 8-2).

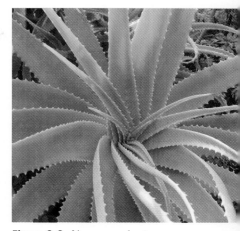

Figure 8-2 Aloe vera plant
Source: © iStockPhoto.com/lubilub

Potential toxicity: Pizzorno and Murray (2000) report that although rare, hypersensitivity reactions have occurred and that aloe vera preparations should not be used for treating deep vertical wounds, such as those produced during cesarean delivery. In these cases, aloe vera may delay wound healing. Individuals who are hypersensitive to aloe vera may experience a burning sensation on the skin. It may be prudent to ask allergy-sensitive individuals if they have a possible allergy to aloe vera or to administer the patch test to ensure that a reaction will not result.

In general, gels are useful for:

- inflamed skin conditions
- muscle aches and pains
- thin or fragile skin (elderly)
- varicose veins
- migraines/headaches
- burns
- wound healing (ulcers)

How to Prepare a Gel

The concentrated aloe vera gel available on the market is able to absorb additional water. To enhance the therapeutic benefits of the gel, add a small amount of hydrosol (e.g., Lavender hydrosol) to desired consistency and then add three to five essential oils at the appropriate dilution. You can also add in herbal and vegetable oils to desired consistency. Combine ingredients in a bowl, stirring with a glass rod or wooden spoon. Place prepared product in a 1 or 2 ounce sterilized jar. This type of gel can be used in localized treatments for muscular aches and pains, varicose veins, headaches, migraines, etc.

Salves

Salves are typically prepared from the combination of beeswax, vegetable oils, herbal-infused oils, and essential oils. They can vary in consistency from quite thick and somewhat hard to soft and semisolid. Salves tend to soften on contact with the skin and require little time to be worked into the skin. Salves provide a healing, emollient, soothing, and protective effect to the skin and are usually used in specific, localized areas.

In general, aromatherapy salves are useful for:

- ▶ dermal inflammation
- ▶ scar therapy: reduces inflammation and improves scar appearance
- ▶ musculoskeletal aches and pains or spasms
- ▶ skin issues: particularly dry, cracked skin conditions
- ▶ wound healing
- ▶ stress/anxiety/emotional conditions

To Make a Salve

Place 1 cup apricot kernel oil (or ¼ cup calendula-infused oil, ¼ cup jojoba, ½ cup apricot kernel oil) with ½ ounce of beeswax. Melt this down in a double boiler at medium temperature. Stir often to ensure the merging of oils with the beeswax. While waiting for the oils and beeswax to melt, create a therapeutic aromatic synergy. Once the oil/beeswax part is melted, remove from the stove and add to small glass jars (usually 1 to 2oz.). Each jar should have 30 to 40 drops of the synergy. Put the lid on the jar and shake, then let stand until hardened. Once hardened, the salve is ready for use.

> **NOTE**
>
> Test the consistency of a salve before blending with essential oils by placing a spoonful of the salve in the refrigerator. Allow the salve to harden. If the salve comes out to hard or thick, you can melt the mixture down again and add more oil. If the salve is too fluid or thin, you can melt it down and mix in some more beeswax. Experiment with different herbal oils or infusions and notice how and when the consistency differs. By working with herbal oils, you are able to increase the potential therapeutic benefits of the salve.

Dilution/Dosage Recommendation

The dosage with salve-making may seem a bit high, but this is due to the fact that a salve holds essential oils differently than a cream or a gel or any other delivery system. My recommended dosage is 30 to 40 drops per ounce of salve.

Facial Creams/Oils

Special facial creams are available from several aromatherapy companies (see appendix 3 for suppliers). A facial cream is more than oil, as it is an oil/water emulsion and is hence capable of delivering moisture to the skin. Creams nourish, soften, and moisturize the skin. The choice between a facial oil or cream would depend on the condition of the client's skin and the goals of the treatment. If a client had dry (lacking oil) and dehydrated (lacking water) skin, then a cream would be appropriate. If, on the other hand, a client had dry skin (lacking oil) but was well hydrated, then a facial oil would be appropriate. The facial skin tends to be more sensitive than the rest of the body, so essential oils may need more consideration and observation regarding client sensitivities (Figure 8-3).

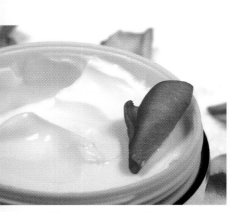

Figure 8-3 Aromatic facial cream
Source: © iStockPhoto.com/ elanathewise

In general, aromatherapy facial oils and creams are utilized to:

- ▶ enhance wound healing
- ▶ influence and slow aging of skin
- ▶ scar reduction and improve appearance
- ▶ support and enhance immune cells of the skin
- ▶ balance sebum production
- ▶ aid the process of detoxification in the skin

▶ increase local circulation
▶ improve tone of skin
▶ encourage hydration of the skin, when used in conjunction with hydrosol/water or cream
▶ soften and soothe the skin
▶ address emotional issues

How to Prepare Facial Oil

Choose three to five essential oils to work with based upon client consultation and the goals of treatment. In a 1 ounce glass bottle, place the appropriate drops for each essential oil. Close the lid and shake the bottle vigorously. The synergy is now ready for the oil to be added. Fill the 1 ounce bottle with the vegetable oil or a combination of vegetable and herbal oils. Place the cap back onto the bottle and shake vigorously for another two or three minutes. The facial oil is now ready for use.

> **Professional Observations: Creams**
>
> It has been my experience and observation that **creams hold essential oils differently than vegetable oils or gel**. Creams need a lower dilution of essential oils than vegetable oils. For face creams, I recommend either less than 1 percent or 1 percent total. There may be times when a higher concentration is indicated, however for general therapeutic care, the lower dilution will be beneficial.

How to Prepare a Facial Cream

For creams, you may wish to use a 1 or 2 ounce jar instead of a bottle. Some creams available on the market will allow you to add hydrosols and herbal oils. If this is the case, add these components to a desired consistency. Add in your choice of essential oils. Stir all ingredients together with a glass stirring rod or a wooden spoon until the essential oils are evenly distributed throughout the base material.

Facial Oil/Cream Dilution Rates

For adults:

Sensitive skin: .5 to 1 percent dilution = 3 to 6 drops per ounce

Normal, healthy skin: 1 to 2.5 percent dilution = 6 to 15 drops per ounce

⤳ UNDILUTED APPLICATION

Undiluted or "neat" application is the use of essential oils applied directly to the skin without a carrier or base oil. In general, undiluted application is only applied to a small specific localized area, most commonly and for acute conditions and for reflex/acupressure work.

Undiluted application is appropriate for the following acute conditions:

▶ acne
▶ cold sore or burn
▶ minor skin trauma or infection
▶ migraines
▶ reflex or acupressure work
▶ lymph congestion

PROFESSIONAL OBSERVATIONS: UNDILUTED APPLICATION

The undiluted application of essential oils is a highly controversial topic in aromatherapy. Practitioners and educators are divided on the issue. Current standards for aromatherapy education in the United States do not prohibit undiluted application.

According to Kurt Schnaubelt, Ph.D. (2004), author of *Advanced Aromatherapy* and *Medical Aromatherapy*: "It appears that most, if not all, of the sweeping generalizations are not inspired by a thorough analysis of potential toxicity, but by a sentiment to err on the side of safety. The aim is to establish simple rules which would prevent a public, often perceived as less than intelligent, from incurring any and all adverse reactions with essential oils" (p. 44). He recommends that a more balanced approach be adopted based upon individual essential oils and their therapeutic efficacy and safety.

To utilize the undiluted application of essential oils effectively, a practitioner must be able to balance their understanding of the therapeutic benefits and applications of a given essential oil with possible concerns. From this knowledge base, a practitioner is empowered to make a responsible professional decision to use undiluted application when deemed necessary or appropriate.

My own experience and practice have taught me that there are indeed times when the undiluted application of essential oils is called for. We certainly should not live in fear but rather should work toward gaining a greater understanding of the potential benefits of this form of application so that it can be used wisely and for therapeutic benefit.

Specific essential oils that tend to be safe to apply undiluted include tea tree (*Melaleuca alternifolia*), lavender (*Lavandula angustifolia*), helichrysum (*Helichrysum italicum*), Roman chamomile (*Chamaemelum nobile*), rose (*Rosa damascena*), and sandalwood (*Santalum album* or *Santalum spicatum*). These oils may be applied undiluted to pimples, cuts and scraps, burns, and cold sores. It is important to only use a small amount (1 to 2 drops) of essential oil. Other essential oils may be used for reflex or acupressure points, however care should be taken in selecting essential oils, and essential oils that can be irritating, sensitizing, or are rich in aldehydes or phenols should be avoided all together for undiluted application.

The undiluted application of essential oils is a highly controversial topic within the aromatherapy industry. Leading authors and educators all differ in their opinions and usually can be found in one of two camps—those who believe the undiluted application of essential oils is extremely beneficial and indeed called upon under specific circumstances and those who believe that essential oils should absolutely not be placed on the skin undiluted and that doing so is not only extremely hazardous but also unprofessional.

➜ INTEGRATING AROMATHERAPY WITH MASSAGE TECHNIQUES

According to the Associated Bodywork and Massage Professionals (n/d) association, "There are more than *200 variations* of massage, bodywork, and somatic therapies and many practitioners utilize multiple techniques. "Whichever modalities you elect to study and master are up to you, and as you continue to explore aromatherapy, you will find innovative new ways of integrating essential oils in your work. Remember that as licensed massage therapists, it is outside our scope of practice to diagnose or prescribe for any physical or emotional illness or injury. When discussing the benefits of aromatherapy with your clients and colleagues, be sure to use terms such as nourishing, supportive, relaxing, or rejuvenating. It is our goal as responsible therapists to enhance the bodywork experience for our clients with the knowledge-able application of quality essential oils and aromatherapy blends.

Aromatic Relaxation Massage

Relaxation massage utilizes basic Swedish massage strokes, such as effleurage, petrissage, friction, percussion, and range of motion. Obviously the goal here is to provide a relaxing experience for the client while massaging away stress and hypertonic muscles (Figure 8-4). Typically when a client requests a "relaxation" massage, they want a good, solid massage with lasting benefit, so it is probably not the time to address that frozen shoulder or dig too deep on the trigger points; the client simply desires to rest and relax. An aromatherapy relaxation massage has as much to do with soothing the mind and calming the spirit as relieving tension in the physical structures. Choose essential oils based on those that would have a relaxing effect on the muscular system itself, as well as work to calm the peripheral nervous system (see Table 8.2). Also take into account the "comfort factor" and include oils that might help sooth any emotional aspects your client may have mentioned in the interview. A typical dilution rate for relaxation aromatherapy massage is 2 to 2.5 percent.

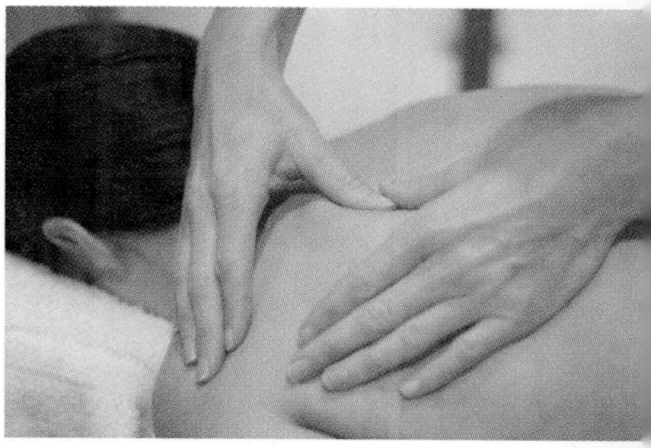

Figure 8-4 Relaxing massage
Source: © iStockPhoto.com/ actionphotonz

Tips for a successful massage:

- ▶ Establish intent for today's session with the client prior to beginning.
- ▶ Keep conversation and any outside noise to a minimum; focus on comfort.
- ▶ Consider dim lighting, relaxing music, and a candle or electric diffuser to scent the room.
- ▶ In a 1 oz. bottle, prepare massage oil, lotion, or gel with essential oils selected for client.
- ▶ Use an aromatic compress, hot towels to massage tight muscles, or add a couple of drops of essential oil to a microwavable rice pack and use it to heat the client's back as you work in other areas.
- ▶ To finish, ask the client to close their eyes and then lightly mist with an aromatic spritzer.
- ▶ Give the client the remaining oil or lotion to use at home following their session.

TABLE 8.2	
Examples of Essential Oils for Relaxation Massage	
Essential Oil	**Latin Name**
Lavender	*Lavandula angustifolia*
Roman chamomile	*Chamaemelum nobile*
Clary sage	*Salvia sclarea*
Frankincense	*Boswellia carterii*
Mandarin	*Citrus reticulata*
Vetiver	*Vetiveria zizanioides*
Ylang ylang	*Cananga odorata*

Aromatic Treatment Massage

Although treatment massage is also effective at relieving stress and tension, it usually focuses on a specific injury or complaint, often chronic, and will most likely employ other, more specific techniques on the part of the therapist. When decreasing pain, tightness, spasms, or inflammation is the goal, we're providing a more "treatment"-based approach to therapy. We may include hydrotherapy (Chapter 9) and Swedish massage techniques as well as myofascial release work, trigger point or acupressure, and range of motion or cross fiber friction to name a few. Including the benefits of aromatherapy in a treatment-based massage can be as simple as a basic blend for sore muscles in the main lotion, gel, or oil. See Table 8.3 for sample essential oils treatment. Other strategies would include using a higher-dilution salve or gel for localized treatment of specific muscles or tender points. See Chapter 10 for specific conditions and corresponding essential oils.

Tips for a successful massage:

▶ Establish intent and treatment goals for today's session with the client prior to beginning.

▶ Communicate with your client on important issues such as breathing, resisting, relaxing, and reporting feedback of sensation to you throughout the treatment session.

▶ Do not add scent to the room if you plan to use more than one blend during the session.

▶ In a 1 oz. bottle, prepare massage lotion, gel, or oil with essential oils selected for client.

▶ In a separate dish, place 1 oz. pre-blended sore muscle salve or add 20 to 30 drops of selected synergy (5%) to 1 oz. massage oil, gel, or cream; use on specific muscles or localized areas.

▶ Use a warm aromatic compress or hot towels to massage tight muscles or add a couple of drops of essential oil to a microwavable rice pack and use it to heat specific areas while you work on others.

▶ Have ice, cold gel packs, or a refreshing compress on hand to complete the treatment session.

▶ Give your client any leftover product for self-massage at home or consider blending a sore muscle Epsom salt soak to add to bathwater for your client to get some relief.

TABLE 8.3

Examples of Essential Oils for Treatment Massage

Therapeutic Action	Essential Oil	Latin Name
Anti-inflammatory	German chamomile	*Matricaria recutita*
Analgesic	Black pepper	*Piper nigrum*
Bruises	Helichrysum	*Helichrysum italicum*
Antispasmodic	Clary sage	*Salvia sclarea*
Warming	Ginger	*Zingiber officinale*

Aromatic Sports Massage

Although most athletes benefit greatly from some form of massage or bodywork, either as a warm-up to or immediately following an event, they probably won't appreciate too much scent on the body while trying to concentrate and compete. Generally speaking, oil and other lubricants aren't usually used in sports massage; instead therapists use methods of compression, pin and stretch, kneading, and gymnastics to warm up, loosen, and cool down muscles to improve flexibility, endurance, and range of motion. The addition of aromatherapy can still be useful and should focus on the physical and mental state of the athlete while being geared toward either the "warm-up" or "cool-down" phase of activity. See Table 8.4 for examples of essential oils for sports massage.

Tips for a successful massage:

- ▶ Establish intent of bodywork for "warm-up" or "cool-down" phase along with client.
- ▶ If working in a private room, use diffuser to scent, either invigorating (warm-up) or relaxing/refreshing (cool down).
- ▶ Pre-event: Create a muscle warming salve or gel at a 5 percent dilution to use on specific, localized muscle groups or areas.
- ▶ Pre-event: Use a warm aromatic compress or hot towels to massage tight muscles or add a couple of drops of essential oil to a microwavable rice pack and use it to heat specific areas while you work in others.
- ▶ Post-event: Have ice, cold gel packs, or a refreshing aromatic compress on hand to relieve sore muscles, minor injuries, and inflammation.
- ▶ Post-event or possibly during the event: Prepare a refreshing aromatic spritzer to use during breaks. Keep chilled in a fridge or cooler for extra benefit.
- ▶ Post-event: Use a cooling gel as a finishing touch for tired muscles. Get all the benefits of a "cool down" rub with no oily residue left on the skin.

Aromatic Reflex Massage

There are many forms of reflex or pressure point massage and bodywork modalities. Each has its own unique history, application, and therapeutic results. For the sake of this book, we will estimate that for the most part, essential oils or

TABLE 8.4	
Examples of Essential Oils for Sports Massage	

Essential Oil	Latin Name
Warm Up	
Black pepper	*Piper nigrum*
Ginger	*Zingiber officinale*
Sweet marjoram	*Origanum marjorana*
Peppermint	*Mentha x piperita*
Cool Down	
Cypress	*Cupressus sempervirens*
Eucalyptus	*Eucalyptus globulus*
Peppermint	*Mentha x piperita*
Rosemary	*Rosmarinus officinalis*

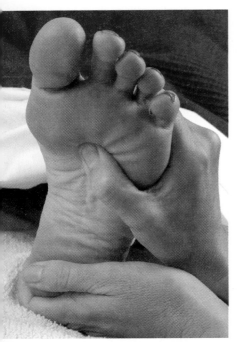

Figure 8-5 Aromatic reflex massage
Source: © iStockPhoto.com/alwekelo

aromatherapy blends can be incorporated in much the same way whether working with foot or hand reflexology (Figure 8-5), acupressure points, Jin Shin Do, or Shiatsu. The oils that you select, however, may change based on the belief system or goals of the particular modality being used.

Tips for a successful massage:

▶ Establish intent and treatment goals for today's session with the client prior to beginning.

▶ Do not add scent to the room if you plan to use more than one blend during the session.

▶ In a 1 oz. bottle, prepare massage lotion, gel, cream, or oil with essential oils at a 2 to 2.5 percent dilution; this will serve as your main blend to use on larger, more general areas.

▶ In a separate dish, place ½ oz. (1 tablespoon) massage oil, gel, or cream. Add 20 to 30 drops of simple synergy consisting of one to three essential oils, forming an 8 to 10 percent dilution; this is your **"point" blend** for use on specific reflex or pressure points.

▶ Occasionally for very specific pressure point work, you may elect to use undiluted essential oils. Only certain oils should be used in this way and in very moderate amounts. Use only one essential oil at a time if combining with other "main" or "point" blends. Combine up to two essential oils if using this method on its own.

How to Create a "Layered" Treatment Effect for a Primary Complaint or Goal

1. Use an undiluted essential oil on very specific reflex or acupressure points; for instance, use fennel essential oil with reflexology points on the bottom of the feet to address constipation and help stimulate peristalsis. Then work "outward" and layer other supporting blends as demonstrated in the following steps.

2. Use a "point blend" on a slightly broader, yet still localized area. With the example of reflexology on the feet, you could massage your point blend into the whole digestive area of the feet to enhance digestion and elimination. Following the example in #1, your point blend could be a combination of grapefruit, fennel and ginger diluted to 8% in jojoba or apricot kernel oil. This same blend could be utilized for abdominal massage.

3. Finish with your core blend, which has been created at a lower dilution with the overall goal of relaxation and wellness in mind. Apply this blend with general massage strokes on a much broader area. In completing our example above, this core blend could be a combination of lavender, sweet orange, and ginger. The blend could be massaged onto both feet and the lower legs as well as for the rest of the body to complete the session.

Remember to limit the number of oils you use in any one blend or for undiluted application when layering your treatments. Be sure that the essential oils you use all work together synergistically, no matter which layer they're being used in, and that they are all selected to achieve the end goal.

Aromatic Hot Stone Massage

Hot stone massage has become very popular in day spas, destination spas, and even private practices (Figure 8-6). If you have ever been fortunate enough to receive a hot stone massage, you know how wonderful it is when the heated stones become an extension of the therapist's hands as they are massaged over tired muscles. If you are a therapist already trained in the art of giving a good hot stone massage, you can now add the many benefits of aromatherapy. Because of the use of heat and cold in these treatments, when combined with the powerful connection to the earth element, there lies a golden opportunity for enhancing the whole process by adding essential oils to the experience. Just have fun and be creative. You will discover new ways to bring aromatherapy into your work. Here are a few ideas to get you started.

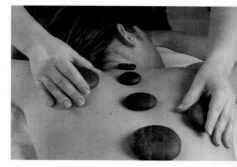

Figure 8-6 Aromatic stone massage
Source: © iStockPhoto.com/alwekelo

Tips for a successful massage:

- ▶ establish intent for today's session with the client prior to beginning.
- ▶ do not use a diffuser or candle burner to scent the room, *instead*;
- ▶ add 3 to 4 drops of essential oil to your pot of rocks and water once they become warm.
- ▶ in a 1 oz. bottle, prepare massage oil with essential oils specifically selected for client (do not use lotion or gel with hot rocks); use this blend as your lubricant for the stones.
- ▶ use a higher dilution blend (5%) on localized areas of the body for acute conditions or when applying to working trigger/acupressure/reflex points.
- ▶ place one large hot stone with 2 to 3 drops of essential oil on a stool or shelf several inches under the face cradle to help clear sinuses.
- ▶ for cleaning stones after treatment: Along with washing stones in hot soapy water, you can also use tea tree and/or lemongrass in a mister to further disinfect stones.
- ▶ avoid the use of clove and thyme essential oils as the heat from the stones may increase dermal irritation.

By combining heat therapy, massage, and aromatherapy as with hot stone massage, you create a powerful, synergistic opportunity for relaxation and healing. Please remember that as with any modality, one *must be trained thoroughly to practice hot stone massage safely and effectively*. Although it is outside the reaches of this book to instruct on specific modalities, we hope that when it comes to learning how to practice hot stone or any other methods discussed, you will continue your education by seeking out quality instruction and training geared toward your specific interests.

Aromatic Facial Massage

Combining massage technique with carefully selected carrier materials and quality essential oils is what makes an aromatic facial treatment so beneficial and enjoyable. It is important to educate your clients as to the purpose of this session and make certain they understand the differences between what you can offer as a licensed massage therapist and what kind of facial they might receive from a licensed esthetician. Estheticians are licensed to perform more in-depth facials that include, extractions and skin typing and are designed to have more dramatic effects. Facials, as performed by estheticians would be outside the scope of practice for licensed massage therapists. Some states may also have different laws that may prohibit you from performing this type of treatment. Check with your local state licensing office to ensure this type of facial massage is within their code of practice for massage therapists.

Therapeutic goals of aromatic facial massage:

▶ improve circulation and nutrient exchange for muscles and skin of the face and head
▶ stimulate healthy lymphatic flow and function
▶ help reduce fluid retention/edema of face and head
▶ support the natural processes of exfoliation and cell renewal
▶ hydrate and enhance the natural appearance of facial skin
▶ stimulate and tonify facial muscles
▶ provide a relaxing and interesting experience with multiple textures, temperatures, etc

Preparing the Materials

Use care when selecting essential oils for the aromatic facial massage. Stay clear of oils that are sensitizing or irritating to the skin (see Chapter 3). Use gentle essential oils and lower dilution rates such as 1 or 2 percent. Additional questions to ask your clients prior to a facial massage are if they know their skin type and if they have any known allergies or sensitivities.

To perform this aromatic facial massage, you will need:

▶ **Hot towels (two hand towels and four washclothes):** These can be made in a hot towel cabinet or by using a Crock-Pot or burner with individual pots for each client. Add 2 to 3 drops of essential oil to the water when preparing the towels.
▶ **Cleanser (½ ounce):** Use a natural, unscented cleansing cream base or create your own with aloe gel and grapefruit seed extract. Some with less sensitive skin can use a low dilution of liquid castile soap in distilled water or aloe. Just don't use standard store-bought bar or liquid soaps as they usually contain unwanted perfumes, dyes, and other chemicals, plus they are often too harsh, stripping the skin's natural ph balance, leaving it dull and dry. Add 3 to 4 drops of essential oils selected for your client's skin type (see Chapter 6) to a natural cleanser.

TABLE 8.5

Examples of Essential Oils for Facial Massage

Essential Oil	Latin Name
Frankincense	*Boswellia carterii*
Lavender	*Lavandula angustifolia*
Roman chamomile	*Chamaemelum nobile*
German chamomile	*Matricaria recutita*
Rose	*Rosa x damascena*
Sandalwood	*Santalum album* or *Santalum spicatum*
Tea tree	*Melaleuca alternifolia*

▶ **Toner (1 ounce):** Mix ½ teaspoon witch hazel with 1 ounce distilled water. Add 6 or 7 drops of essential oils selected for your client's skin type. Mix or shake well. Chill just before using.

▶ **Massage oil (½ ounce):** Create a blend of vegetable-based oils and include herbal-infused oils for their various healing properties if desired. Add 3 to 5 drops of essential oil or synergy based on your client's skin type, consultation, and goals of treatment. Mix or shake well. See Chapter 6 for more on the properties of individual carrier oils.

▶ **Mask (1 ounce):** Mix 2 tablespoons plain yogurt, 1 teaspoon white clay, 1 teaspoon ground (not too fine) oats, and 7 to 10 drops of essential oil or synergy based on your client's skin type, consultation, and goals of treatment. Mix well and chill just before using.

▶ **Lotion or cream (½ ounce):** Use a low dilution blend of nonirritating, gentle essential oils that can comfortably be used on sensitive skin, as this facial lotion or cream is applied last and left on the skin to moisturize and hydrate. Add 1 to 3 drops of essential oil to ½ ounce natural, unscented face lotion or cream and mix well (Figure 8-7).

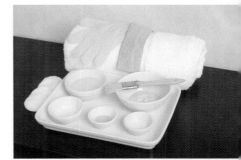

Figure 8-7 Facial massage supplies
Source: © Dennis Gallaher

In addition to the blended materials previously discussed, you will also need to have on hand:

1 bath towel

1 exfoliating glove (light)

1 headband

4 round cotton pads

1 one-inch paintbrush

Practicing the Technique

Besides the obvious skin softening, smoothing, and moisturizing benefits of the aromatic facial massage are the wonderful aromas (as the name would imply) and the interesting variations of temperature and texture that make for an amazing tactile experience.

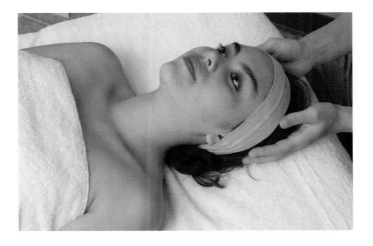

Figure 8-8 Prepare client
Source: © Dennis Gallaher

1. Ask your client to arrive without face makeup on if possible. Provide the fabric headband or tie to hold hair away from the face and out of the way. Place the bath towel at the head of the table (under the client's head) and make sure your client is positioned comfortably supine (Figure 8-8).

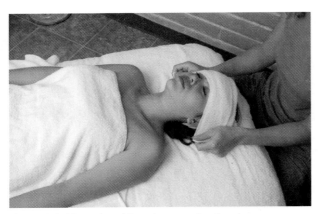

Figure 8-9 Warm head towel across forehead
Source: © Dennis Gallaher

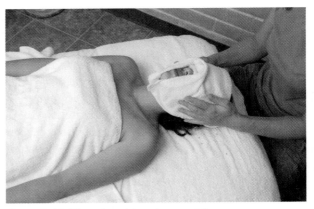

Figure 8-10 Warm hand towel around face
Source: © Dennis Gallaher

2. Apply one hand towel across the forehead (Figure 8-9) and then down each side of the face (Figure 8-10); press/massage and hold gently. Make sure the towel is thoroughly wrung out and not too hot.

Figure 8-11 Gentle cleanser and exfoliate
Source: © Dennis Gallaher

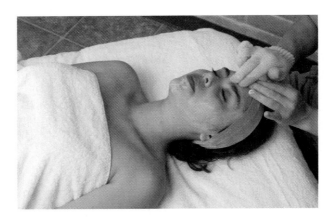

3. Put on exfoliating glove and lightly moisten fingertips with warm water and cleanser. Apply cleanser with other hand using gentle upward strokes, followed close behind with small circular strokes of the gloved hand. Cover the whole face with gentle strokes and avoid the eye area. Remove the glove (Figure 8-11).

Figure 8-12 Warm wash clothes to remove cleanser
Source: © Dennis Gallaher

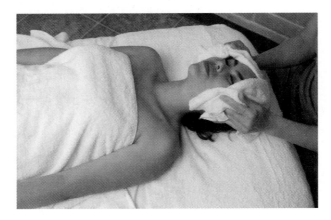

4. Use two warm/wet washcloths to remove the cleanser by placing one on each side of the face (leaving the nostrils exposed to breathe); press/massage and hold gently (Figure 8-12).

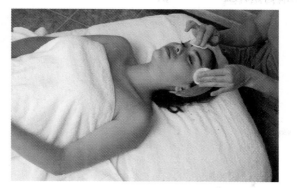

Figure 8-13 Apply chilled toner
Source: © Dennis Gallaher

5. Moisten two cotton pads in the chilled toner. With one in each hand, use light, upward strokes beginning at the chin, cheeks, and then forehead to remove excess dirt or cleanser from the skin. Avoid the eye area (Figure 8-13).

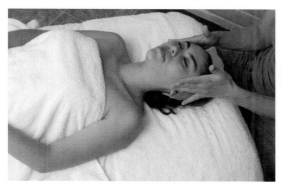

Figure 8-14 Massage with facial oil
Source: © Dennis Gallaher

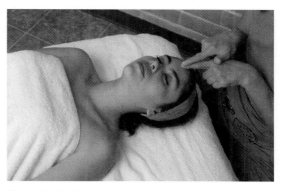

Figure 8-15 Acupressure points
Source: © Dennis Gallaher

6. Apply massage blend to the face and neck using various techniques, such as effleurage, petrissage, small circular friction, and acupressure or trigger points. Consider incorporating some lighter lymphatic strokes for the face and head as well. Massage approximately ten minutes, avoiding the eye area (Figure 8-14 and 8-15).

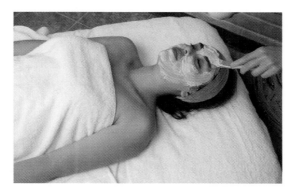

Figure 8-16 Apply mask with brush
Source: © Dennis Gallaher

7. Use the paintbrush to carefully apply the chilled mask. Load the brush and begin each stroke by placing the brush and cold mask at a common point, such as the chin, cheek, or forehead, then spreading the mask outward along the stroke. Make sure you use plenty of mask, but just like painting, it is better to go over each area twice than to apply too much on the first pass and risk dripping. Avoid the eye area. Leave mask on until it is almost dry or about 10 to 12 minutes (Figure 8-16).

Figure 8-17 Massage shoulders
and arms whole mask dries
Source: © Dennis Gallaher

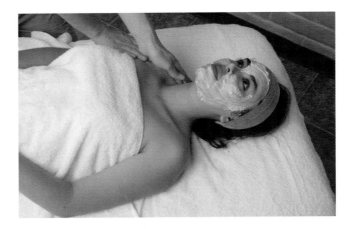

8. While the mask is on, use the remainder of the massage oil to massage the arms, hands, and scalp. When combining the aromatic facial massage with a regular full-body massage, opt to do the full-body massage first, leaving the arms, hands, and head for treatment during the facial massage portion (Figure 8-17).

Figure 8-18 Remove mask with
warm wash clothes
Source: © Dennis Gallaher

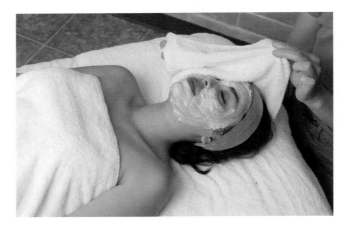

9. Use two warm/wet washcloths to remove the mask by placing one on each side of the face (leaving the nostrils exposed to breathe); press/massage and hold gently. Scoop up and lightly wipe off any leftover mask. Use an extra set of washclothes if needed (Figure 8-18).

Figure 8.19 Warm hand towel
around face
Source: © Dennis Gallaher

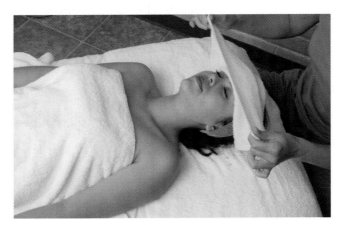

10. Apply one hand towel across the forehead and then down each side of the face; press/massage and hold gently. Make sure the towel is thoroughly wrung out and not too hot before placing! (Figure 8-19).

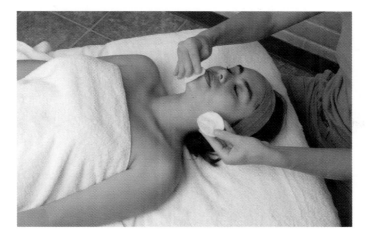

Figure 8-20 Apply chilled toner
Source: © Dennis Gallaher

11. Moisten two cotton pads in the chilled toner. With one in each hand, use light, upward strokes beginning at the chin, cheeks, then forehead to remove excess dirt or mask from the skin. Avoid the eye area (Figure 8-20).

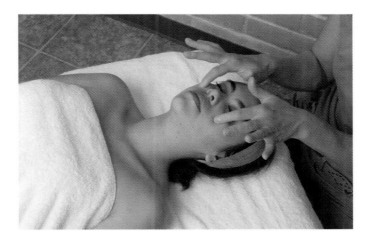

Figure 8-21 Massage with light lotion
Source: © Dennis Gallaher

12. Apply a small amount of moisturizing lotion or facial cream with gentle soothing strokes. Don't use too much or your client may be left feeling "greasy." This should be a lighter textured cream or lotion with a low dilution (Figure 8-21).

SUMMARY

- The integration of essential oils with massage and bodywork techniques can enhance the effects on the body via their therapeutic actions, the mind via their aroma, and the spirit via their energetic nature.
- The basis of holistic aromatherapy is to customize aromatherapy blends based upon the individual goals and needs.
- Pre-blended aromatherapy products are most often created for generalized purposes. They can be individualized by adding 1 or 2 essential oils based upon the client's needs.
- The term "aromatherapy blend" typically implies the dilution of essential oils within a base or carrier product, such as a vegetable oil, lotion, gel, or cream.

- The term "aromatherapy synergy" typically implies the combination of two or more essential oils without a base or carrier product.
- The use of fragrance products should be avoided in the practice of aromatherapy as it increases the likelihood of adverse dermal or emotional reactions and negates the very foundations of aromatherapy.
- A point blend is usually one or more essential oils diluted in a base or carrier product at a higher dilution. It is used for specific reflex or pressure points.

NEW TERMINOLOGY

Aromatherapy blends	PET bottle
Aromatherapy synergies	Pre-blended synergies
Massage delivery systems	Point blend

REFERENCES

Associated Bodywork and Massage Professionals (AMBP). (n/d). *Introduction to Massage*. Retrieved on June 20, 2006, from http://www.massagetherapy.com/learnmore/index.php.

Pizzorno, J., and Murray, M. (2000). *Textbook of Natural Medicine*. London: Churchill Livingstone.

Schnaubelt, K. (1999). *Medical Aromatherapy*. Berkeley, CA: Frog, Ltd.

Schnaubelt, K. (2004). *Aromatherapy Lifestyle*. San Rafael, CA: Terra Linda Scent and Image.

Tappan, F., and Benjamin, P. (1998). *Tappan's Handbook of Healing Massage Techniques*. Stamford, CT: Appleton and Lange.

Aromatic Applications (Part I)

Name: _____   Date: _____

Making Massage Lotions and Gels

1) Using the instructions in this chapter, select your base oils and make a massage lotion or gel. Leave unscented for future blends or add essential oils of your choosing.
2) Vegetable oils used: _____
3) How did it turn out? Are you happy with the texture, consistency, scent, etc.?
   _____

4) Would you do anything differently in the future?
   _____

Aromatic Facial Massage

5) Determine your facial skin type from the list below. Discuss your needs with your partner.

How would you classify your skin type? *(more than one may apply!)*

❏ Mature: slightly older, thinner skin, some fine lines or wrinkles, less elasticity, and possibly sun or age spots

❏ Normal: skin is soft and supple, has firm texture and good color. Doesn't usually suffer from blemishes or dry patches

❏ Normal to Oily: an overproduction of sebum (or oil) in at least the T-zone area, shiny nose, prone to breakouts

❏ Normal to Dry: generally soft skin with some tightness, dry or flaky patches, usually around the mouth and on cheeks or under eyes

❏ Sensitive: skin often turns red or blotchy after washing or applying certain products, reacts to hot and/or cold, chemicals, and the environment

❏ Acne Prone: frequent breakouts and blemishes, pores clog easily causing pimples and blackheads, may be due to hormones, diet, or stress

Key Notes

_____

_____

Aromatic Applications (Part II)

Aromatic Facial Massage

6) Based on the information provided, blend the materials necessary for the aromatic facial massage as given in this chapter. List the ingredients used below.

% or # Drops	Cleanser	Toner	Massage Oil	Mask	Lotion/Cream
Base Material					
Essential Oils					

7) Following the steps outlined on page 171, take turns and exchange aromatic facial massages with your partner.
8) Following today's treatment, how do your skin/facial muscles feel?

_____

9) What would you tell a friend or prospective client about this treatment?

_____

CHAPTER TEST

1. Massage blends are when essential oils are combined with:

   a. sitz baths

   b. lotions, gels, or oils

   c. a compress

   d. additional essential oils

2. In a massage oil, a _____ dilution is recommended for infants and young children.

   a. 3 percent

   b. 2.5 percent

   c. .5 to 1 percent

   d. 15 percent

3. Facial oils differ from face creams because they do not contain:

   a. heat

   b. an aroma

   c. vitamins

   d. water

4. Gels are typically derived from:

   a. sea salt

   b. aloe vera

   c. water

   d. oil

5. The following essential oils are widely accepted as being safe for undiluted application:

   a. cinnamon bark and clove bud

   b. lemongrass and ginger

   c. tea tree and lavender

   d. peppermint and sassafrass

6. Salves are excellent for:

   a. facial massage

   b. depression

   c. scar therapy

   d. constipation

7. A point blend is used:

   a. on the full body

   b. only on reflex points

   c. in a localized area

   d. specifically for sports massage

8. Use aromatherapy during relaxation massage to:

   a. decrease stress and anxiety

   b. relieve trigger points

   c. work reflexively

   d. heat the skin

9. The goal of an aromatic facial massage is to:

   a. clear up blemishes

   b. decrease wrinkles or age spots

   c. extract the pores

   d. enhance circulation, skin texture, and underlying musculature

10. Facial creams can use a dilution of _____ percent because cream holds essential oils differently from other carrier or base products.

    a. 5 percent

    b. 2.5 percent

    c. 1 percent

    d. 25 percent

REVIEW QUESTIONS

1. Discuss the undiluted application of essential oils and under what circumstances this method would be best employed.

2. Discuss how you would explain the differences and benefits of an aromatic facial massage versus a full esthetic facial treatment.

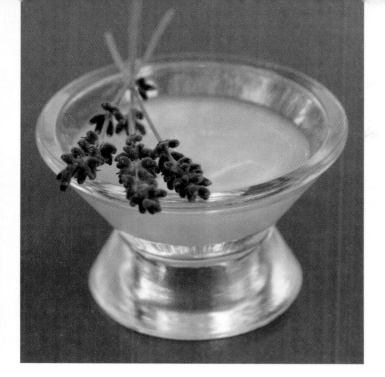

The Healing Properties of Water and Salt

→ LEARNING OBJECTIVES

After reading this chapter, you will be able to

1. Explain the difference between a hydrosol and an aromatic spritzer.
2. List by common and Latin name seven hydrosols and describe their therapeutic benefits.
3. Describe four physiological effects of hydrotherapy.
4. List conditions which should have heat applied and which should have cold applied.
5. List seven potential water-based methods of application and their potential therapeutic benefits.
6. Discuss the value of salt and water in bodywork and massage practice.
7. Create a salt scrub and perform a salt glow treatment.

INTRODUCTION

Water and salt have been used since antiquity for their healing abilities on the body, mind, and spirit. Massage therapists and bodyworkers often incorporate the use of water and salt for a variey of purposes, including hydrotherapy and spa treatments. The first half of this chapter is designed to cover the basics of hydrotherapy and the integration of hydrosols and essential oils. The second half covers the potential benefits of adding salt into one's practice. The subject of hydrotherapy is vast but attempts have been made to include only the necessary information relevant to the integration of aromatherapy with bodywork and massage.

BACK TO BASICS: WATER

Throughout the ages, the energy and mysteries of water have touched our bodies, minds, hearts, and imaginations (Figure 9-1). Nearly all cultures have revered water as healing and precious while also holding great respect for its ability to give life as well as to take life away. Humans have used water for its healing powers most commonly in the form of baths. Baths have been employed for their health benefits since ancient times. The earliest writings regarding the therapeutic benefits of bathing are attributed to the Indian Vedas that date from approximately 1500 B.C. The ancient Greeks revered bathing where it was often prescribed along with exercise, nutrition, and intellectual stimulation. They utilized both hot and cold submersion therapies along with massage and scented oils in their famous public baths.

When the Romans conquered the Greeks, they absorbed much of their culture, especially in regard to philosophy, medicine, the arts, and sciences. The public bath became a pillar of the Roman community. The Romans are perhaps best known for creating elaborate bathhouses for people to use for their health benefits. Hippocrates, the famed Greek physician, employed "hydrotherapy" with aromatic oils and deemed baths as essential to good health. The history of medicinal baths is extensive, and it would appear that they are experiencing a renaissance in the modern world due to their benefits for the body, mind, and spirit.

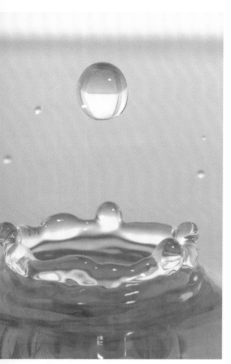

Figure 9-1 Water drop
Source: © iStockPhoto.com/Trout55

Body

Water accounts for approximately 75 percent of our total body weight. Our organs and muscles are comprised mainly of water, and even bones are nearly one-fourth water in composition. Water also makes up the majority of our bodily fluids, including blood, saliva, lymph, and urine. Water, known as the "universal solvent," moves throughout the body in the form of blood plasma, carrying with it water soluble nutrients, oxygen, and wastes that are exchanged with tissue cells by passing through the watery interstitial fluid. Water helps regulate body temperature and chemical reactivity within the body. It is also the primary component of synovial fluid in joints, serous fluids that lubricate internal organs, and cerebrospinal fluid that helps to protect and cushion the brain and spinal cord. During pregnancy, the amniotic fluid serves to surround and protect the growing fetus within the mother's body. This is our first experience of the warm, nurturing, life-giving qualities of water.

Our Bodies Need for Water

We have all heard the standard recommendation of consuming at least 8 eight-ounce glasses of water a day, and even though we know it's good for us, how many of us really drink enough on a daily basis?

If you are not taking in enough water, your body will limit how much water certain organs get to have. Lack of hydration can contribute to headaches, fatigue, chemical imbalances, and low concentration, to name a few. One of the places we notice poor hydration first is in the skin. This is the body's largest organ, and it looks and functions its best, like the rest of the body, when there's plenty of water to go around.

We suggest to our clients that they properly hydrate following their massage or bodywork sessions in an effort to continue flushing the system and replenishing the tissue after increasing circulation and lymphatic flow *(though hopefully we're not "prescribing" water here— take a look at how you phrase this to your clients!)*

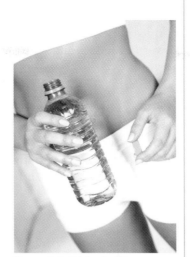

Figure 9-2 Water bottle
Source: © iStockPhoto.com/dashek

In an effort to encourage proper hydration, consider providing your clients with a free bottle of water for the road immediately following their session! They will feel better, thank you for thinking of it, and appreciate your ongoing concern for their health and well-being.

Mind

Water is a soother, a healer, a purifier, and a source of rejuvenation. The molecules of which we are comprised as human beings carry a certain electrical charge that emits and receives energy, thus creating a pulsing, wave-like force that extends outside our physical body. When this "aura" reflects an even, balanced pattern, we feel happy and content in our emotional body. But when we are experiencing emotions of sadness, resentment, anxiety, or confusion, this "aura" will reflect a different energy. Because of its molecular makeup, water is eager to bond with all things hydrogen. Water, by its very nature, wants to bond and absorb; therein lies its unique, transformative characteristics. As the great "universal solvent," water absorbs the excess energy created by our emotions, offering purification, comfort, and healing. Even the sound of water rushing over rocks, crashing against the shore, or moving down a waterfall has the ability to calm and soothe and even excite and energize. In large part, we relate to the soothing quality of water because we *are* water.

Spirit

The nature of water is known to be absorbent and easily influenced by outside energies, and many cultures and religions hold the belief that water can be infused by the vibration of prayer, chanting, medicine songs, or decrees. In his book, *The Message from Water*, Japanese photographer Masuro Emoto demonstrates the effects that positive and negative words and thoughts have on water. By exposing the water to either beautiful, positive words and energies, such as love or peace, or negative words and energies, such as anger or hate, then freezing the exposed water and photographing the resulting crystals, Emoto has captured what would appear to be striking results. The negative words and energies formed ugly, unpleasant-looking formations while the positive words or prayers created beautiful, delicate formations. His work reveals the ability of water to be imbued with different energies, and although his work is contested by some as being unscientific, we may find comfort by looking to the very history of water and the many beliefs and rituals among ancient and indigenous peoples regarding its ability to heal, purify, and act as a conductor of subtle energies. Beyond spoken words or thoughts, water is capable of absorbing and conducting the energies of gemstones, moonlight, a holy place or temple, plants, such as with Bach Flower Remedies, and, of course, essential oils and hydrosols.

Types of Water and Uses

Water is a hot topic these days for a variety of reasons, from concern over polluted and toxic water to the growing decrease in water availability. Since water is an important and vital aspect of life, the quality and kind of water we use, whether for drinking, bathing, etc., is important. To learn more about water, see references and other resources at the end of this chapter. Table 9.1 outlines common types of

	TABLE 9.1
Common Types of Water	

Type of Water and *Usage*	Information
Artesian Water *Drinking* *Aromatherapy bathing*	Also known as artesian well water, FDA regulations require that this water must come from a well in a confined aquifer. The water level in the well must extend at some point above the top of the aquifer.
Distilled Water *Drinking* *Aromatherapy products*	Distillation of water, similar to essential oils. Impurities and electrolytes are removed. It is used in the manufacturing of pharmaceuticals and cosmetics. Because trace elements and minerals have been removed, some refer to this as "dead water." There are ongoing debates about whether humans should drink distilled or purified water.
Purified Water *Drinking* *Aromatherapy bathing* *Aromatherapy products*	Like distilled water, purified water is "de-mineralized." It is produced by deionization, reverse osmosis, or other processes that meet the legal definition of "purified water."
Fluoridated Water *Drinking*	Fluoride is added within FDA guidelines. The adding of fluoride to water is a highly controversial health issue. Some springs have naturally occurring fluoride in trace amounts.
Mineral Water *Aromatherapy bathing* *Drinking*	Mineral water may contain any number of minerals, most commonly magnesium and calcium. The mineral sulphur may cause the water to smell somewhat like rotten eggs, and water rich in iron (ferruginous) will be orange/red. Water rich in minerals is typically referred to as "hard water." For drinking, mineral water must contain no less than 250 parts per million total dissolved solids (minerals in the water), and it must come from a geologically and physically protected underground water source.
Spring Water *Aromatherapy bathing* *Aromatherapy* *Drinking*	Emanates from beneath the earth's crust. Lightly mineralized springs close to air temperature tend to be shallower, while heavily mineralized springs tend to be hotter and originate from deeper within the earth's strata. Thermal or "hot" springs are extremely beneficial for bathing depending on which core minerals are present at a given location. For drinking water, the FDA requires that spring water must come from an underground formation and flow naturally to the earth's surface. Must be collected at the spring or through a bore hole tapping the underground formation/spring.
Well Water *Drinking* *Aromatherapy bathing*	Comes from a hole in the ground that is mechanically bored or drilled, thus tapping the water of an aquifer. Some wells are shallow and can run low on water or pick up contaminates, while others are very deep and have a strong supply. Well water is often rich in minerals of magnesium and calcium (hard water).

water that you may use in your practice for external (hydrotherapy) or internal (drinking) applications.

Aromatic Waters: Hydrosols

Aromatic waters could be considered a type of water that can be used for hydrotherapy applications. **Hydrosols**, also known as hydrolats, are the by-product of the distillation process and are extracted from specified botanical species.

	TABLE 9.2
Hydrosols and Their Therapeutic Benefits	

Hydrosol / Stability	Therapeutic Benefits
German chamomile *Matricaria recutita* Stable: Can last up to two years.	• Anti-inflammatory and cooling properties make it useful for various skin conditions, such as eczema, psoriasis, rashes, acne, sunburns, and other inflammatory conditions • Calming and balancing to the autonomic nervous system; soothes or reduces feelings and symptoms of stress • German chamomile, like lavender, can be added to the bath for its sedative and soothing properties • Muscular aches and pains, sprains, strains, spasms, whiplash
Roman chamomile *Chamaemelum nobile* Stable: Can last up to two years.	• #1 hydrosol for infants and young children: diaper rash, calm and soothe, and help with sleeping • Calming and soothing effects on the mind: insomnia, stress relief, mildly euphoric • Anti-inflammatory and antiseptic for the skin: rashes, acne • Beneficial for reducing anxiety, anger, and childhood hyperactivity
Clary sage *Salvia sclarea* Stable: Can last up to two years.	• Astringent and can be used on oily skin types • Mild antispasmodic, muscle spasms, cramps • Antidepressant and euphoric qualities • Female tonic: cramps, PMS symptoms, emotional upsets, hot flashes • Emotional trauma, heartache
Lavender *Lavandula angustifolia* Stable: Can last up to two years.	• Relaxing, soothing, and comforting: headaches, stress-related conditions • Anti-inflammatory and antiseptic • For infants in the bath or as a spritzer for diaper rash, sleep problems • Muscular aches and pains, sprains, strains, sore or stiff muscles
Orange flower *Citrus aurantium* var. *amara* Stable: Can last up to two years.	• Antidepressant, euphoric • Stress relieving, insomnia, mild sedative • Toner for acne and oily skin due to mild astringent effect
Peppermint *Mentha* x *piperita* Unstable: Lasts under one year and must be refrigerated.	• Digestive tonic: constipation, colic, indigestion • Muscular aches and pains, sprains, strains, spasms, shin splints, sore or stiff muscles • Mentally stimulating, energizing
Rose *Rosa damascena* Stable: Can last up to two years.	• Astringent, useful for acne, varicose veins, oily skin, normal-to-dry, mature, sensitive, and devitalized skin • Calming, soothing, nurturing • Strong affinity with the heart, useful for individuals who are grieving or are in need of emotional support, heartache • Female tonic: cramps, PMS symptoms, emotional upsets, hot flashes, menopause symptoms

Hydrosols contain the *water-soluble constituents* of the aromatic plant and retain a small amount of essential oil. According to Catty (2001), "every liter of hydrosol contains between 0.05 and 0.2 milliliter of dissolved essential oil, depending on the water solubility of the plant's components and the distillation parameters" (p.12).

Hydrosols are sometimes inaccurately called floral waters. I say inaccurate because most hydrosols are not from flowers and most hydrosols do not smell flowery. The term hydrosol is a much more accurate term. Hydrosols are also very different than a blend of essential oils in water. When water and essential oils are mixed, with or without a dispersing agent, this would be called an **aromatic spritzer**, and its therapeutic benefits would be slightly different from that of a true hydrosol.

To keep hydrosols fresh, it is important to keep them cool and away from direct light or heat. The average shelf life for most hydrosols is twelve to twenty-four months. I have found that storing hydrosols in the refrigerator ensures freshness and liveliness of aroma. Be sure to smell your hydrosols from time to time to ensure they are still good.

Hydrosols can play a valuable role in the application of hydrotherapy, in baths, sprays, compresses, and internal applications. Hydrosols can also be used for salt scrubs, gels, lotions, and creams. Hydrosols, like essential oils, can be combined together for a variety of different therapeutic purposes. Table 9.2 covers the more commonly used hydrosols and their therapeutic benefits.

Hydrosols as Hydrating Agents

Modern skin suffers tremendously at the hands of environmental conditions, excessive coffee use, low water intake, and nutritional deficiencies. When the skin is in need of hydration, besides consuming water internally, the application of hydrosols is incredibly beneficial. Neither essential oils nor vegetable carrier oils contain water and hence are not hydrating to the skin. Hydrosols and all natural skin care creams are able to deliver the necessary moisture to the skin (along, of course, with dietary measures and increased water consumption).

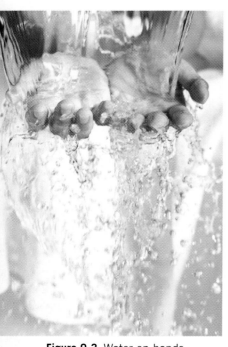

Figure 9-3 Water on hands
Source: © iStockPhoto.com/alephxol

⟳→ WATER AS THERAPY

It seems almost obvious that since our own bodies are so incredibly similar in makeup to that of ocean or seawater that we would desire to replenish and restore our body, mind, and spirit by immersing ourselves within this life-giving element (Figure 9-3). **Hydrotherapy** is the use of water in any form (solid, liquid, vapor) for the treatment of disease or injury as well as for the maintenance of good health. It is commonly employed by massage therapists and bodyworkers either as part of treatment work, for spa sessions, or as a part of self-care for the client and practitioner.

Thalassotherapy is a type of hydrotherapy that refers specifically to the therapeutic use of seawater, seaweeds, or various other seawater extracts. Later in this chapter we will discuss salt in more depth. **Balneotherapy** refers to the use of baths that aim to enhance the immune system; stimulate the circulatory process, including lymph and blood circulation; accelerate cell activity, by dilating tissue and vessels; and activating the self-healing potential naturally (www.balneotherapy.com).

Some of the general therapeutic benefits of hydrotherapy include:

 ▸ relief from pain
 ▸ reduction in swelling from injuries

- ▶ elimination of toxins
- ▶ improved lymphatic flow
- ▶ relief of spasms
- ▶ improve immune functioning
- ▶ cultivate and nurture emotional well-being

In our therapeutic use of water, we can also include other beneficial ingredients, such as herbs and essential oils, each of which provides their own benefits and powerful healing affects on the body, mind, and spirit.

Effects of Hydrotherapy

Significant physiological changes that occur with the use of hydrotherapy can be classified as:

■ **Mechanical:** The effects produced by the impact of water on the surface of the body, e.g., water sprays, frictions, and whirlpools. For example, in a deep bath, the hydrostatic pressure of water against the body actually increases blood and lymph flow and increases urine output and detoxification.

■ **Reflexive:** The effects produced by the influence of water on the nervous system in response to the application; for example, heat applied to one foot can cause corresponding changes in blood flow in the opposite foot.

■ **Chemical:** The effects produced by taking water internally; for example, drinking water to flush out toxins.

■ **Thermal:** The effects produced by the application of water at temperatures above or below actual body temperature. This is of primary concern when applying hydrotherapy. Water temperatures may vary from very cold to very hot as indicated in Table 9.3.

TABLE 9.3	
Water Temperatures	
Description	**Temperature**
Very cold	32° to 55°F
Cold	55° to 65°F
Cool	65° to 80°F
Tepid	80° to 92°F
Warm	93° to 99°F
Hot	100° to 104°F
Very hot	104°F and above
Warning: During pregnancy the core body temperature should not be raised above 102°F, therefore hot baths, saunas, full body steam, and wraps should be avoided.	

General considerations that affect the desired outcome of hydrotherapies include:

- ▸ temperature of the water
- ▸ difference between skin and water temperatures (the greater the difference the greater the reaction)
- ▸ amount of surface area covered (via method of application)
- ▸ duration and frequency of application (short, sudden exposure or prolonged)
- ▸ client's weight, age, and general health condition

The therapist can adjust his or her treatment to achieve specific results according to these variables. The following guidelines help to determine when hot or cold applications should be used and when they are contraindicated.

Heat is indicated for:

- ▸ chronic conditions
- ▸ the subacute and maturation phases of healing
- ▸ the reduction of pain and stiffness
- ▸ the relief of contracture and muscle spasms
- ▸ the increase of circulation and waste removal
- ▸ improved range of motion and flexibility

Do not use heat therapy (*contraindicated*) for:

- ▸ recently injured tissue (within seventy-two hours of trauma)
- ▸ prenatal clients: core body temperature should not be raised above 102°F
- ▸ active tuberculosis
- ▸ any disorder in which decreased circulation impairs the client's ability to respond to increased temperatures
- ▸ anyone who is high risk for heart attack due to history or unresolved chest pain should avoid steam rooms, saunas, and hot baths
- ▸ any malignant conditions. Clients suffering from cancer should obtain prior consent from their treating physician before receiving hydrotherapy
- ▸ clients with a medical history of diabetes, vascular problems, severe hypertension, or who are on daily medication should consult with their primary care provider prior to receiving thermotherapy

Cold is *indicated* for:

- ▸ recently injured tissue (within seventy-two hours of trauma)
- ▸ the acute stage of the healing process
- ▸ reduction of sharp pain and/or spasm
- ▸ the control of swelling and inflammation
- ▸ RICE: rest, ice, compression, elevate

Do *not* use cold therapy (*contraindicated*) for:

- ▸ Raynaud's syndrome, due to systemic vasoconstriction in response to cold.
- ▸ Areas of the body with a medical history of frostbite.
- ▸ Clients with decreased sensation in which they are unable to accurately report temperature-induced sensations.
- ▸ Any malignant conditions. Clients suffering from cancer should obtain prior consent from their treating physician before receiving hydrotherapy.

IN PRACTICE 9.1

RICE Method Review

To help ease the pain and inflammation often associated with joint and soft tissue damage, try using the RICE method immediately following an injury.

R Rest. For most injuries it is best to give the body a break and rest the area until a decrease in pain is achieved.

I Ice. Apply ice to the injured area as soon as possible immediately following injury. This will help reduce pain and inflammation by reducing the amount of blood and fluid buildup in the injured area.

C Compress. Wrap the injury with an elastic bandage to help reduce swelling and provide support to the damaged limb or area. Begin distill and work proximal, using care not to wrap too tightly.

E Elevate. Use pillows or propping to raise the injured area above the heart. This will help move extra fluid and reduce swelling.

▶ Clients with a medical history of diabetes, vascular problems, severe hypertension, or who are on daily medication should consult with their primary care provider prior to receiving cold therapy.

▶ Certain conditions, such as lupus erythematosus, rheumatic arthritis, and progressive scleroderma are at high risk for unfavorable outcomes using cold therapy.

Contrast Therapy

An extremely beneficial method of hydrotherapy treatment, contrast therapy involves the altering of hot and cold application to the same area of the body. The main physiological effects of this method are the alternating vasodilation and vasoconstriction of localized blood vessels that creates a vascular pump of sorts. This benefits injured tissue and facilitates the healing process by bringing nutrient-rich blood into the local area and also pushing wastes and stagnant blood out of the injured site.

Contrast therapy is a valuable tool in treating the subacute phase of an injury and in resolving edema or hematoma (bruises). Contrast therapy can be done with hot and cold packs or localized submersion.

An example of a basic contrast session may be:

5 minutes heat

5 minutes cold

2 minutes heat

4 minutes cold

2 minutes heat

6 minutes cold

Actual times may very slightly depending on case-by-case factors, for example, the part of the body being treated and/or the general condition of the client, but times should be kept in similar proportions. It doesn't matter so much whether you start with cold or with heat, but in every case *be sure to end with cold!*

Unfavorable Reactions to Hydrotherapy

Hydrotherapy treatments are generally considered helpful and mild in nature. Occasionally an individual may suffer some degree of adverse effect due to their own physiological response or a treatment that was not thought out or properly applied. If any of the following reactions occur, treatment should be stopped immediately and counteractive measures taken to resolve the issue.

In the case of client chilliness, always act quickly to warm the person with plenty of blankets and/or warm packs on hands:

> ▶ Headaches: sometimes appear with failure to apply a cool compress to the head during a full-body heat therapy or with resulting mild dehydration of heat therapy
> ▶ Uncontrolled shivering: if cold applications are left on too long or are not followed by appropriately covering and warming the body
> ▶ dizziness or lightheadedness
> ▶ heart palpations
> ▶ skin sensitivity
> ▶ hyperventilation
> ▶ nausea
> ▶ insomnia

Side effects are possible during, immediately following, or up to twenty-four hours after a treatment. It is important for therapists to take the time to explain the treatment, possible side effects, and actions to be taken by the client should any concerns arise. If you are recommending the client do a home treatment, complete instructions need to be given, preferably in writing, for their safe and effective use.

WATER-BASED METHODS OF APPLICATION

Since this is not a book dedicated solely to the practice of hydrotherapy or spa treatments, we will focus on a few of the most common and simplest to use of these techniques and combine them with the remarkable healing qualities of essential oils and hydrosols. With the exception of full-body baths, which therapists can recommend to their clients for home use, these techniques can, for the most part, be easily incorporated into any bodywork practice, even those without the luxury of a wet room. The choice of essential oils and/or hydrosols to use for each method will depend on the goals and purpose of treatment (Figure 9-4).

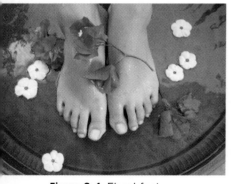

Figure 9-4 Floral feet
Source: © iStockPhoto.com/liewy

Full-Body Baths

A full-body bath is defined as "the complete immersion of the body in a fluid or in a vaporous medium such as steam" (Green, 2000, p. 254). The effects of a full-body bath will vary according to the temperature of the water and the duration of time the individual will be immersed. The average time for a full-body hot bath (100° F) is twenty minutes or less. Epsom/sea salt baths are highly effective in aiding and supporting the body in detoxifying, both physically and emotionally. See Aromatic Baths with Epsom or Sea Salts in the section on salt therapies.

In general, aromatherapy full-body baths are useful to:

> ▶ reduce stress/anxiety
> ▶ alleviate muscular aches, pains, and tension
> ▶ soothe mental or physical fatigue
> ▶ stimulate circulation

▶ enhance lymph circulation
▶ reduce pain and stiffness
▶ increase local circulation
▶ improve tone and health of skin
▶ aid detoxification

Therapeutic Dilution Recommendation

The number of drops of essential oil to place into a bath will depend upon the essential oil(s) being utilized. On average, one can place 5 to 10 drops of essential oil into a full-body bath. However, there are some oils, such as jasmine, when 1 to 2 drops would be sufficient and other oils, like lavender, when 10 to 15 drops would be fine. Avoid essential oils that are dermal irritants, dermal sensitizers, and mucus membrane irritants in baths. Combine essential oils with dispersant prior to adding to bathwater. See In Practice 9.2 for possible dispersing agents.

Adding hydrosols: According to Catty (2001), "for babies up to six months add 1 teaspoon of chosen hydrosol to an infant bathtub or 2 teaspoons for an adult tub filled to baby depth. For children up to twelve years of age, add 1 teaspoon of hydrosol per year of age, up to a maximum of 8 teaspoons. Adults can use from 30 to 250 milliliters (or 1 to 8 ounces per tub)." (p.171)

How to Prepare a Bath

The water should be at the desired temperature, and the essential oils or hydrosols should be added to the bath once the individual is in it. Placing essential oils in the bath prior to immersion can lose some of the desired effects, as well as increase the chance of irritation to the mucus membranes of the vaginal/rectal area. Once the individual is in the bath, add the appropriate essential oil/synergy drops (that have been combined with a dispersant) and agitate the water to disperse the concentration throughout the bathwater. Essential oils are lipophilic and hydrophobic, so most often the essential oils will quickly seek to be absorbed by the skin.

Foot and Hand Baths

A hand or footbath means the complete or partial immersion of only the hands or feet in water. Green (2000) comments that "the sole of the foot is one of the most important areas in the body, having direct connection with the nerve centers that control the

> **CAUTION**
>
> If an individual gets red blotches or irritation on the skin while bathing, this means that too much essential oil was added to the bath, a dispersant should have been used, or the client has experienced an idiosyncratic or allergic reaction. Should irritation occur, recommend a light cream or aloe vera gel without essential oils; the irritation should dissipate within an hour.

IN PRACTICE 9.2

Dispersing Agents

Water Dispersant: Polysorbate 20
Polysorbate 20 is a non-ionic surfactant that is used to disperse essential oils into water emulsions, such as baths, lotions, spritzers, and body mists. According to Essential Wholesale (n/d), polysorbate 20 is made from oleic acid (olive oil source) connected to a sugar (sorbitol). This compound is then ethoxylated (grain-based alcohol) to make it water dispersable.

Other Bath Dispersants:

Honey

Milk: fresh whole milk or dried milk

Coconut milk

Sea or Epsom salts

Vegetable oils

TABLE 9.4

Synopsis of Hot/Cold Foot and Hand Baths

Temperature	Therapeutic Actions
Hot Foot/Hand Bath 100 to 110°F	• Useful for balancing the circulation by the dilation of the blood vessels of the legs • Relieves congestion of the brain and other organs in the upper half of the body • Stimulates the involuntary muscles of the uterus, intestines, bladder, and other pelvic and abdominal viscera • Insomnia, lung congestion, dysmenorrhea, suppressed menstruation, ovarian congestion • Early stages of mucous congestion and local congestion of the head, chest, or abdomen
Cold Foot/Hand Bath 45 to 55°F	• Produces reflex, or counterirritant, effects • Contraction of the vessels and muscles of the uterus and the organs connected with it • Intestinal peristalsis and contraction of bladder is stimulated • Blood vessels of the brain, stomach, liver, bladder, and intestines contract at the same time

circulation of the pelvic and abdominal viscera" (p. 272). Foot and hand baths can be used as an aspect of reflexology or bodywork treatment. Table 9.4 summarizes the therapeutic effects of different temperatures, according to Green (2000).

In general, aromatherapy foot and hand baths are useful for:

- ▶ stress/anxiety
- ▶ poor circulation
- ▶ low energy
- ▶ foot or hand aches and pains
- ▶ arthritis and rheumatism (subacute phase)
- ▶ nail and toe fungal infections
- ▶ comfort therapy

How to Make a Foot/Hand Bath

Fill basin with water at the desired temperature and add in chosen essential oils and/or hydrosols. A dispersant such as vegetable oil or milk may be used but is not necessary in a hand or footbath. Place feet or hands in the basin. Let feet or hands soak for 5 to 10 minutes. Add ½ cup of Epsom or sea salts for enhanced benefits.

Therapeutic Dilution Recommendation

5 to 10 drops of essential oil in a basin of warm/hot water

1 to 3 tablespoons of chosen hydrosol

Steam Inhalation

Steam inhalation is used specifically for the respiratory system and can be effectively applied to support the expectorating properties of essential oils (Figure 9-5). Boyd and Sheppard (1968) report that steam inhalation can affect the output and composition of respiratory tract fluid. They also point out that low dilutions of aromatics for short periods of time are most effective. Longer exposure times can reduce the efficacy of steam inhalations so short durations and low concentration are the keys to optimal results.

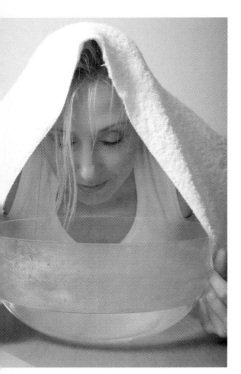

Figure 9-5 Steam inhalation
Source: © iStockPhoto.com/lovleah

Steam inhalations are indicated for:

- ▶ congestion in upper respiratory tract (cold or flu)
- ▶ sinus infection or sinusitis
- ▶ enhancing respiratory function

How to Make a Steam Inhalation

Bring 2 cups of water to boil, reduce heat, and let water cool for 5 to 10 minutes. Pour water into a glass bowl and place on a table so the individual can sit or stand over the bowl. Add 2 to 5 drops of essential oil or synergy. Inhale vapors for 3 to 5 minutes. A towel can be placed over the head to increase the concentration of inhalation. Inhalations can be used 2 or 3 times a day in the treatment of specific respiratory disorders.

Therapeutic Dilution Recommendation

A low concentration of 2 to 5 drops of essential oil or a synergy in approximately 2 cups of steaming hot water is sufficient.

> **CAUTION**
>
> Keep eyes closed to avoid irritation. Avoid mucus membrane irritating essential oils (see Chapter 3).

Compress

A compress is when a cotton or flannel cloth, soaked in cold/hot water, is applied directly to the skin. Compresses are usually for the treatment of a small localized area. A cold compress can be used to prevent or relieve congestion, reduce blood flow to an area, and inhibit inflammation. Cold aromatic compresses can be applied with the RICE technique for the relief of recent sprains, strains, and bruising. A hot compress is applied for pain relief for such conditions as menstrual cramps. A hot compress can also increase blood flow to a particular part of the body.

In general, aromatherapy compresses are useful for:

- ▶ muscular aches and pains (hot or cold as indicated)
- ▶ sprains and strains (hot or cold as indicated)
- ▶ menstrual cramps (warm/hot)
- ▶ respiratory congestion (warm/hot)
- ▶ bruises (cold/warm)
- ▶ skin inflammations (cold)
- ▶ varicose veins (cold)
- ▶ comfort care (warm)

How to Make a Compress

Fill a sink or large bowl with approximately 1 liter of hot or cold water as desired. Place 5 to 10 drops of selected essential oils along with a dispersant (if desired) in the water. Place cotton or flannel cloth in the water and swish around the water. Wring out the cloth to the desired amount of moisture and place on the area to be treated. At this point, if indicated, you can drop an additional 1 to 3 drops of your chosen synergy directly to the compress, then apply compress to the appropriate location. A hot compress should be left on until it has cooled to body temperature, then repeat directions above for soaking and reapply. Repeat 3 to 4 times. A cold compress can be refreshed every 5 to 7 minutes.

Therapeutic Dilution Recommendation

To 1 liter of water, place 5 to 7 drops of essential oil/s or 1 to 3 drops of essential oil directly on the compress.

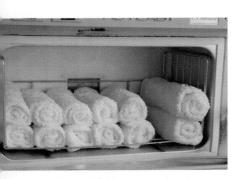

Figure 9-6 Hot towel cabinet
Source: © Dennis Gallaher

> **CAUTION**
>
> When removing towels from the cabinet, be careful not to touch the inner walls with your hands as you may get burned. Also, unfold the towels and test them on your inner forearm just prior to using on your client. Although professional grade cabinets are supposed to maintain a safe temperature, you may need to allow the towel to cool for just a moment before applying to your client's skin.

Adding hydrosols: According to Catty (2001), for adults add 3 to 5 tablespoons of hydrosols to 1 liter of water at the desired temperature; for children add 2 to 3 teaspoons of hydrosols per 1 liter of water.

Hot Towel Cabinet

A hot towel cabinet is a simple addition to any treatment room. This small metal box heats to a regulated temperature and has a UV bulb inside to help inhibit bacterial growth and maintain sanitization. Easy to use, the hot towel cabinet simply requires an electrical outlet and a shelf that is out of the way. By preparing aromatic towels ahead of time, you can include the use of moist heat even during your basic massage sessions (Figure 9-6).

In general, aromatic hot towels are useful to:

- ▶ relax tight or sore muscles
- ▶ increase overall relaxation
- ▶ improve local circulation
- ▶ remove salt glows, scrubs, or masks
- ▶ use as a welcoming or departing ritual, just prior to or immediately following the massage session

How to Prepare Hot Towels

Fill sink or small tub with hot water. Add 3 to 5 drops of your chosen essential oil and mix. Add 5 to 10 small hand towels. Soak towels for a few minutes, wring out well, and roll or fold. Place in the towel cabinet and let heat for at least 30 minutes prior to treatment.

Aromatic Spritzers

An aromatic spritzer is a combination of essential oils and water. Often a dispersant such as Polysorbate 20 is used to diffuse the essential oils within the water. Aromatic spritzers can be sprayed on face cradles to keep respiratory passages clear or sprayed on the body prior to applying the massage oil. This will enhance the therapeutic benefits of massage and the aromatherapy blend.

AAAAHH!

An aromatic spritzer can be used to refresh and rehydrate both the skin and the emotions. To make a spritzer you will need:

1 4-ounce glass or PET bottle
1 atomizer spray top
1 tablespoon witch hazel
20 drops essential oil
Mineral/distilled or spring water

Make sure the bottle is new and/or sterilized. Pour witch hazel into the bottle. Add essential oils of choice. Fill with distilled water. Cover with spray top and shake well. Eyes should be closed when misting face, and always remember to shake well before each use. Keep in the fridge prior to use for an extra cool and refreshing treat! Store away from direct light or heat.

In general, aromatic spritzers are useful for:

- ▷ room and air freshener
- ▷ body sprays over which an aromatic blend will be applied
- ▷ reducing undesirable odors in the air
- ▷ enhancing breathing
- ▷ soothing a variety of emotional states

BACK TO BASICS: SALT

Throughout history, salt has been a long-standing, necessary element of life. There have been stories, fables, customs, commerce, and even warfare surrounding this miraculous substance. In what is most likely the earliest known publication on pharmacology, the **Peng-Tzao-Kan-Mu** from China dated 2,700 BC, more than forty different kinds of salt and the processes of extraction are discussed. Egyptians record salt making as early as 1450 BC, and in ancient Greece, salt was used in trade for slaves, demonstrating its value and economic importance.

Sodium chloride or salt as we know it can be found throughout the world, especially in seawater, a seemingly inexhaustible supply; salt represents approximately 77 percent of the total dissolved solids seawater contains (Figure 9-7). Salt also appears elsewhere on earth as mixed evaporates in salt lakes and as surface salt deposits (a reminder of ancient seas) as well as man-made salt flats. Salt is available in various sizes (gradation), colors, quality, and elemental makeup, depending on the end use.

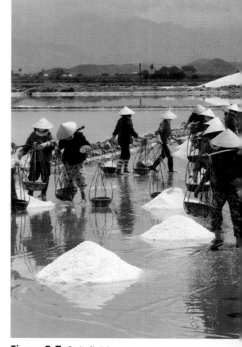

Figure 9-7 Salt field
Source: © iStockPhoto.com/dzalcman

Body

Salt is an essential element of life that the human body cannot exist without. The majority of salts found in the body are those containing calcium and phosphorus and are primarily in bones and teeth. Salts are also found in body fluids. Salts are **electrolytes**, which means they conduct an electrical current in solution. Proper electrolyte balance is vital for the body to function. In the United States, it is estimated that the consumption of sodium is on average about 3 grams a day, which would be equivalent to consuming about 7 to 8 grams of salt per day. It is reported that the National Academy of Sciences recommends Americans consume a minimum of 500 mg salt per day. As you can see, we usually tend to get more than enough in our daily diets. There is some controversy and debate among scientists as to the real or imagined dangers of excess salt in the diet. Though we do need it for survival and optimal function, it would appear that, like anything, too much is never a good thing.

Mind

We really can not separate the body/mind connection and, for the most part, what's good for one is good for the other. Salt with its cleansing, detoxifying, and healing properties can have a similar effect on our mind and emotions. Coupled with the benefits of water, a nice warm soak in aromatic bath salts will go a long way in helping to relieve tension, sadness, anxiety, and stress. Excess adrenalin due to chronic stress is believed to drain the body of magnesium and other vital minerals. **Magnesium** is a necessary component in the body's ability to form adequate amounts of serotonin, a chemical within the brain that elicits feelings of well-being and relaxation. Epsom salts offer increased magnesium levels and sulfates that are readily absorbed through the skin, helping to improve digestion and detoxification. Let us not forget that simply taking time out of our hectic, stressful schedules and dedicating that time to the ritual of the bath or an aromatic, salt-inspired bodywork session, is the first step in quieting the mind and preparing a place within for true healing to occur.

Spirit

Throughout the ages, salt has had a significant role in religious beliefs, customs, and rituals. Primarily used as a symbol of unbridled purity, salt was used by Greek worshippers in their rituals. Jewish temple offerings included salt, and salt is mentioned on several occasions in both the Old and New Testaments. The Catholic Church has used salt in a variety of purification rituals including baptisms. There is something to be said of salt in the word "salvation." As in many religions, the Buddhists believe salt drives away evil spirits. You can find the concept of throwing salt over your shoulder or sprinkling it around a home for purity and protection in several different belief sets. Even today, a gift of salt in India is a welcomed symbol of good luck and represents Mahatma Gandhi's liberation of the nation, which in 1930 included a symbolic 200-mile march to the Arabian Ocean to collect untaxed salt for India's poor.

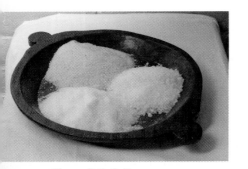

Figure 9-8 Salts
Source: © Dennis Gallaher

Types of Salt

Table 9-5 illustrates the various types of salt along with their therapeutic uses. See Figure 9-8 for types of salt.

			TABLE 9.5
Types of Salt			
Name	**Description**	**Sizes**	**Uses**
Sea Salt (Sal Del Mar, Sale Marino) Common Sources: Mediterranean Sea, North Sea, France (Atlantic Ocean), Pacific Ocean	A general classification that refers to salt derived directly from a living ocean or sea. It is harvested naturally via the sun and wind. Sea salt is typically not as refined as other salts so it maintains trace elements of iron, magnesium, calcium, potassium, and zinc, to name a few.	Coarse Fine Extra-fine	Bath Salts Salt Scrubs Salt Compress Therapeutic Treatments Cooking
Table Salt Common Source: Local salt mines	Salt most commonly found in the kitchen. Usually produced from salt mines, it is refined and processed until almost all trace elements are removed and it is pure sodium chloride. In the case of iodized salt, iodine is added as a dietary supplement. Sea salt is a healthy replacement for table salt.	Fine Course	Cooking *Not recommended for body treatments as it can be drying and irritating to those with sensitive skin. *Doesn't dissolve as well in scrubs and salt glows.
Dead Sea Salt Common Source: Only found in the Dead Sea	Total salt concentration in the Dead Sea is about 33 percent verus the 3 percent found in your average ocean. Dead Sea salt also contains magnesium, potassium, calcium chlorides, and a high concentration of bromides. Because of its unique makeup, water of the Dead Sea has been praised for its healing abilities since the time of Cleopatra. For over 2000 years, travelers have sought the waters for relief of skin and rheumatic disorders, wound healing, and beauty treatments.	Fine Coarse	Bath Salts Salt Scrubs Salt Compress Therapeutic Treatments

TABLE 9.5   (Continued)

Name	Description	Sizes	Uses
Celtic Gray Sea Salt (Fleur de Sel) Common Source: France	This special sea salt is gray in color and usually considered organic. It is generally harvested by hand and receives no treatment after harvesting. It is unwashed and unrefined and maintains its trace elements and nutrients.	Fine Medium Coarse	Bath Salts Salt Scrubs Salt Compress Therapeutic Treatments
Haleakala Red Common Source: Hawaii	Red Alaea is considered a medicinal clay that is reddish in color and high in trace minerals and iron oxide. It is only found in the Hawaiian Islands. The clay is added to sea salt and used to create a one-of-a-kind salt.	Fine Coarse	Cooking Bath Salts Salt Scrubs Therapeutic Treatments Native Healing Rituals
Kilauea Black Common Source: Hawaii	This sea salt undergoes a process in which the highest quality activated charcoal forms a bond with the salt and becomes a unique, glistening black mixture, with luxurious flavor and the proven anti-toxin health benefits of activated charcoal.	Fine Coarse	Cooking Salt Scrubs *(small amount)* Therapeutic Treatments Native Healing Rituals
Bali Sea Salts Common Source: Bali	Famous for the traditional method in which Bali sea salts are created, production is only possible during the dry months and can take weeks to complete, as sea water is channeled through canals of tree trunks and hand-dried in a grass hut. For the Balinese people, the sea is revered as sacred with the power to purify. Because of the unique hand-crafted process, these salt crystals are coarse and geometric in appearance.	Coarse	Bath Salts Salt Compress Therapeutic Treatments
Epsom Salt Common Source:	Magnesium sulfate or Epsom salt is often called for in healing recipes for the bath and body. Besides being the best choice for relieving muscular aches and pains, it is thought that raising magnesium levels in the body may improve circulation, reduce irregular heartbeats, prevent hardening of the arteries, reduce blood clots, and lower blood pressure. Epsom salt is also touted for improving the body's ability to use insulin, flushing toxins and heavy metals from cells, and improving nerve function by regulating electrolytes.	Coarse	Bath Salts Salt Compress Therapeutic Treatments *Doesn't dissolve as well in scrubs and salt glows.
Himalayan Pink Common Source: Himalayan Mountains	A naturally occurring, pure salt that is hand-mined deep inside the Himalayan Mountains. These crystals are pink to deep-red due to their high content of iron and eighty-four other trace elements. Two hundred fifty million years old, this remarkable salt is known for its many health benefits, such as stimulating circulation and helping to remove toxins from the body. This is a very dry salt, which makes it excellent for aromatherapy.	Fine Small Medium Large	Bath Salts Salt Scrubs Salt Compress Therapeutic Treatments

⟶ INCORPORATING SALTS IN YOUR TREATMENTS

Traditional Salt Glow

The salt glow or scrub is a well-known, highly effective body treatment for stimulating circulation and removing dirt and dead surface layer skin cells while leaving the skin soft and glowing, making it capable of both producing its own natural secretions and of better accepting the essential oils that are applied during the massage or other body treatments immediately following the salt glow. In creating a salt scrub, it is best to use a fine-to-medium-sized sea salt. Stay away from anything too coarse as you don't want to scratch or damage the skin. If you intend to remove the scrub with a sponge or hot towels, it is best to use sea salt because Epsom salts do not seem to evaporate as well, making removal more difficult.

Begin by placing a plastic liner under the bottom sheet to protect your table. Add a layer of bath towels under the client (on top of the bottom sheet) if you will be providing massage services on the same table immediately following the salt scrub. This way the towels can be carefully rolled up and slipped out from under your client before beginning the massage.

Use a couple of large bath towels to drape your client. Be sure to have plenty of extra towels handy:

- ▸ In a small bowl, mix 2 cups of sea salt + ½ cup of natural vegetable oil (almond, apricot, sunflower oil).
- ▸ Add 10 drops of essential oil or synergy; stir well.
- ▸ Wet the skin, either in the shower (then turn off water) or by using a hydrosol or aromatic spritzer.
- ▸ Apply salt glow mixture beginning at the feet and working up the legs toward the torso. Use quick, vigorous strokes or make it more relaxing with longer, slower strokes, but the important thing is to keep the mixture and circulation moving.
- ▸ Remove or rinse mixture from lower body.
- ▸ Continue with the same process for the arms, working from the hands toward the heart.
- ▸ Remove or rinse and conclude with the same process on the back and shoulders.
- ▸ Avoid using salt scrubs on the face as this skin is too delicate and prone to scratching.
- ▸ Be sure to conclude your salt glow with at least a minimal massage application of natural moisturizing oil or lotion to feed and replenish the newly exfoliated, thirsty skin.

Variations on the traditional salt glow can be achieved by incorporating dried herbs, ground nuts, seaweeds, and other natural ingredients. Just remember, what you put on the body, so must you get off the body! In the case of no wet room or shower, sea salt is the only thing that will mostly dissolve or evaporate with the use of hot moist towels.

In any case, this is a great opportunity to create three different aromatherapy blends for your client: one for the spritzer (wetting of the skin), one for the salt glow itself, and one for the moisturizing massage to finish. Make sure that these three blends work together and are not overwhelming. Keep them simple and look to address different aspects of the client's primary complaint or general wellness through each blend and step of the process.

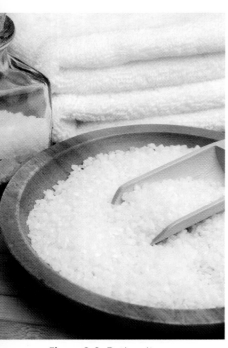

Figure 9-9 Bath salts

Source: © iStockPhoto.com/Rebecca Picard

Precautions:

▶ Never apply salt scrub to broken skin.

▶ To avoid possible irritation, wait 24 to 48 hours after shaving or waxing.

▶ Occasionally, salt or essential oils may be irritating to moles or skin conditions.

▶ Always check in with your client; be prepared to remove the mixture in a hurry if necessary.

Aromatic Baths with Epsom or Sea Salts

Epsom/sea salt baths are highly effective in aiding and supporting the body in detoxifying, physically and emotionally (Table 9.6). Epsom salts, in particular, enhance the elimination of waste material from the skin and reduce muscular aches and pains by aiding the elimination of uric acid buildup. The use of salts in a bath can support and enhance the body's immune response by stimulating lymph and blood circulation. Sea salt or Epsom salt baths can also be incredibly useful for energetic/emotional cleansing (Figure 9-9).

Recommended essential oil dilution: 5 to 7 drops of essential oils per cup of salt.

IN PRACTICE 9.3

An Aromatic Footbath

Consider offering your clients an aromatic footbath and/or salt scrub prior to the massage or bodywork session (Figure 9-10). Footbaths are a perfect addition before a massage or reflexology session, and they are a great way to introduce your clients to the many benefits of aromatherapy.

Refreshing Aromatic Footbath

1. Fill basin with warm/hot water.
2. Add fresh orange slices to footbath.
3. Add 3 drops of peppermint e/o and 5 drops of orange e/o.
4. Allow client to soak feet for 5 to 10 minutes prior to massage.

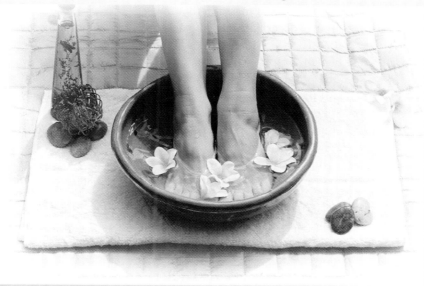

Figure 9-10 A foot soak

Source: © iStockPhoto.com/lovleah

TABLE 9.6

Different Types of Salts in Baths

Type of Salt	Therapeutic Purpose
Epsom Cleansing, detoxifying, flushs toxins, relieves muscular aches and pains, replaces magnesium	To detoxify the system, go for about 3 cups of Epsom salt with 1 tablespoon of white clay and approximately 10 to 20 drops of essential oil in a warmer temperature bath. Consume plenty of water before, during, and after the bath. Rinse in cool water after soaking for 15 to 20 minutes. For localized treatment of sore muscles, add ½ cup Epsom salt to the water used in making a hot or cold compress.
Sea Salt Skin healing, cleans pores, purifying, restores trace minerals	For strong detoxification, use up to 1½ pounds of sea salt or dead sea salt with 10 to 20 drops of essential oil. For general health maintenance or relaxation, use 1 to 2 cups of salt with 10 to 15 drops of essential oil. Soak 15 to 20 minutes in moderately warm water.
Combination Benefits of both	For muscular aches and pains, relaxation, and replacing nutrients, mix equal parts Epsom and sea salts.
*Add 1 tablespoon baking soda if you have "hard water" or itchy skin. Salt baths can be drying, so if this is a problem be sure to rinse off after soaking and use a moisturizing lotion or cream afterward.	

SUMMARY

- Water and salt have been utilized throughout history for their therapeutic benefits for the body, mind, and spirit.
- Hydrotherapy is the use of water in any form (solid, liquid, vapor) for the treatment of a variety of conditions. It is easily integrated into various forms of bodywork and massage therapy.
- Hydrosols are aromatic waters produced from a specified botanical species via the process of distillation. They are valuable additions to a wide range of hydrotherapy applications.
- The physiological effects of hydrotherapy are mechanical, reflexive, chemical, and thermal.
- Specific water temperatures are indicated or contraindicated for a variety of conditions and purposes. It is crucial to know when to use hot and when to use cold applications.
- Aromatic water-based methods of application that can be easily integrated into massage and bodywork include foot and hand baths, steam inhalation, compresses, hot towels, and aromatic spritzers.
- There are many different kinds of salt that can be used in various body spa treatments. Table salt, however, should not be used on the body.
- The traditional salt glow treatment is an effective body treatment for stimulating circulation, removing surface dead skin cells, and revitalizing the skin.
- Aromatic baths with Epsom and/or sea salts are highly effective in reducing muscular aches and pains, detoxifying the body, and enhancing the immune response.

NEW TERMINOLOGY

Aromatic spritzer

Balneotherapy

Contrast therapy

Dispersant

Electrolytes

Haleakala Red

Hard water

Himalayan Pink

Hydrosol

Hydrotherapy

Magnesium

Peng-Tzao-Kan-Mu

Sodium chloride

REFERENCES

Boyd, E.M., and Sheppard, E.P. (1968). The effect of steam inhalation of volatile oils on the output and composition of respiratory tract fluid. *Journal of Pharmacology and Experimental Therapeutics, 163* (1), 250–256.

Catty, S. (2001). *Hydrosols: The Next Aromatherapy*. Rochester, VT: Healing Arts Press.

Essential Wholesale (n/d). Blending Base (Polysorbate 20). Retrieved on December 20, 2006 from http://www.essentialwholesale.com/shop/shopexd.asp?id=225.

Green, J. (2000). *The Herbal Medicine-Maker's Handbook*. Freedom, CA: Crossing Press.

WORKSHEET

Water and Salt (Part I)

Name: _____   Date: _____

Water: Hydrosols and Spritzers

1) Choose your favorite hydrosol covered in this chapter. Then create a 2oz aromatic spritzer using the instructions in this chapter. Based upon your favorite hydrosols (e.g. lavender) use the essential oil of the same (e.g. lavender e/o) to make your spritzer with. Spray some hydrosol into the air and smell/experience the aroma. Then spray the aromatic spritzer you made and smell/experience the aroma. Compare the differences.

Spritzer is: _____

Hydrosol is: _____

Water: Foot Soaks

1) Working with a partner, first determine whether a cold, warm, or contrast foot soak would be most appropriate for them. Ask basic questions to create an aromatherapy blend for their soak.

❑ Cold Therapy

❑ Heat Therapy

❑ Contrast Therapy

Total Essential Oil Blend: _____ *drops*

Essential Oil—Common Name	Essential Oil—*Latin Name*	Drops	Why Chosen?

2) Prepare your water and exchange doing foot soaks with your partner. Remember you can massage their feet a little while they're soaking!

3) Did you enjoy this treatment? How was the temperature?

_____

4) Do you think your clients would enjoy this as part of their sessions with you?

_____

WORKSHEET

Water and Salt (Part II)

A Salt Glow

5) Working with your partner, blend a salt scrub using salt, vegetable oils, and essential oils based on their skin type or personal preferences. Prepare all your materials and supplies. Use the spritzer you made earlier to moisten the skin prior to applying the scrub.

Salt Glow Ingredients

Salt: _____

Vegetable Oils: _____

Essential Oils: _____

Other Ingredients: _____

6) Following the steps provided in this chapter, take turns and exchange aromatic salt glows with your partner.

7) Following the steps provided in this chapter, take turns and exchange aromatic salt glows with your partner. Choose to work with the arms, legs, back, feet or hands.

_____

8) What would you tell a friend or prospective client about this treatment?

_____

9) What would you do differently (if anything) next time?

_____

CHAPTER TEST

1. Hydrosols are the by-product of distillation and do not contain any essential oil.

    _____ True

    _____ False

2. Water accounts for about _____ percent of our total body weight:

    a. 55 percent

    b. 65 percent

    c. 75 percent

    d. 85 percent

3. Which hydrosol has the strongest affinity with the heart?

    a. Roman chamomile

    b. rose

    c. peppermint

    d. German chamomile

4. An unfavorable reaction to hydrotherapy could include:

    a. increased lymphatic flow

    b. enhanced respiratory function

    c. nausea

    d. increased hydration

5. The best salts for soaking muscular aches and pains are:

    a. table salt and sea salt

    b. Epsom salt and Dead Sea salt

    c. table salt and Epsom salt

    d. Dead Sea salt and table salt

6. Use heat therapy for:

    a. a chronic muscle spasm

    b. a recently sprained ankle

    c. clients with severe diabetes

    d. prenatal clients

7. Use cold therapy for:

    a. rheumatic arthritis

    b. recent or acute injury

    c. Raynaud's syndrome

    d. malignant conditions

8. Very hot hydrotherapy would be considered:
    a. 93 to 99°
    b. 100 to 105°
    c. 105 to 110°
    d. 120° and above

9. When using contrast therapy you should:
    a. always end with cold
    b. always end with heat
    c. mix hot and cold together
    d. always include salt

10. It is best to just use table salt for scrubs and soaks.
    _____ True
    _____ False

REVIEW QUESTIONS

1. Discuss how salt and water each play important roles in the body/mind/spirit connection.

2. Discuss how you would best phrase the recommendation of drinking water to your clients.

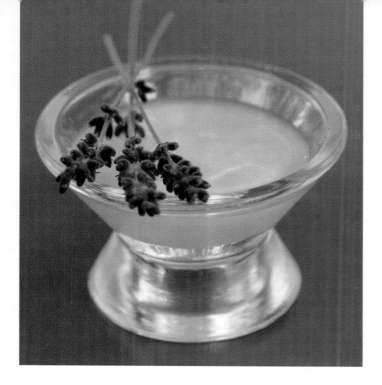

Essential Therapeutics

Enhancing Massage Therapy with Aromatherapy

➔ LEARNING OBJECTIVES

After reading this chapter, you will be able to

1. Identify the characteristics of common complaints/ailments that may affect the seven systems of the body covered in this chapter.

2. List and describe core therapeutic actions essential oils have on the seven systems covered.

3. Describe potential aromatic applications for a variety of ailments for the seven systems covered.

4. Create massage blends for a range of conditions.

5. Identify, set, and reach effective goals for treatment for a wide range of conditions.

6. Identify specific actions of at least five essential oils on the various systems of the body.

7. Know when and how to utilize essential oils in the phases of healing.

INTRODUCTION

> **NOTE**
>
> The common names have been listed in the Essential Oil Therapeutics table for each system. All essential oils listed refer to the specific essential oils covered in this book in the Essential Oil Datasheet section. Please refer to these sheets for correct Latin binomials.

The integration of bodywork and massage therapy techniques with aromatherapy can have profound benefits for clients. Ongoing research and years of practice have shown that massage can reduce or manage pain; increase circulation; increase lymphatic flow in superficial lymphatic capillaries; improve respiratory function; clear mucus in respiratory system; increase the activity of the immune system; reduce stress, anxiety, depression, and much more. Though not intended to suggest massage therapists or bodyworkers should diagnose or prescribe, this chapter covers some of the common conditions a therapist may encounter, as well as therapeutic goals and essential oils that can be incorporated to enhance bodywork or massage techniques, thus helping to increase therapeutic effects.

TABLE 10.1

Essential Oil Therapeutics for the Musculoskeletal System

Therapeutic Action	Essential Oils
Analgesic: a substance that relieves or reduces pain	Black pepper, Birch, Cinnamon leaf, Clove bud, Eucalyptus globulus, Ginger, Lemongrass, Sweet marjoram, Myrrh, Peppermint, Rosemary ct. camphor and cineole
Anti-inflammatory: a substance that soothes and reduces inflammations	German chamomile, Frankincense, Helichrysum, Lavender, Myrrh, Patchouli, Sandalwood
Antirheumatic: a substance that helps to relieve the symptoms of rheumatism	Black pepper, German chamomile, Juniper berry, Lemon, Rosemary ct. camphor, Vetiver
Antispasmodic: a substance that relieves smooth/skeletal muscle spasms	Angelica root, Bay laurel, German chamomile, Roman chamomile, Clary sage, Cypress, Fennel, Ginger, Lavender, Sweet marjoram, Neroli, Peppermint, Petitgrain, Sage
Detoxifier: a substance that enhances the removal of toxic substances from the body	Carrot seed, Cypress, Fennel, Grapefruit, Juniper berry, Lemon
Nervine: a substance that relaxes the nervous system and can reduce nervous disorders	Angelica root, Bergamot, German chamomile, Roman chamomile, Frankincense, Lavender, Mandarin, Sweet marjoram, Melissa, Neroli, Sweet orange, Petitgrain, Rose, Sandalwood, Vetiver, Ylang ylang
Rubefacient: a substance that increases cutaneous blood flow to a local area; causes reddening and warming of the skin	Black pepper, Ginger, Juniper berry, Sweet marjoram, Rosemary ct. camphor, Thyme

MUSCULOSKELETAL HEALTH

Fibromyalgia

The Fibromyalgia Network (n/d) defines the fibromyalgia syndrome (FMS) as a widespread musculoskeletal pain and fatigue disorder for which the cause is still unknown. Fibromyalgia means pain in the muscles, ligaments, and tendons of the soft fibrous tissues in the body. Some symptoms of FMS include chronic pain, fatigue, stiffness, sleeping disorders, headaches, restless leg syndrome, anxiety, and depression. Massage treatments help to reduce stress levels, stiffness, fatigue, and pain resulting in overall improvement in the client's condition (Rattray and Ludwig, 2000) Cold/ice hydrotherapy and deep work are contraindicated as they can exacerbate symptoms or increase pain.

> Grace (2001) recommends a blend of nine essential oils, including ylang ylang complete, Roman chamomile, neroli, bergamot, melissa, black pepper, ravensara, sandalwood, and ginger. She calls this blend "Fibromix." This blend has been successfully used to reduce pain and stress and to increase the ability to sleep.

Therapeutic goals:

▶ reduce pain
▶ reduce stress and/or anxiety
▶ improve quality of sleep
▶ address emotional or physical issues that are either causing the condition or are a reaction to it

Essential Oils

Angelica root, Bergamot, Birch, Black pepper, German chamomile, Roman chamomile, Ginger, Helichrysum, Laurel, Lavender, Mandarin, Sweet marjoram, Neroli, Ravensara, Rose, Rosemary, Sandalwood, Spearmint, Vetiver, Ylang ylang, Arnica and St. John's wort herbal infusion.

Aromatherapy applications:

▶ massage blend with 2.5 to 5 percent dilution
▶ Epsom/sea salt bath
▶ hydrotherapy
▶ diffusion (for emotional aspects)

Spasms or Cramps

Spasms and cramps are both the involuntary contraction of a muscle. The main difference between the two is that spasms tend to be longer lasting but of a lower grade than cramps, which tend to be of short duration yet acute. Massage is indicated for spasms and subacute cramps.

Therapeutic goals:

▶ reduce pain and spasm
▶ enhance detoxification

Essential Oils

Birch, German chamomile, Clary sage, Cypress, Eucalyptus, Fennel, Juniper berry, Lavender, Lemon, Sweet marjoram, Peppermint, Petitgrain, Sage, Spearmint.

Aromatherapy applications:

- ▶ massage blend with 5 percent dilution
- ▶ gel
- ▶ compress

Plantar Fasciitis

Plantar fasciitis is the pain and inflammation caused by injury to the plantar fascia of the foot. Massage is indicated and can help release tension in deep calf muscles that put strain on the plantar fascia.

Therapeutic goals:

- ▶ reduce pain and inflammation
- ▶ improve the thixotropic state or pliability of fascia
- ▶ address emotional states that are either causing the condition or are a reaction to it

Essential Oils

Birch, Cardamom, German chamomile, Roman chamomile, Clary sage, Clove bud, Eucalyptus, Helichrysum, Laurel, Lavender, Sweet marjoram, Peppermint, Rosemary ct. camphor or ct. cineol, Spearmint, Arnica and St. John's wort herbal infusion.

Aromatherapy applications:

- ▶ Epsom salt footbath
- ▶ massage oil or cream with 5 percent dilution
- ▶ hydrotherapy
- ▶ reflexology
- ▶ myofascial release

Whiplash

Whiplash refers to a number of potential injuries to the cervical vertebrae. These injuries include sprained ligaments, strained muscles, misaligned or fractured vertebrae, TMJ problems, and central nervous system damage. Massage is indicated for the subacute stage of whiplash (Werner and Benjamin, 1998).

Therapeutic goals:

- ▶ reduce pain, inflammation, and swelling
- ▶ reduce edema
- ▶ relax muscles and maintain mobility
- ▶ soothe individual from trauma of whiplash

Essential Oils

Birch, Black pepper, Cardamom, German chamomile, Roman chamomile, Clary sage, Clove bud, Cypress, Frankincense, Ginger, Helichrysum, Juniper berry, Laurel, Lavender, Sweet marjoram, Neroli, Peppermint, Petitgrain, Rosemary ct. camphor, Spearmint, Vetiver, Arnica and St. John's wort herbal infusion.

Aromatherapy applications:

- ▸ massage oil with 5 to 10 percent dilution for localized application
- ▸ gel
- ▸ compress
- ▸ hydrotherapy

Sciatica

According to Werner and Benjamin (1998), sciatica is a term used to describe any situation that causes the sciatic nerve to become irritated and inflamed, resulting in pain, numbness, or reduced sensation from the buttocks down to the legs. Massage is indicated for sciatica brought about by muscular or ligamentous forces.

Therapeutic goals:

- ▸ reduce pain and inflammation
- ▸ relax muscles that may be chronically contracted, causing nerve impingement
- ▸ soothe individual emotions that may arise from coping with pain

Essential Oils

Birch, Cardamom, German chamomile, Roman chamomile, Cinnamon leaf, Clary sage, Clove bud, Cypress, Frankincense, Helichrysum, Juniper, Laurel, Lavender, Sweet marjoram, Neroli, Peppermint, Rosemary ct. camphor, Spearmint, Arnica and St. John's wort herbal infusion.

Aromatherapy applications:

- ▸ massage oil with 5 to 10 percent dilution for localized application
- ▸ gel or massage oil with arnica and St. John's wort infusions (20 percent dilution) plus 5 to 10 percent essential oil dilution

Sprains and Strains

Sprains are tears to the ligaments that can cause pain, redness, heat, swelling, and loss of joint function in the acute stage. In the subacute stage of sprains, these symptoms are reduced although pain will be present at all stages. Sprains are considered to be more serious than strains or tendinitis. Strains, on the other hand, are injured muscles resulting in pain, stiffness, and occasionally palpable heat and swelling are present. Massage is indicated for subacute sprains and for muscle strains (Werner and Benjamin, 1998).

Therapeutic goals:

- ▸ reduce pain and inflammation
- ▸ reduce edema
- ▸ maintain local circulation
- ▸ soothe emotions
- ▸ increase range of motion (strains)

Essential Oils

Birch, Black pepper, Cardamom, German chamomile, Roman chamomile, Clove bud, Cypress, Eucalyptus, Grapefruit, Helichrysum, Juniper berry, Laurel, Lavender, Lemon, Lemongrass, Sweet marjoram, Peppermint, Spearmint, Arnica and St. John's wort herbal infusion.

Aromatherapy applications:

▶ compress
▶ RICE technique
▶ lymphatic massage
▶ massage (subacute and maturation phase)
▶ hydrotherapy (cold/warm contrast)

Carpal Tunnel Syndrome or Tendenitis

Carpal tunnel syndrome (CTS) is an irritation of the median nerve in the wrist that can be caused by edema or repetitive movements. CTS can cause pain, tingling, numbness, and weakness in part of the hand (Werner and Benjamin, 1998). Horrigan (2004) reports that "aromatherapy can help reduce compression by passive exercises and massage with essential oils aimed at fluid reduction" (p. 117).

Therapeutic goals:

▶ reduce pain
▶ reduce edema
▶ support range of motion
▶ address emotional states that are either causing the condition or are a reaction to it

Essential Oils

Birch, Black pepper, Cardamom, Clary sage, Clove bud, Cypress, Eucalyptus, Fennel, Geranium, Helichrysum, Juniper berry, Laurel, Lavender, Lemon, Peppermint, Rosemary ct. camphor or ct. cineole, Arnica and St. John's wort herbal infusion.

Aromatherapy applications:

▶ massage oil with 5 to 10 percent dilution
▶ gel or cream
▶ hand/wrist baths

Bursitis

Bursitis is an inflammation of the bursae and is commonly called by such names as "housemaid's knee and student's elbow." Bursitis involves inflammation, excess fluid, pain, and reduced mobility of the area involved. Massage is recommended during the subacute phase and for the rest of the body during the acute phase (Werner and Benjamin, 1998). According to Horrigan (2004), "aromatherapy aims at natural drainage and return to normal function by massage with analgesic and diuretic essential oils with gradual, passive movement of the joint through full range, until it is returned to its original ability" (p. 116).

IN PRACTICE

Case Study 10.1

Carpal Tunnel Syndrome

M. is thirty-three years old and a successful tattoo artist. He decided to visit an aromatherapy massage practitioner, upon referral from a friend, to address chronic pain in his wrists caused by the repetitive motions of tattooing. He also complained of chronic lower back pain from leaning over to tattoo. M. considers himself to be in good health and good physical condition. He did mention feeling stressed due to ongoing relationship difficulties, which may be adding to his back stiffness and pain.

Massage Blend: 1oz, bottle, 5 percent dilution

Arnica herbal oil 10 percent

St. John's wort herbal oil 10 percent

Apricot kernel 80 percent

Peppermint (*Mentha* x *piperita*) to reduce pain and increase range of motion: 4 drops

Lemon (*Citrus limon*) to reduce edema: 8 drops

Juniper berry (*Juniperus communis*) to reduce pain and edema: 7 drops

Lavender (*Lavandula angustifolia*) to reduce pain and relieve stress: 11 drops

Gel for Pain Relief to Be Used at Home: 2oz, 5 percent dilution

Aloe vera concentrated gel blended with lavender hydrosol. All essential oils have been chosen for their ability to relieve pain.

Peppermint (*Mentha* x *piperita*): 11 drops

Bay laurel (*Laurus nobilis*): 14 drops

Birch (*Betula lenta*): 8 drops

Lavender (*Lavandula angustifolia*): 27 drops

M. received localized massage work on the hands, wrists, arms, and back two times a month for four months. He reported a decrease in the pain in his wrists and lower back after two sessions. M. is committed to having one massage per month. He also reported using the gel at home on a regular basis and is pleased with the results. He has made a ritual of using the gel each night when he comes home from work and reports feeling less stressed and less pain in his back and wrists.

Therapeutic goals:

▶ reduce pain and inflammation
▶ reduce edema
▶ increase mobility

Essential Oils

Birch, Cardamom, German chamomile, Cypress, Eucalyptus, Grapefruit, Helichrysum, Juniper berry, Lavender, Lemon, Peppermint, Rosemary ct. camphor, Arnica and St. John's wort herbal infusion.

Aromatherapy applications:

▶ massage oil with 5 to 10 percent dilution
▶ gel
▶ compress (warm)
▶ hydrotherapy

Osteoarthritis

Osteoarthritis is joint inflammation brought on by the cumulative wear and tear that occurs throughout an individual's lifetime. Joints that are affected by osteoarthritis are stiff, painful, and potentially inflamed. It is a condition most commonly affecting the knees, hips, and fingers. Massage is indicated in the subacute phase.

Therapeutic goals:

- reduce inflammation and pain
- relax muscles
- increase mobility
- address emotional states that are either causing the condition or are a reaction to it

Essential Oils

Birch, German chamomile, Clove bud, Cypress, Eucalyptus, Grapefruit, Helichrysum, Juniper berry, Laurel, Lavender, Lemon, Sweet marjoram, Palmarosa, Peppermint, Rosemary ct camphor, Spearmint.

Aromatherapy applications:

- massage oil with 5 to 10 percent dilution
- gel
- compress
- hydrotherapy

Rheumatoid Arthritis

Rheumatoid arthritis is an inflammatory, destructive, chronic, autoimmune disease of multiple joints and connective tissue throughout the body. It often starts in the hands and wrists. The condition causes the affected joints to be hot, puffy, and swollen, and range of motion is reduced due to pain and stiffness (Rattray and Ludwig, 2000). Massage is recommended during the subacute stages to reestablish mobility and to reduce stress that could trigger another flare-up of symptoms.

Therapeutic goals:

- reduce pain and inflammation
- reduce stress
- maintain and/or increase mobility
- address emotional states that are either causing the condition or are a reaction to it

Essential Oils

Birch, Black pepper, German chamomile, Clove bud, Cypress, Eucalyptus, Frankincense, Ginger, Grapefruit, Helichrysum, Juniper berry, Laurel, Lavender, Lemon, Sweet marjoram, Palmarosa, Peppermint, Rose, Rosemary ct. camphor, Spearmint, Thyme, Vetiver, Ylang ylang.

Aromatherapy applications:

- ▶ massage oil with 5 to 10 percent dilution
- ▶ gel
- ▶ hydrotherapy

Temporomandibular Joint Disorder

Temporomandibular joint disorder (TMJ) refers to a multitude of problems in and around the jaw resulting from constant strain, stress, and malocclusion of the jaw. Symptoms of TMJ include head, neck, and shoulder pain, ear pain, mouth pain, clicking or locking in the jaw, and loss of range of motion in the jaw (Werner and Benjamin, 1998). Massage is recommended for TMJ.

Therapeutic goals:

- ▶ reduce pain and inflammation
- ▶ reduce stress
- ▶ maintain and/or increase range of motion
- ▶ address emotional states that are either causing the condition or are a reaction to it

Essential Oils

Bergamot, Birch, Black pepper, German chamomile, Roman chamomile, Clove bud, Eucalyptus, Frankincense, Ginger, Helichrysum, Juniper berry, Laurel, Lavender, Lemon, Mandarin, Neroli, Peppermint, Rose, Rosemary ct. camphor, Spearmint, Vetiver, Ylang ylang.

Aromatherapy applications:

- ▶ massage oil with 5 to 10 percent dilution
- ▶ gel or cream
- ▶ compress

↳ NERVOUS SYSTEM HEALTH

Multiple Sclerosis

Multiple sclerosis (MS) is a condition in which demyelination of the nerves occurs. MS begins with an inflammatory process, followed by the loss of myelin that surrounds the nerve axons. Symptoms of MS vary from person to person but may include fatigue, muscle spasms and weakness, numbness, tingling or burning sensations, cold extremities, sweating abnormalities, mood swings, and a host of others. MS is a chronic degenerative disease accompanied by remission periods and acute attacks (Rattray and Ludwig, 2000). Massage is indicated during the subacute or remission periods. Caution is expressed when using heat, which could exacerbate symptoms.

TABLE 10.2

Essential Oil Therapeutics for the Nervous System

Therapeutic Action	Essential Oils
Analgesic: a substance that relieves or reduces pain	Black pepper, Birch, Cinnamon leaf, Clove bud, Eucalyptus globulus, Ginger, Lemongrass, Sweet marjoram, Myrrh, Peppermint, Rosemary ct. camphor and cineole
Antidepressant: a substance that relieves depression	Bergamot, Clary sage, Grapefruit, Jasmine, Mandarin, Melissa, Neroli, Orange, Patchouli, Petitgrain, Rose, Ylang ylang
Anti-inflammatory: a substance that soothes and reduces inflammations	German chamomile, Frankincense, Helichrysum, Lavender, Myrrh, Patchouli, Sandalwood
Antispasmodic: a substance that relieves smooth/skeletal muscle spasms	Angelica root, Bay laurel, German chamomile, Roman chamomile, Clary sage, Cypress, Fennel, Ginger, Lavender, Sweet marjoram, Neroli, Peppermint, Petitgrain, Sage
Nervine: a substance that relaxes the nervous system and can reduce nervous disorders	Angelica root, Bergamot, German chamomile, Roman chamomile, Frankincense, Lavender, Mandarin, Sweet marjoram, Melissa, Neroli, Sweet orange, Petitgrain, Rose, Sandalwood, Vetiver, Ylang ylang
Sedative: a substance that has a calming effect, relieving anxiety, tension, insomnia	German chamomile, Roman chamomile, Lavender, Sweet marjoram, Melissa

Therapeutic goals:

▶ reduce spasticity
▶ maintain range of motion
▶ provide emotional support
▶ encourage relaxation, reduce stress

Essential Oils

Bergamot, Birch, Cardamom, Roman chamomile, German chamomile, Clary sage, Clove bud, Eucalyptus, Frankincense, Grapefruit, Helichrysum, Juniper berry, Laurel, Lavender, Lemon, Melissa, Neroli, Palmarosa, Peppermint, Petitgrain, Pine, Ravensara, Rose, Rosemary ct. camphor or ct. cineole, Sandalwood, Spearmint, Vetiver, Ylang ylang.

Aromatherapy applications:

▶ massage with 2.5 to 5 percent dilution
▶ hydrotherapy (temperature based on client needs)
▶ reflexology

Headaches/Migraines

Headaches are a common problem and are typically caused by muscular tension, bone misalignment, TMJ disorders, or other muscular problems. Massage is indicated for such tension headaches. Rarely, a headache may indicate a more serious underlying pathology. Massage is contraindicated when headache is accompanied by fever, infection, or Central Nervous System disturbances (Werner and Benjamin,

1998). According to the AMTA (2005), individuals suffering with headaches have found that therapeutic massage has lessened or relieved the condition.

Migraines, on the other hand, are considered to be more severe than simple tension headaches. A migraine begins with extreme vasoconstriction in the affected hemisphere, which can leave the individual feeling euphoric for a short time. This is followed by a huge vasodilation into the same hemisphere. This incredible increase of blood flow causes excess pressure against the meninges, which then causes the excruciating pain (Werner and Benjamin, 1998). Typically a migraine sufferer will have feelings of nausea, extreme sensitivity to light and heat, and may have blurred vision. The causes of a migraine are numerous and may include hormonal imbalances, food allergies, extreme stress/tension, and alcohol. Massage is typically contraindicated during the acute stage of a migraine. Massage can be used in the subacute stage or for preventative care for individuals who suffer with recurring migraines.

Therapeutic goals:

- ▶ reduce pain
- ▶ reduce stress

Essential Oils

Bergamot, Roman chamomile, Grapefruit, Ginger, Lavender, Lemon, Neroli, Sweet orange, Peppermint.

Aromatherapy applications:

- ▶ scalp massage (for headaches or migraines)
- ▶ gel (to be applied on temples and neck)
- ▶ baths (to reduce stress, for headaches only)
- ▶ full-body massage (for headaches only)
- ▶ cold compress (for migraines)

Anxiety

The National Institute of Mental Health (2001) defines a generalized anxiety disorder (GAD) as constant, exaggerated, worrisome thoughts and tension about everyday routine life events and activities, lasting at least six months. Individuals suffering with GAD are almost always anticipating the worst, even though there is little reason to expect it; it is accompanied by physical symptoms, such as fatigue, trembling, insomnia, muscle tension, headache, or nausea.

Therapeutic goals:

- ▶ provide emotional support
- ▶ encourage relaxation, reduce stress
- ▶ reduce muscle tension

Essential Oils

Angelica root, Bergamot, Cardamom, Cedarwood, Roman chamomile, German chamomile, Clary sage, Frankincense, Geranium, Ginger, Grapefruit, Jasmine, Lavender, Lemon, Mandarin, Melissa, Myrrh, Neroli, Peppermint, Petitgrain, Pine, Rose, Sandalwood, Vetiver, Ylang ylang.

IN PRACTICE

Case Study 10.2

Anxiety

B. is a fifty-three-year-old woman, vibrant and healthy. She leads a healthy lifestyle that includes exercise three times a week, a well-balanced diet, dietary supplements, and annual medical checkups. She seems satisfied with those aspects of her life. Her professional life, however, is a bit challenging. She works for herself as a life coach, a job that fulfills her but causes her stress. After the events of September 11, B. experienced a significant drop in client numbers. This, coupled with the effects of a sluggish economy on her investments, has left B. feeling very anxious. She's very worried about her finances.

This past summer, B.'s anxiety seems to have escalated to such levels that she started experiencing anxiety attacks. Her symptoms consisted of shortness of breath, pressure on her chest, and rapid heartbeat. She visited the doctor who could not find anything physically wrong with her. She then contacted me in hopes that massage and aromatherapy would be able to relieve her anxiety She believes that investing in her health is a good investment.

My aim was to provide a full-body general relaxation massage coupled with the use of relaxing, calming, and comforting essential oils.

Massage Blend: 1oz., 2.5 percent dilution

Jojoba, 25 percent

Sunflower, 25 percent

Apricot kernel, 50 percent

Sandalwood (*Santalum spicatum*): calming, centering, inner awareness: 4 drops

Rose (*Rosa damascena*): nurturing, comforting: 2 drops

Tangerine (*Citrus reticulata*): uplifting, comforting: 7 drops

Vetiver (*Vetiveria zizanioides*): grounding, strengthening: 2 drops

Synergy for Home Use:

Lavender (*Lavandula angustifolia*): calming, soothing: 20 drops

Vetiver (*Vetiveria zizanioides*): grounding, strengthening: 5 drops

Tangerine (*Citrus reticulata*): uplifting, comforting: 18 drops

Rose geranium (*Pelargonium graveolens* var. *roseum*): balancing: 7 drops

B. absolutely loved the aromatic massage and commented on feeling very relaxed and ready for a good night's sleep. B. made a point to have a massage at least once every four to six weeks. She used her home synergy regularly between massage appointments and feels that it helps tremendously with reducing the severity of her anxiety attacks, if not preventing them all together. She is feeling more centered within herself and feels confident in the future.

Aromatherapy applications:

▶ massage with 2.5 to 5 percent dilution

▶ hydrotherapy (temperature based on client needs)

Neuralgia

Neuralgia or nerve pain is usually a sign or symptom of some other nervous system disorder or condition in which pain travels along a sensory peripheral nerve path. A most common neuralgia is trigeminal neuralgia that involves cranial nerve five and produces sharp, severe pain or burning sensations. Other common neuralgias include a version that is a complication of the herpes zoster infection or neuralgia as a symptom of nerve inflammation caused by herniated discs or other structural impingement. Massage is locally contraindicated during an acute episode, but is otherwise appropriate within the client's comfort zone. Ice or cold therapy is recommended to reduce inflammation and numb the area to reduce pain.

Therapeutic goals:

- ▶ reduce pain
- ▶ reduce inflammation
- ▶ encourage relaxation

Essential Oils

Birch, German chamomile, Cinnamon leaf, Clove bud, Laurel, Lavender, Lemongrass, Eucalyptus, Sweet Sweet marjoram, Melissa, Neroli, Palmarosa, Pine, Ravensara, Spearmint, Vetiver.

Aromatherapy applications:

- ▶ massage with 2.5 to 5 percent dilution
- ▶ hydrotherapy (usually cold)

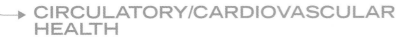

CIRCULATORY/CARDIOVASCULAR HEALTH

	TABLE 10.3
Essential Oil Therapeutics for the Circulatory System	

Therapeutic Action	Essential Oils
Astringent: a substance that causes cells to shrink; contracts, tightens, and binds tissues	Cedarwood, Cypress, Geranium, Lemon, Patchouli, Rose
Anti-inflammatory: a substance that soothes and reduces inflammations	German chamomile, Frankincense, Helichrysum, Lavender, Myrrh, Patchouli, Sandalwood
Circulatory Stimulant: a substance that enhances or increases blood circulation	Carrot seed, Black pepper, Juniper berry, Laurel, Lemon, Lemongrass, Scots pine, Rosemary ct. camphor or cineole
Detoxifier: a substance that enhances the removal of toxic substances from the body	Carrot seed, Cypress, Fennel, Grapefruit, Juniper berry, Lemon
Hypertensive: a substance that raises blood pressure	Black pepper, Rosemary ct. camphor or cineole, Thyme ct. thymol
Hypotensive: a substance that lowers blood pressure	German chamomile, Lavender, Sweet marjoram, Neroli, Ylang ylang
Nervine: a substance that relaxes the nervous system and can reduce nervous disorders	Angelica root, Bergamot, German chamomile, Roman chamomile, Frankincense, Lavender, Mandarin, Sweet marjoram, Melissa, Neroli, Sweet orange, Petitgrain, Rose, Sandalwood, Vetiver, Ylang ylang

Raynaud's Syndrome

Raynaud's syndrome is defined by episodes of vasospasm of the arterioles, usually in the fingers and toes. The blood vessels in the extremities experience a spasm of smooth muscle tissue that makes the skin appear white to blue. Massage is indicated for Raynaud's syndrome when it is not associated with any other underlying pathology (Werner and Benjamin, 1998). Horrigan (2005) says "regular, gentle massages in a warm environment with warmed oils are so beneficial as to be almost essential as part of the care protocol."

Therapeutic goals:

▶ reduce spasm
▶ enhance circulation
▶ provide warmth

Essential Oils

Black pepper, Cardamom, Cinnamon leaf, Clary sage, Eucalyptus, Fennel, Juniper berry, Laurel, Lemon, Peppermint, Petitgrain, Rosemary ct. camphor or ct. cineol.

Aromatherapy applications:

▶ massage with 2.5 to 5 percent dilution
▶ hydrotherapy (temperature based on client needs)
▶ reflexology

Varicose Veins

Varicose veins are distended or dilated veins commonly found in the legs. They are caused by the impaired function of the venous valves (Rattray and Ludwig, 2000). Massage is locally contraindicated for extreme varicose veins and anywhere distal to

IN PRACTICE

Case Study 10.3

Poor Circulation

J. is a forty-five-year-old manager at a local natural foods store. She has been familiar with the benefits of aromatherapy and came to see if aromatherapy and massage could be of benefit to poor circulation in her hands and feet. She spends much of her day sitting at a desk but says she also works out two or three times a week. She is quite happy with her job and home life and has a healthy diet.

Massage Blend: 1oz., 3 percent dilution
Apricot kernel, 100 percent
Rosemary (*Rosmarinus officinalis*): stimulate circulation: 5 drops

Black pepper (*Piper nigrum*): warming, stimulate circulation: 6 drops

Lemon (*Citrus limon*): detoxing, stimulating: 7 drops

J. scheduled a regular massage appointment for once a month. I saw her over a period of three months before she began to see results. J. commented that at first she was not sure this was going to help but after three months of regular massage and aromatherapy treatments she was feeling a great improvement in her circulation. She plans on continuing her massage appointments and looks forward to trying new aromatherapy blends.

them. Mild varicose veins contraindicate deep, specific work, but are otherwise safe for massage (Werner and Benjamin, 1998).

Therapeutic goals:

▷ enhance circulation
▷ prevent varicose veins from getting worse
▷ reduce pain

Essential Oils

Cedarwood, German chamomile, Cypress, Frankincense, Geranium, Helichrysum, Lavender, Lemon, Lemongrass, Patchouli, Peppermint, Sandalwood, Vetiver.

Aromatherapy applications:

▷ gel
▷ light massage for mild varicose veins
▷ compress: cold/warm

Hypertension

Hypertension is the elevation of blood pressure above the normal range for a prolonged period of time (Rattray and Ludwig, 2000). According to Werner and Benjamin (1998), massage for borderline or mild high blood pressure may be useful to control stress and increase general health. Massage for high blood pressure due to underlying pathologies is contraindicated.

Therapeutic goals:

▷ reduce stress
▷ improve general health and wellness

Essential Oils

Angelica root, Bergamot, Roman chamomile, German chamomile, Clary sage, Frankincense, Geranium, Grapefruit, Lavender, Mandarin, Sweet marjoram, Neroli, Sweet orange, Patchouli, Petitgrain, Sandalwood, Vetiver, Ylang ylang.

Aromatherapy applications:

▷ massage with 2.5 to 5 percent dilution

Hypotension

While most people are concerned with hypertension or high blood pressure, hypotension refers to low blood pressure and is usually considered to be a systolic blood pressure below 100 mm Hg. In most cases, low blood pressure isn't much cause for concern and usually reflects a well-conditioned body. Occasionally there are other health factors to consider, such as age, pregnancy, medications, or poor circulation. When working with clients who report having low blood pressure, therapists should use care and help clients sit up off the table or recommend they get up slowly after treatment.

Therapeutic goals:

- ▶ enhance circulation
- ▶ improve muscle tone
- ▶ encourage relaxation, relieve exhaustion

Essential Oils

Black pepper, Grapefruit, Ginger, Juniper, Palmarosa, Peppermint, Rosemary, Spearmint, Thyme.

Aromatherapy applications:

- ▶ massage with 2.5 to 5 percent dilution

LYMPH AND IMMUNE HEALTH

Edema

Edema is the accumulation of fluid between cells and is sometimes associated with inflammation or poor circulation. In either case, the stagnant fluid needs to be pulled into the lymphatic capillaries and processed by the lymph system. Massage is indicated when the edema is related to a subacute musculoskeletal injury, bed confinement, or partial immobility (Werner and Benjamin, 1998). Horrigan (2005) reports that edema and lymphatic congestion can be successfully treated with essential oils and the use of lymphatic drainage massage or manual lymphatic drainage.

Therapeutic goals:

- ▶ increase circulation
- ▶ aid fluid movement or detoxification

Essential Oils

Black pepper, Carrot seed, Cypress, Fennel, Grapefruit, Geranium, Juniper berry, Laurel, Lemon, Lemongrass, Patchouli, Peppermint, Pine, Rosemary ct. camphor.

TABLE 10.4

Essential Oil Therapeutics for the Lymphatic/Immune System

Therapeutic Action	Essential Oils
Anti-inflammatory: a substance that soothes and reduces inflammations	German chamomile, Frankincense, Helichrysum, Lavender, Myrrh, Patchouli, Sandalwood
Circulatory Stimulant: a substance that enhances or increases blood circulation	Carrot seed, Black pepper, Juniper berry, Laurel, Lemon, Lemongrass, Scots pine, Rosemary ct. camphor or cineole
Detoxifier: a substance that enhances the removal of toxic substances from the body	Carrot seed, Cypress, Fennel, Grapefruit, Juniper berry, Lemon
Immune Enhancer: a substance that enhances immunity, either by stimulating the immune system or by destroying microbes	Frankincense, Bay laurel, Lemon, Niaouli, Ravensara, Tea tree, Thyme

IN PRACTICE

Case Study 10.4

Edema

R. is a forty-five-year-old nurse who works four twelve-hour shifts a week at a local hospital. She has been a nurse for sixteen years. She complains of edema in her legs and feet. She also has chronic pain in her feet. R. has never had massage but is hoping it helps her to feel better.

We began our session together with the following:

Footbath

Juniper berry (*Juniperus communis*): detoxing: 2 drops

Rosemary (*Rosmarinus officinalis* ct. camphor): circulatory tonic: 3 drops

Lemon (*Citrus limon*): enhance detoxing, elimination: 3 drops

R. soaked her feet in a warm-water aromatic footbath for approximately ten minutes. After drying her feet, we moved into the massage room. She received a full-body massage treatment with some manual lymphatic drainage techniques.

The following aromatic blend was used for the massage:

Apricot kernel oil, 50 percent

Organic sunflower oil, 50 percent

Juniper berry (*Juniperus communis*): detoxing: 6 drops

Grapefruit (*Citrus paradisi*): detoxing: 8 drops

Bay laurel (*Laurus nobilis*): increases lymphatic circulation: 4 drops

Foot Cream for Home Use

Peppermint (*Mentha × piperita*): analgesic, soothing: 7 drops

Lavender (*Lavandula angustifolia*): soothing: 10 drops

2 oz. cream

Directions for use: Apply each night to feet and ankles.

I worked with R. for four months, one or two massages a month. R. was delighted with the results. She experienced some reduction in the edema in her legs and feet but mostly she loved the foot cream that she says "makes her feel like dancing." She also remarked that her body feels much better, not so tight and achy. We have decided to begin some reflexology sessions along with aromatherapy to further address her sore feet.

Aromatherapy applications:

- ▶ massage with 2.5 to 5 percent dilution
- ▶ manual lymphatic massage
- ▶ sea salt baths
- ▶ dry brushing
- ▶ reflexology

Infections and Immunity

Massage is contraindicated with a systemic infection, if a fever is present, or if edema is present due to a localized infection. Once the client has sufficiently recovered, massage and aromatherapy can help encourage the rebuilding of a strong, healthy immune system.

Therapeutic goals:

- ▶ support the body's natural ability to heal
- ▶ enhance function of the immune system

    ▸ Aid fluid movement or detoxification

    ▸ Introduce antimicrobial substance to help rid the body of unwanted bacteria or viruses

Essential Oils

Cinnamon leaf, Eucalyptus, Geranium, Grapefruit, Juniper berry, Laurel, Lavender, Lemon, Lemongrass, Niaouli, Ravensara, Rosemary, Tea tree, Thyme.

Aromatherapy applications:

    ▸ massage with 2.5 to 5 percent dilution

    ▸ localized (spot) application in high dilution, 5 to 10 percent

    ▸ Epsom and sea salt baths

    ▸ dry brushing

    ▸ compress (warm or cool)

    ▸ diffuser or aromatic spritzer for cleaning the air/environment

Cellulite

According to Cellulite.com (n/d), cellulite results from adipose tissue (fat) in the uppermost layers projecting into the dermis and causing bumps, "dimples," and pitting. It is believed to result from the destruction of collagen associated with fatty tissue as well as altered blood and lymph circulation resulting in a buildup of toxic elements. Women are more prone to have cellulite than men due to the differences in fatty tissue makeup.

Therapeutic goals:

    ▸ support and enhance lymphatic circulation

    ▸ aid detoxification

Essential Oils

Cypress, Eucalyptus, Ginger, Grapefruit, Juniper berry, Lemon, Lemongrass, Myrrh, Neroli, Patchouli, Rosemary ct. camphor or cineole.

Aromatherapy applications:

    ▸ massage with 2.5 to 5 percent dilution

    ▸ Epsom and sea salt baths

    ▸ dry brushing

↪ REPRODUCTIVE HEALTH

Dysmenorrhea

Dysmenorrhea is the technical term for menstrual pain that is severe enough to interfere with and limit the activities of women of childbearing age. Massage is indicated unless underlying pathology indicates otherwise or during heavy menstrual flow (Werner and Benjamin, 1998).

	TABLE 10.5

Essential Oil Therapeutics for the Reproductive System

Therapeutic Action	Essential Oils
Analgesic: a substance that relieves or reduces pain	Black pepper, Birch, Cinnamon leaf, Clove bud, Eucalyptus globulus, Ginger, Lemongrass, Sweet marjoram, Myrrh, Peppermint, Rosemary ct. camphor and cineole
Antidepressant: a substance that relieves depression	Bergamot, Clary sage, Grapefruit, Jasmine, Mandarin, Melissa, Neroli, Orange, Patchouli, Petitgrain, Rose, Ylang ylang
Antispasmodic: a substance that relieves smooth/skeletal muscle spasms	Angelica root, Bay laurel, German chamomile, Roman chamomile, Clary sage, Cypress, Fennel, Ginger, Lavender, Sweet marjoram, Neroli, Peppermint, Petitgrain, Sage
Aphrodisiac: a substance that increases sexual stimulation and excitement	Cardamom, Cinnamon leaf, Clary sage, Ginger, Jasmine, Ylang ylang
Hormonal Balancer: a substance that helps balance the endocrine system	Clary sage, Geranium, Lavender, Rose, Sage
Nervine: a substance that relaxes the nervous system and can reduce nervous disorders	Angelica root, Bergamot, German chamomile, Roman chamomile, Frankincense, Lavender, Mandarin, Sweet marjoram, Melissa, Neroli, Sweet orange, Petitgrain, Rose, Sandalwood, Vetiver, Ylang ylang
Sedative: a substance that has a calming effect, relieving anxiety, tension, insomnia	German chamomile, Roman chamomile, Lavender, Sweet marjoram, Melissa

Therapeutic goals:

▶ reduce pain
▶ soothe emotions
▶ balance hormones

Essential Oils

Angelica root, Birch, Black pepper, Roman chamomile, Cinnamon leaf, Clary sage, Fennel, Frankincense, Geranium, Ginger, Helichrysum, Lavender, Sweet marjoram, Mandarin, Neroli, Sweet orange, Patchouli, Peppermint, Spearmint, Vetiver, Ylang ylang.

Aromatherapy applications:

▶ massage with 2.5 to 5 percent dilution
▶ compress
▶ hydrotherapy

Amenorrhea

Amenorrhea is a condition in which there is an absence or cessation of menstruation. Stress is one of the most common causes of amenorrhea. Other causes may include a disorder of the hypothalamus, pituitary or thyroid gland deficiency, stress, excessive exercise, deficiency of ovarian hormone, anorexia nervosa, and removal of the womb or ovaries.

Therapeutic goals:

- ▶ reduce stress, soothe emotions
- ▶ balance hormones
- ▶ address individual emotional issues that are either causing the condition or are a reaction to it

Essential Oils

Angelica root, Bergamot, Roman chamomile, Clary sage, Fennel, Geranium, Jasmine, Lavender, Sweet marjoram, Mandarin, Neroli, Sweet orange, Patchouli, Vetiver, Ylang ylang.

Aromatherapy applications:

- ▶ massage with 2.5 to 5 percent dilution
- ▶ inhalations/Diffusion
- ▶ hydrotherapy

Premenstrual Syndrome

Premenstrual syndrome (PMS) is a multifaceted disorder that women all over the world suffer. Symptoms can include swelling of breasts, water retention, bloating, aches and pains, nervousness, irritability, emotional disturbances, headaches, depression, fatigue, tension, anxiety, loss of concentration, etc. The symptoms experienced vary so much from individual to individual that it is very important to have a clear understanding of each case presented.

Therapeutic goals:

- ▶ reduce water retention and bloating
- ▶ relieve cramping
- ▶ balance hormones
- ▶ reduce stress and/or anxiety

Essential Oils

Angelica root, Bergamot, Black pepper, Cardamom, Roman chamomile, Clary sage, Fennel, Frankincense, Geranium, Ginger, Helichrysum, Jasmine, Juniper berry, Laurel, Lavender, Sweet marjoram, Mandarin, Melissa, Neroli, Sweet orange, Patchouli, Peppermint, Petitgrain, Spearmint, Vetiver, Ylang ylang.

Aromatherapy applications:

- ▶ massage with 2.5 to 5 percent dilution
- ▶ compress
- ▶ hydrotherapy

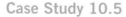

IN PRACTICE

Case Study 10.5

Premenstrual Syndrome

S. is a twenty-nine-year-old woman who has come in for an aromatherapy massage to relieve stress and potentially address hormonal issues. S. gets very irritable seven or eight days before her period. She becomes very emotional and has zero tolerance for friends and family and is easily angered or frustrated. She also notices a change in her sleep pattern at this time as well. Once her period arrives, she has uncomfortable cramping. Her period is regular.

Massage Blend: 2 oz, bottle, 3 percent dilution

Apricot kernel, 100%

Geranium (*Pelargonium graveolens*): balancing: 6 drops

Clary sage (*Salvia sclarea*): antispasmodic, balancing: 6 drops

Bergamot (*Citrus bergamia*): stress relieving, soothing: 10 drops

Lavender (*Lavandula angustifolia*): soothe frustration and anger: 14 drops

Full-body massage

S. loved the massage and the aromatherapy. She commented that she felt much more relaxed and would like to continue using the blend at home. She took the remaining blend home. I encouraged her to use the blend five days prior to menstruation and then as needed throughout her period. S. continued to receive massage once a month. After five months she remarked that frustration and irritability had not been an issue for two months, and her period was no longer causing such painful cramping. She also bought some lavender to use in baths and feels this helps her to sleep better at night.

Infertility

The inability of a couple to become pregnant is referred to as infertility. The causes of infertility are vast and varied; sometimes due to weak or low sperm counts in the male or a woman's body not ovulating or rejecting the sperm, waiting until later in life to start a family, or it can even just be a case of poor timing. In any event, couples struggling with infertility issues usually also have a lot of stress and anxiety around the situation and conventional treatments. Because of this, they may end up on your treatment table.

Therapeutic goals:

▶ balance hormones
▶ reduce stress and/or anxiety surrounding or causing the condition
▶ unconditional comfort and support

Essential Oils

Bergamot, Cardamom, Roman chamomile, Clary sage, Cypress, Fennel, Geranium, Jasmine, Melissa, Neroli, Rose.

Aromatherapy applications:

▶ massage with 2.5 to 5 percent dilution
▶ full-body baths
▶ compress
▶ hydrotherapy

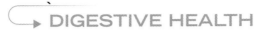

DIGESTIVE HEALTH

Constipation

Constipation is the slow, difficult, or infrequent movement of feces through the bowel. The causes of constipation are numerous and range from lifestyle factors, such as poor diet, stress, and postural imbalances, to physiological factors, such as medication side effects, gastrointestinal conditions, and poor muscle control (Rattray and Ludwig, 2000). Massage is indicated unless a medical condition, such as bowel obstruction or inflammatory bowel disease, contraindicates it.

Therapeutic goals:

▶ reduce stress
▶ decrease pain
▶ aid elimination

Essential Oils

Angelica root, Cardamom, Carrot seed, Black pepper, Clary sage, Fennel, Ginger, Grapefruit, Juniper berry, Lavender, Mandarin, Sweet orange, Peppermint, Petitgrain, Spearmint.

Aromatherapy applications:

▶ massage with 5 percent dilution
▶ abdominal compress

TABLE 10.6

Essential Oil Therapeutics for the Digestive System

Therapeutic Action	Essential Oils
Analgesic: a substance that relieves or reduces pain	Black pepper, Birch, Cinnamon leaf, Clove bud, Eucalyptus globulus, Ginger, Lemongrass, Sweet marjoram, Myrrh, Peppermint, Rosemary ct. camphor and cineole
Antispasmodic: a substance that relieves smooth/skeletal muscle spasms	Angelica root, Bay laurel, German chamomile, Roman chamomile, Clary sage, Cypress, Fennel, Ginger, Lavender, Sweet marjoram, Neroli, Peppermint, Petitgrain, Sage
Carminative: a substance that relieves flatulence or excess gas in stomach	Black pepper, Cardamom, Carrot seed, Clove bud, Fennel, Ginger, Peppermint, Spearmint
Detoxifier: a substance that enhances the removal of toxic substances from the body	Carrot seed, Cypress, Fennel, Grapefruit, Juniper berry, Lemon
Digestive: a substance that aids digestion, serves as a tonic to digestive system	Angelica root, Black pepper, Cardamom, Carrot seed, Fennel, Lemon
Nervine: a substancethat relaxes the nervous system and can reduce nervous disorders	Angelica root, Bergamot, German chamomile, Roman chamomile, Frankincense, Lavender, Mandarin, Sweet marjoram, Melissa, Neroli, Sweet orange, Petitgrain, Rose, Sandalwood, Vetiver, Ylang ylang

IN PRACTICE

Case Study 10.6

Constipation and Stress

K. is a thirty-eight-year-old business owner who has been experiencing bouts of constipation and high levels of stress from her work. She is currently looking to change her diet and to drink more water. She would like to have an aromatherapy massage that addresses her constipation and stress levels.

Massage Blend: 1oz. bottle, 3 percent dilution

Apricot kernel, 100%

Sweet fennel (*Foeniculum vulgare*): digestive tonic: 3 drops

Cardamom (*Elettaria cardamomum*): digestive tonic: 4 drops

Lemon (*Citrus limon*): cleansing, supportive: 4 drops

Lavender (*Lavandula angustifolia*): stress relief: 7 drops

Full-body massage

K. felt much better after the initial massage session. She called three days after her appointment to remark that not only did she feel much calmer but she had experienced regular bowel movements. She would like to continue the massage and aromatherapy sessions.

▶ reflexology
▶ hydrotherapy

Irritable Bowel Syndrome

Irritable bowel syndrome (IBS) is a common condition of the digestive system that is often attributed to prolonged anxiety or stress-related states. It can also be brought on by food intolerances (e.g., wheat, coffee, fruits, and dairy products) and/or sugar lactose intolerance. The individual may experience extended periods of constipation and/or diarrhea (also known as the spastic colon type of IBS or pain-less diarrhea) often accompanied by abdominal pain. Other symptoms include bloating, flatulence, and headaches. According to the AMTA (2005), therapeutic massage has lessened or relieved gastrointestinal disorders such as spastic colon and constipation.

Therapeutic goals:

▶ reduce stress
▶ reduce spasms and gas pains
▶ stimulate peristalsis movement, if needed
▶ aid elimination
▶ address emotional issues that are either causing or a cause of

Essential Oils

Bergamot, Black pepper, Cardamom, Carrot seed, Clary sage, Fennel, Ginger, Grapefruit, Juniper berry, Lavender, Mandarin, Neroli, Sweet orange, Peppermint, Petitgrain, Spearmint.

Aromatherapy applications:

▸ massage with 5 percent dilution
▸ abdominal compress

Nausea or Upset Stomach

Generally not a disease or condition in itself, nausea or an upset stomach are common symptoms of something else, such as motion sickness, influenza, pregnancy, or poor digestion. It is always important for a therapist to ask questions and understand any potential underlying contraindications, but if it is appropriate to work with the client, then consider incorporating a low dilution of essential oils to help bring relief.

Therapeutic goals:

▸ reduce stress
▸ improve digestion and absorption
▸ reduce spasms and gas pains
▸ address emotional issues that are either causing or a cause of

Essential Oils

Cardamom, Carrot seed, Roman chamomile, Fennel, Ginger, Grapefruit, Lavender, Mandarin, Peppermint, Rosemary, Spearmint.

Aromatherapy applications:

▸ massage with 1 to 2.5 percent dilution
▸ abdominal massage with 5 percent dilution
▸ abdominal compress
▸ acupressure points
▸ reflexology
▸ inhalation

↪ RESPIRATORY HEALTH

Bronchitis

Chronic bronchitis is a condition that results in the production of bronchial mucus for at least three months in a row over two consecutive years. Airways can become chronically inflamed and potentially obstructed due to an increase in bronchial mucous (Rattray and Ludwig, 2000). According to the AMTA (2005), therapeutic massage has lessened or relieved many of the symptoms of asthma and bronchitis.

Therapeutic goals:

▸ reduce bronchial inflammation
▸ enhance immune system

TABLE 10.7

Essential Oil Therapeutics for the Respiratory System

Therapeutic Action	Essential Oils
Anti-inflammatory: a substance that soothes and reduces inflammations	German chamomile, Frankincense, Helichrysum, Lavender, Myrrh, Patchouli, Sandalwood
Antimicrobial: a substance that destroys or resists pathogenic microorganisms	Roman chamomile, Cinnamon leaf, Clove bud, Eucalyptus, Lemon, Lemongrass, Tea tree, Thyme
Antispasmodic: a substance that relieves smooth/skeletal muscle spasms	Angelica root, Bay laurel, German chamomile, Roman chamomile, Clary sage, Cypress, Fennel, Ginger, Lavender, Sweet marjoram, Neroli, Peppermint, Petitgrain, Sage
Antitussive: a substance that helps to relieve coughs	Cypress
Balsamic: a substance that soothes the lungs	Frankincense, Sandalwood
Decongestant: a substance that reduces or relieves nasal congestion	Eucalyptus, Scots pine, Rosemary ct. camphor
Expectorant: a substance that aids the removal of phlegm or mucus	Cardamom, Eucalyptus, Fennel, Bay laurel, Niaouli, Scots pine, Peppermint, Ravensara, Rosemary ct. cineole or camphor, Sage, Tea tree
Immune Enhancer: a substance that enhances immunity, either by stimulating the immune system or by destroying microbes	Frankincense, Bay laurel, Lemon, Niaouli, Ravensara, Tea tree, Thyme
Mucolytic: a substance that dissolves mucus or breaks down mucus. Mucolytics are used to treat chest conditions involving excessive or thickened mucus secretions	Cedarwood, Helichrysum, Rosemary ct. camphor or cineole or verbenon, Sage

  ▸ aid elimination of excess mucous
  ▸ support health of respiratory system
  ▸ encourage relaxation

Essential Oils

Cardamom, Cedarwood, German chamomile, Cinnamon leaf, Clove bud, Cypress, Eucalyptus, Fennel, Frankincense, Ginger, Helichrysum, Laurel, Lemon, Niaouli, Peppermint, Pine, Ravensara, Rosemary ct. camphor or cineole, Tea tree, Thyme.

Aromatherapy applications:

  ▸ massage with 5 to 10 percent dilution
  ▸ salve
  ▸ reflexology
  ▸ hydrotherapy
  ▸ steam inhalation

IN PRACTICE

Respiratory Congestion and Relaxation

Recently one of my regular clients came in for a much needed massage session. As I spoke with her before her treatment, I could tell she had some congestion with an occasional cough. She told me she hadn't been in for awhile because she had been quite ill. It seems some out-of-town guests had come to stay for a couple of weeks and brought their pet, which my client referred to as a "fur dog." During this time my client had an increased number of asthma attacks. Combined with the fact that they had just moved into a newly constructed home, she was also dealing with the dust and fibers from construction, carpeting, etc. that contributed to the attacks and finally led to an infection and chronic bronchitis. Though the majority of concern had already passed, she still complained of body aches and pain around her chest, ribs, and diaphragm from coughing so much over the past few weeks. She wanted primarily to relax and relieve the aches and pains.

Massage Blend: l oz., 2.5 percent dilution

Apricot kernel, 50 percent

Sunflower, 50 percent

Eucalyptus (*Eucalyptus globulus*): decongesting, breathe easy: 7 drops

Lavender (*Lavandula angustifolia*): stress relieving, chest tightness: 9 drops

*Used for abdominal and chest massage to open bronchioles and relieve tightness. Gave remaining blend to her to take home and use.

Aromatic Spritzer: 1 oz.

Distilled water

Peppermint (*Mentha × piperita*): open sinuses: 5 drops

Eucalyptus (*Eucalyptus globulus*): open sinuses: 8 drops

*Sprayed face cradle.

Massage Oil for Full-Body Massage: 1 oz., 2 percent dilution

Apricot kernel, 100 percent

Lavender (*Lavandula angustifolia*): relax and soothe: 10 drops

Rose (*Rosa damascena*): self-care comfort, relax: 2 drops

Following the massage this client found the soreness around her chest had been relieved, her sinuses were more open, and most of the aches and pains had subsided. She was well on her way to feeling stronger and better. She rescheduled for the following week and no longer allows "fur dogs" to visit.

Asthma

Asthma is a chronic inflammatory disorder of the lungs characterized by bronchial spasms or narrowing of the airways in the lungs making breathing difficult (Rattray and Ludwig, 2000). There are two types of asthma: extrinsic asthma and intrinsic asthma. Extrinsic asthma results from irritating agents outside the body, such as cigarette smoke, allergens (pollen), animal dander, and allergic reactions to food. Intrinsic asthma tends to be more difficult to reverse and can be caused by genetics, structural problems, infections, pollutants, and stress. Intrinsic asthma is the most common type of asthma. Werner and Benjamin (1998) report that massage is indicated for asthma to reduce stress and deal with muscular problems that accompany difficulty with breathing. Massage is contraindicated when the client is in the throes of an asthma attack.

Therapeutic goals:

▶ reduce spasms
▶ aid elimination of excess mucus

- support health of respiratory system
- reduce stress and encourage relaxation

Essential Oils

Bergamot, Cardamom, Cedarwood, German chamomile, Roman chamomile, Clary sage, Eucalyptus species, Myrrh, Neroli, Patchouli, Peppermint, Petitgrain, Pine, Ravensara, Rosemary ct. camphor or cineole, Ylang ylang.

Aromatherapy applications:

- massage with 2.5 to 5 percent dilution
- reflexology
- hydrotherapy

Common Cold

The common cold is an upper respiratory infection caused by any one of hundreds of possible viruses. According to Werner and Benjamin (1998), colds are seldom dangerous unless they complicate other more serious conditions. We're all aware of the usual symptoms: stuffy nose, sneezing, sore throat, maybe a headache. During the worst of a cold, it is usually quite uncomfortable and massage is contraindicated, but it is recommended in the recovery or subacute stages of healing.

Therapeutic goals:

- enhance immune system
- aid elimination of excess mucus
- support health of respiratory system
- encourage rest and relaxation
- relieve muscular aches and pains

Essential Oils

Cardamom, German chamomile, Roman chamomile, Cinnamon leaf, Cypress, Eucalyptus, Fennel, Frankincense, Ginger, Helichrysum, Laurel, Lavender, Lemon, Myrrh, Niaouli, Peppermint, Pine, Ravensara, Rosemary ct. camphor or cineole, Sandalwood, Tea tree, Thyme.

Aromatherapy applications:

- massage with 5 to 10 percent dilution
- Epsom or sea salt bath
- salve
- reflexology
- hydrotherapy
- steam inhalation

SUMMARY

- The main therapeutic actions of essential oils on the musculoskeletal system include analgesic, anti-inflammatory, antirheumatic, antispasmodic, detoxifier, nervine, and rubefacient.
- The main therapeutic actions of essential oils on the nervous system include analgesic, antidepressant, anti-inflammatory, antispasmodic, nervine, and sedative.
- The main therapeutic actions of essential oils on the circulatory system include astringent, anti-inflammatory, circulatory stimulant, detoxifier, hypertensive, hypotensive, and nervine.
- The main therapeutic actions of essential oils on the lymphatic/immune system include anti-inflammatory, circulatory stimulant, detoxifier, and immune enhancer.
- The main therapeutic actions of essential oils on the reproductive system include analgesic, antidepressant, antispasmodic, hormonal balancer, nervine, and sedative.
- The main therapeutic actions of essential oils on the digestive system include analgesic, antispasmodic, carminative, detoxifier, digestive, and nervine.
- The main therapeutic actions of essential oils on the respiratory system include anti-inflammatory, antimicrobial, antispasmodic, antitussive, balsamic, decongestant, expectorant, immune enhancer, and mucolytic.
- Essential oils are capable of enhancing massage and bodywork applications for a wide range of common conditions.

NEW TERMINOLOGY

Amenorrhea

Bursitis

Carpal tunnel syndrome

Dysmenorrhea

Edema

Fibromyalgia

Irritable bowel syndrome

Neuralgia

Plantar fasciitis

Raynaud's syndrome

Tempuromandibular joint disorder

↳ REFERENCES

AMTA. (2005). *Massage Therapy Facts for Physicians*. Evanston, IL: American Massage Therapy Association. Retrieved on August 10, 2005, from www.amtamassage.org.

Cellulite.com. (n/d). *What is cellulite?* Retrieved on March 12, 2006, from http://www.cellulite.com/what_is_cellulite.htm.

Fibromyalgia Network. (n/d). *Fibromyalgia Basics*. Retrieved on April 13, 2006, from http://www.fmnetnews.com/pages/basics.html.

Grace, U. (2001). Treating Fibromyalgia Syndrome with Essential Oils. *International Journal of Aromatherapy 11* (1), 20–25.

Horrigan, C. (2004). Aromatherapy in the management and treatment of rheumatoid and musculoskeletal autoimmune disorders. *International Journal of Aromatherapy 14* (3), 110–118.

Horrigan, C. (2005). Aromatherapy in the management and treatment of rheumatoid and musculoskeletal autoimmune disorders, Part III. *International Journal of Aromatherapy 15* (1), 15–23.

National Institute of Mental Health. (2001). *Facts about anxiety disorders.* Retrieved on April 10, 2006, from http://www.nimh.nih.gov/publicat/adfacts.cfm.

Rattray, F., and Ludwig, L. (2000). *Clinical Massage Therapy.* Toronto, Ontario: Talus Incorporated.

Werner, J., and Benjamin, B. (1998). *A Massage Therapist's Guide to Pathology.* Baltimore, MD: Williams and Wilkins.

WORKSHEET

Essential Therapeutics (Part I)

Enhancing the Session with Aromatherapy

1) Read the client profiles below. Based on the information given, determine which essential oils and method of application you would choose when creating a blend for each.

   a) Mary is a 37 year old, self-employed individual who is currently experiencing high levels of stress due to a large project she is working on. She feels she is holding much tension in her neck and shoulders. Currently she has a low grade headache and at night has difficulty sleeping. She has come for an aromatherapy massage in hopes that it helps alleviate or lessen the stress she is feeling. She has no known allergies and is not on any medication.

Method of application_____

Base: _____ Dilution: _____

Essential Oils	Number of Drops	Why Chosen?

Method of application_____

Base:_____ Dilution: _____

Essential Oils	Number of Drops	Why Chosen?

   b) Tom tripped stepping off a curb and twisted his ankle three days ago. He immediately used the RICE technique and stayed off of it for a day. Currently the ankle appears to have only slight-to-moderate swelling with a little residual bruising and tenderness when weight is applied. Tom is back at work and walking without crutches. He has come in for massage to relieve the tension in the rest of his body and keep the ankle from losing mobility.

Method of application_____

Base: _____Dilution: _____

Essential Oils	Number of Drops	Why Chosen?

WORKSHEET

Essential Therapeutics (Part II)

2) Complete the following intake form and exchange with a partner. Conduct a brief interview for each individual, then design a blend appropriate for addressing their specific complaint or treatment goal. Exchange treatments with your partner.

List any current medications and the conditions they're used for. Include aspirin, ibuprofen, herbal supplements

_____

Surgeries, Major Illnesses, Hospitalizations, or Accidents

_____

Previous Health History

Please mark any of the following that you now have or have had in the past. Circle the applicable condition where two or more are listed on the same line. Please indicate right or left side where appropriate.

Now	Past	Condition	Now	Past	Condition
		Nervous System			**Digestive System**
☐	☐	Shingles	☐	☐	Chronic Pain
☐	☐	Numbness/Tingling	☐	☐	Constipation/Diarrhea
☐	☐	Trigeminal Neuralgia	☐	☐	Gas/Bloating
☐	☐	Bell's Palsy	☐	☐	Diverticulitis
☐	☐	Sciatica	☐	☐	Irritable Bowel Syndrome
☐	☐	Pinched Nerve	☐	☐	Ulcers
☐	☐	Other:_____	☐	☐	Other:_____
		Musculoskeletal System			**Other Conditions/Comments**
☐	☐	Bone or Joint Disease	☐	☐	_____
☐	☐	Tendonitis/Bursitis	☐	☐	_____
☐	☐	Arthritis/Gout			
☐	☐	Sprains/Strains			**Circulatory System**
☐	☐	Low Back Pain	☐	☐	Heart Condition:_____
☐	☐	Hip/Leg Pain	☐	☐	Phlebitis/Varicose Veins
☐	☐	Neck Pain	☐	☐	Blood Clots
☐	☐	Shoulder/Arm Pain	☐	☐	High/Low Blood Pressure
☐	☐	Spasms/Cramps	☐	☐	Lymphedema
☐	☐	Jaw Pain/TMJ	☐	☐	Thrombosis/Embolism
☐	☐	Lupus	☐	☐	Other:_____
☐	☐	Osteoporosis			
☐	☐	Other:_____			**Respiratory System**
			☐	☐	Breathing Difficulty/Asthma
		Skin Conditions	☐	☐	Emphysema
☐	☐	Allergies:_____	☐	☐	Allergies
☐	☐	Rashes	☐	☐	Sinus Problems
☐	☐	Athletes Foot	☐	☐	Other:_____
☐	☐	Herpes/Cold Sores			**Reproductive/Urinary Systems**
☐	☐	Warts	☐	☐	Pregnant: stage_____
☐	☐	Other:_____	☐	☐	Ovarian Problems:_____

Now	Past	Condition	Now	Past	Condition
☐	☐	Menstrual Problems:_____	☐	☐	Chronic Fatigue
☐	☐	PMS	☐	☐	Sleep Disorders
☐	☐	Prostate Problems:_____	☐	☐	Depression
☐	☐	Bladder/UTI Infections	☐	☐	Anxiety/Stress Syndrome
☐	☐	Kidney Ailments:_____	☐	☐	Inflammation/Swelling
☐	☐	Other:_____	☐	☐	Fever
			☐	☐	Infection:_____
		Misc. Conditions	☐	☐	Infectious Disease:_____
☐	☐	Cancer/Tumors	☐	☐	Contact Lenses: soft or hard
☐	☐	Diabetes	☐	☐	Oral Bite Guard/Braces
☐	☐	Drug/Alcohol Use	☐	☐	Foot Problems:_____
☐	☐	Caffeine/Tobacco Use			

CHAPTER TEST

1. The following group of essential oils is considered to be anti-inflammatory:

    a. frankincense, laurel, lemon

    b. German chamomile, helichrysum, lavender

    c. grapefruit, juniper berry, ylang ylang

    d. lemongrass, Scots pine, rosemary ct. camphor

2. The following group of essential oils is considered to be analgesic:

    a. black pepper, birch, clove bud

    b. lemon, lavender, jasmine

    c. neroli, carrot seed, grapefruit

    d. sandalwood, vetiver, ylang ylang

3. Strains and sprains should be addressed with massage:

    a. as early as possible in the acute phase

    b. in the subacute or maturation phases

    c. primarily with aromatic inhalations

    d. in an emergency room

4. TMJ is a condition that:

    a. never involves stress

    b. is strictly structural in nature

    c. almost always requires surgery

    d. can include head and neck pain

5. Constipation could potentially be relieved with the following essential oils:

    a. ylang ylang, Roman chamomile

    b. jasmine, neroli

    c. fennel, ginger

    d. sandalwood, German chamomile

6. Generally speaking, edema:

    a. cannot be helped with massage techniques

    b. should not be interfered with or reduced

    c. can be successfully aided by essential oils and lymphatic massage techniques

    d. is caused when an individual drinks too much water

7. The following group of essential oils can be used to alleviate the symptoms of PMS:

   a. eucalyptus, laurel, tea tree

   b. pine, ravensara, lemon

   c. peppermint, rosemary ct. camphor, black pepper

   d. lavender, geranium, clary sage

8. The following group of essential oils is considered to be immune enhancers:

   a. ylang ylang, neroli, peppermint

   b. ginger, cardamom, carrot seed

   c. niaouli, tea tree, thyme

   d. German chamomile, Roman chamomile, clary sage

9. The following group of essential oils is considered to be expectorants:

   a. eucalyptus, ravensara, rosemary ct. cineole

   b. angelica root, bergamot, German chamomile

   c. ylang ylang, vetiver, grapefruit

   d. black pepper, ginger, juniper berry

10. The following group of essential oils could be used to help stimulate circulation:

    a. ginger, bergamot

    b. rosemary, black pepper

    c. lavender, clary sage

    d. tangerine, veranium

REVIEW QUESTIONS

1. Discuss how you might go about incorporating essential oils in your therapeutic sessions for specific client complaints.

2. What would you say to a client who came to you looking for a cure or remedy?

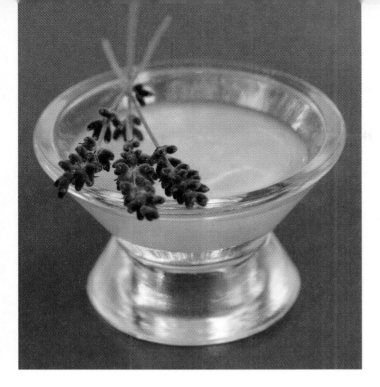

11

Aromatherapy in Practice
Special Populations and Settings

 LEARNING OBJECTIVES

After reading this chapter, you will be able to

1. List and describe four special populations who would benefit from the integration of bodywork and aromatherapy.

2. Identify at least five prenatal/postpartum conditions/symptoms and describe potential essential oils, methods of application, and special precautions or considerations.

3. Identify at least five infant and childhood conditions/symptoms and describe potential essential oils, methods of application, and special precautions or considerations.

4. Identify at least five conditions experienced by the aging/elderly population and describe potential essential oils, methods of application, and special precautions or considerations.

5. Identify at least five hospice/end-of-life care conditions and describe potential essential oils, methods of application, and special precautions or considerations.

6. Discuss the importance of self-care as a massage or bodywork professional and describe various methods that could be incorporated into one's lifestyle to accomplish this.

7. Describe potential methods of incorporating aromatherapy and essential oils in a variety of practice settings.

INTRODUCTION

Professional bodyworkers and massage therapists have a wide range of options when it comes to what type of clientele they would like to work with and in what kind of environment or facility. Throughout this chapter we will look at ideas on how to incorporate the benefits of essential oils when working with special client populations and in various locations and/or settings. In addition to properly incorporating aromatherapy, it is highly recommended that you seek the proper training required for your particular modality of bodywork in order to safely and effectively work with the client populations that interest you, as most will have very specific needs and contraindications related to each group.

→ AROMATHERAPY AND SPECIAL POPULATIONS

Prenatal and Postpartum

Pregnancy and childbirth are major landmarks in a woman's life (Figure 11-1). There are many physical, psychological, and spiritual changes that take place, affecting not only a woman's body shape and size but also her hormone levels, which can affect skin texture and tone, digestion, circulation, and emotional states. Even in the most positive of situations, we know that change often creates stress, and stress can contribute to psychological and physical unease. Discomforts of pregnancy are vast and varied, with different concerns arising at different times throughout the process.

According to Tiffany Field, Ph.D., founder of the Touch Research Institute at the Miami School of Medicine, prenatal clients who received regular massage had a decreased level of uterine stress hormone (norepinephrine) as well as fewer complications during labor. Prenatal clients also experienced a reduction in anxiety, improved mood, better sleep, and less back pain. Their infants had fewer postnatal complications, and fewer babies were born prematurely (Field et al., 1998). Integrating aromatherapy with massage for prenatal clients can potentially enhance these benefits of massage. According to Buckle (2003), "aromatherapy can be helpful for many symptoms of pregnancy including general tiredness, aches and pains, nausea, insomnia, and backache" (p. 324).

Whether it be pre-conception, early, mid, or late pregnancy, labor, delivery, or postpartum, there are certain essential oils generally considered safer than others, those to be avoided, and those to be selected for more specific complaints (see Tables 11.1 and 11.2). As a general rule, you may want to avoid using essential oils (with perhaps the exception of lavender) as well as some forms of bodywork and energy modalities until the pregnancy is well established, usually by the twelfth week. All essential oils should be used with care, consideration, and moderation during pregnancy. Remember that every woman and every pregnancy is different. If there is a questionable health history or cause for concern, always opt for safety and stick to the more gentle oils, refer to a well-trained aromatherapist, or just wait until after the birth to resume using essential oils with your client.

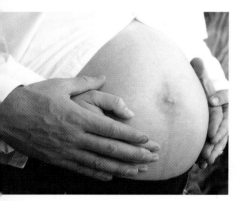

Figure 11-1 Pregnant belly
Source: © iStockPhoto.com/ BigPoppa

TABLE 11.1

Common Conditions, Methods of Application, and Essential Oils During Pregnancy, Labor, and Postpartum	
Condition	**Method of Application: Essential Oils**
Anxiety	*Inhalation, Massage oil, Diffusion, Bath*: Lavender, Frankincense, Mandarin, Sandalwood, Neroli and Rose
Back pain	*Gel, Massage oil, Salve*: Lavender, Rosemary ct. camphor or cineole, Peppermint, Clary sage, Sweet marjoram
Constipation	*Inhalation, Footbaths, Massage oil*: Peppermint, Ginger
Depression	*Inhalation, Massage oil, Diffusion, Bath*: Jasmine, Patchouli, Rose, Mandarin, Neroli
Edema	*Footbath*: Lemon, Juniper berry, Rosemary ct. cineole or camphor
Indigestion	*Inhalation, Massage oil*: Peppermint, Ginger
Leg pain/cramps	*Gel, Massage oil, Salve*: Lavender, German Chamomile, Roman Chamomile
Nausea	*Inhalation*: Peppermint, Ginger
Postpartum "baby blues"	*Inhalation, Massage oil*: Patchouli, Rose, Neroli, Mandarin/Tangerine, Sweet orange
Slow or difficult labor	*Inhalation, Diffusion, Massage oil*: Lavender, Clary sage, Jasmine, Rose
Stretch marks	*Salve, Massage oil*: Lavender, Frankincense
Varicose veins	*Gel, Massage oil*: Cypress, Lemon, Geranium, German chamomile

Therapeutic Dilution

For pregnant and lactating women we generally recommend a 2% dilution (9–10 drops per ounce of carrier) or 3–7 drops essential oil in baths or 4 drops per quart of water for warm or cool compress.

TABLE 11.2

Essential Oils to Avoid Throughout Pregnancy, Labor, and During Breastfeeding	
Essential Oil	**Latin Name**
Aniseed	*Pimpinella anisum*
Basil ct. estragole	*Ocimum basilicum*
Birch	*Betula lenta*
Camphor	*Cinnamomum camphora*
Hyssop	*Hyssopus officinalis*
Mugwort	*Artemisia vulgaris*
Parsley seed or leaf	*Petroselinum sativum*
Pennyroyal	*Mentha pulegium*
Sage	*Salvia officinalis*
Tansy	*Tanacetum vulgare*
Tarragon	*Artemisia dracunculus*
Thuja	*Thuja occidentalis*
Wintergreen	*Gaultheria procumbens*
Wormwood	*Artemisia absinthium*

PRENATAL AND POSTPARTUM AROMATIC RECIPES

Gentle Massage Oil 1 oz / 2 percent dilution

Tangerine	5 drops
Lavender	5 drops

Base Oils: Calendula 10 percent
Apricot kernel 70 percent

Jojoba   20 percent

Stretch Mark Blend/Salve 1 ounce / 2 percent dilution

Frankincense   7 to 10 drops
               or
Neroli   3 to 5 drops is sufficient.

Jojoba oil/Shea butter/Vitamin E

Hydrosol Spritzer 2 oz. bottle

Third trimester and labor

Rose hydrosol 50 percent

Roman chamomile hydrosol 50 percent

Spritz room just before beginning massage or chill and use to refresh during labor

Back Pain Blend 1oz. / 2 percent dilution

Lavender	7 drops
Roman chamomile	3 drops
or	
Frankincense	5 drops
Lavender	5 drops

Base Oils: Apricot kernel 80 percent Jojoba   20 percent

Anxiety and Depression Blend 1oz. / 2 percent dilution

Rose	3 drops
Mandarin	5 drops
Vetiver	2 drops

Or just Rose: 5 drops per one ounce should be sufficient.

Base Oils: Calendula	10 percent
Apricot kernel	70 percent
Jojoba	20 percent

Reflexology Digestive Tonic Blend 1oz. / 2 percent dilution

Fennel	4 drops
Peppermint	3 drops
Lavender	3 drops

Aromatic application ideas:

- ▶ lotions, oils, or gels for massaging sore or fatigued muscles
- ▶ Aloe gel for light massage on cramping or "tired" legs and varicose veins
- ▶ diffuser, nebulizer, cotton pads, or aromatic spritzers can be used to ease nausea, anxiety, depression, and slow/difficult labor
- ▶ moisturizing cream or rich massage oil to replenish and restore elasticity to dry, overstretched skin
- ▶ reflexology combined with essential oils to enhance digestion, support labor, or simply to soothe aching and tired feet
- ▶ postpartum sitz baths to ease discomfort and help facilitate healing of tears or episiotomy
- ▶ warm compress or light massage oil for sore or engorged breasts
- ▶ refreshing cool compress and/or unique massage blends specific to supporting the process of labor and delivery

Precautions and Special Considerations

Use only the more gentle essential oils throughout pregnancy, and avoid oils that may directly affect uterine contractions until it's time for the delivery. As mentioned previously, it is best to wait until the pregnancy is well established before implementing prenatal blends. Be aware that due to an increase in the odor sensitivity during pregnancy, some aromas may induce nausea or elicit strong emotions/reactions, even at low dilutions. When it comes to incorporating aromatherapy, keep your dilutions light, and remember the primary goal when working with prenatal and postpartum moms is to simply provide comfort, unconditional support, rest, relaxation, and relief from the basic discomforts that accompany this life transition. Seek the proper training in your particular bodywork modality in order to work safely and effectively with this special population.

Infants and Children

The experiences we have as infants and young children greatly impact our physical, emotional, and memory bodies throughout the duration of our lifetime, as each contributes to our critical development into adulthood. Many of us have children of our own and have been witness to their remarkable growth and amazing ability to adapt. For those of us fortunate enough to work with children in our bodywork practices, we appreciate the pliability of these formative years, their sensitivities, and how quickly and readily their little bodies respond to treatment (Figure 11-2).

Little ones have stresses and strain patterns held in the body just as we do, with one of the most intense stresses of life, the birth process, being much more recent for them. They too possess the ability to develop a particular scent memory and in fact can begin doing so while still in the womb. Children have smaller bodies and much greater sensitivities both mentally and physically, as their senses have usually yet to become dulled, impaired, or ignored.

According to Field (2001), "infant massage therapists say that massaging healthy infants helps the parent-infant bonding; reduces the infant's distress following painful procedures such as inoculations; reduces pain from colic, constipation, and teething; reduces sleep problems; and makes the parents feel good while they are massaging their infants" (p. 118). The addition of aromatherapy for infant massage can increase these and other benefits as listed in Table 11.3.

Therapeutic Dilution

It is probably best to wait on using essential oils directly on newborns until the age of six weeks. If there is a really good reason for doing so, one might utilize a method of diffusion such as with a nebulizer or by placing a bowl of steaming water on the floor of the baby's room and adding 1 or 2 drops of essential oil as a method of releasing the molecules into the environment.

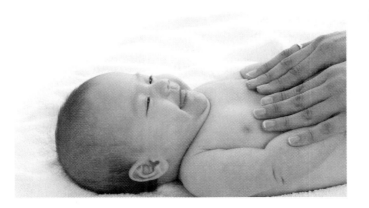

Figure 11-2 Infant massage
Source: © iStockPhoto.com/ Bennewitz

	TABLE 11.3

Common Conditions, Methods of Application, and Essential Oils for Infants and Children

Condition	Method of Application: Essential Oils
Sleeplessness	*Baths, Massage oil, Diffusion*: Lavender, Roman chamomile
Diaper rash	*Baths*: Hydrosols of Lavender, Roman chamomile *Baths, Creams, Salves*: Lavender, Roman chamomile
Colic	*Baths, Diffusion, Massage oil*: Lavender, Roman chamomile, Neroli, Rose
Cradle cap	*Massage oil*: Lavender, Rose
Hyperactivity	*Massage oil, Baths, Diffusion, Inhalation*: Lavender, Roman chamomile, Neroli, Sandalwood
Scrapes/bruises	*Massage oil, Salve, Cream*: Lavender, Tea tree, German chamomile, Helichrysum
Growing pains	*Massage oil, Salve, Cream, Lotion*: Rosemary ct. cineol or camphor, *Eucalyptus smitthi* or *radiata*, Lavender, Roman chamomile
Colds	*Massage oil, Salve, Inhalation, Diffusion*: Lemon, Rosemary ct. cineol or camphor, *Eucalyptus smitthi* or *radiata*, Tea tree

Infants 6 weeks to 12 months—.5 percent dilution: 3 drops of essential oil per ounce of carrier. Try one or two drops of essential oil for a full baby's bath, but make certain to blend into an emulsifier such as milk before placing baby in the tub.

Children 1 to 7 years—.75 to 1 percent dilution: 4 to 6 drops of essential oil per ounce of carrier.

Children 7 to 12 years—2 to 2.5 percent dilution: 12 to 15 drops of essential oil per ounce of carrier.

Aromatic application ideas:

▶ lotions, oils, or gels for relaxing massage to encourage better sleep, decrease overactivity, aid in digestion, and help relieve colic
▶ baby salve for irritated or chaffed skin
▶ diffuser, nebulizer, cotton pads, or aromatic spritzer to help ease sinus congestion, aid sleep, or clear the environment of unwanted odors (Remember not to let a small child spray the spritzer, as they may get essential oil in their eyes.)
▶ Blend a low dilution of essential oils in a natural, unscented bubble-bath base, whole milk, or light oil for bath time.
▶ Give parents or caregivers any leftover bath blend, massage oil, or lotion along with some basic instructions on how to give an aromatic bath or gentle massage at home.

Precautions and Special Considerations

Use only all-natural base materials and gentle essential oils for infants and children. Avoid the use of carriers that contain unknown chemical compounds, sulfates, artificial color, perfumes, or fragrance. Avoid using essential oils during the first six weeks unless truly needed to treat the environment. Make certain you are using safe and gentle

	TABLE 11.4
Essential Oils for Infants and Young Children	

Age	Safe Essential Oils
Infants 6 weeks to 6 months	German chamomile, Roman chamomile, *Eucalyptus smitthi*, Lavender, Mandarin/Tangerine, Neroli, Sweet orange, Rose, Sandalwood
Infants 6 months to 1 year	Add: Frankincense, Grapefruit, Tea tree, Patchouli
Children 1 year to 2 years	Add: Bergamot, Clary sage, Cypress, Geranium, Ginger, Lemon, Rosemary ct. camphor or cineole
Children 2 to 7 years	Add: Helichrysum, Peppermint after thirty months of age only, Vetiver, Ylang ylang

essential oils (See Table 11.4), lower dilutions, and don't overdo it for these sensitive ones. According to Harris (2005), it is best to avoid the routine, regular/daily dermal application of essential oils on babies and young children which may lead to allergies later in life. Infants and toddlers have greater skin permeability so use low dilutions (under 1%) until at least the age of 7. The use of hydrosols and aerial dispersion is recommended.

Keep all essential oils and aromatherapy products out of reach of children. If essential oils are accidentally ingested by a child, seek medical care immediately. When applying topical aromatherapy blends to infants, always avoid the hands, eyes, nose, and mouth areas. If irritation occurs, apply unscented vegetable-base oil to the area and discontinue use.

Aging and Elderly

Just as we were all infants and children at one time, the majority of us will also experience the other end of the spectrum and eventually reach our full maturity. As the years pass, they often take a certain toll on our bodies, and by our mid-to-late

INFANT MASSAGE BLEND
6 WEEKS TO 6 MONTHS

Hydrosols for Bathing and Room Spritzers

Roman chamomile
Orange flower
Lavender

Baby's First Massage Oil 1 oz. / .5 percent dilution

Roman chamomile	1 drop
Lavender	2 drops
Or just Lavender	3 drops
Or just R. chamomile	3 drops

In 100 percent Jojoba, sweet almond, or kukui oil

Childhood Massage Blend

1 to 7 years old

Soothe Hyperactivity 1 oz. / 1 percent dilution

Mandarin	3 drops
Roman chamomile	1 drops
Lavender	2 drops

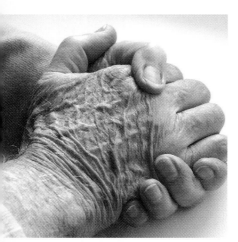

Figure 11-3 Senior hands
Source: © iStockPhoto.com/trigga

forties and onward we may begin to experience a general slowing of bodily systems, decreased mobility, changing connective tissue, thinner skin with less elasticity, and the lifelong effects of prolonged stress on the body (Figure 11-3). In addition to the physical changes, quite often a degree of mental and emotional change also takes place, such as memory loss, a decrease in thought processing, or even mild dementia.

In the process of aging, it is also common to experience the loss of a spouse, partner, or friends that may leave an elderly individual feeling more alone, dependent on others, limited in options, and quite often starved for personal connection or even human touch. According to Nelson (2001), "my observation and experience working with the elderly has shown that those who are deprived of nurturing physical contact experience a diminishing quality of life, a lessening of their desire to relate to others and a weakening of what may already be a fragile relationship with physical reality."

Massage and other bodywork modalities can be pivotal in countering many of the physical and emotional aspects of aging and can be an aspect of enhancing the quality of life, providing comfort care, and promoting the concept of healthy aging. Incorporating aromatherapy in these sessions can prove even more beneficial and enjoyable for both you and your elderly clients. See Table 11.5 for a list of common conditions, methods of application, and essential oils for the elderly population.

"In the aged especially, the need for tactile stimulation is a hunger which has so often remained unsatisfied that, in their disappointment, its victims tend to become uncommunicative concerning their need for it."

(MONTAGU, 1986, P. 396)

TABLE 11.5

Common Conditions, Methods of Application, and Essential Oils for the Elderly

Condition	Method of Application: Essential Oils
Anxiety	*Inhalation, Baths, Massage oil, Diffusion*: Angelica root, Bergamot, German chamomile, Roman chamomile, Frankincense, Lavender, Mandarin, Sweet marjoram, Melissa, Neroli, Sweet orange, Petitgrain, Rose, Sandalwood, Vetiver, Ylang ylang
Bedsores/Ulcers	*Baths, Gel*: German chamomile, Frankincense, Helichrysum, Lavender, Myrrh, Neroli
Depression	*Inhalations, Baths, Massage oil, Diffusion*: Bergamot, Clary sage, Frankincense, Jasmine, Lavender, Sweet orange, Mandarin/Tangerine, Rose, Ylang ylang
Sluggish Digestion	*Baths, Massage Oil, Reflexology*: Angelica root, Black pepper, Cardamom, Carrot seed, Fennel, Grapefruit, Lemon
Insomnia	*Inhalations, Baths, Massage oil, Diffusion*: German chamomile, Roman chamomile, Lavender, Sweet marjoram
Lowered Immunity	*Inhalations, Baths, Massage oil, Diffusion*: Eucalyptus globulus, Frankincense, Bay laurel, Lemon, Niaouli, Ravensara, Tea tree, Thyme
Muscular Aches and Pains	*Baths, Massage oil, Salves, Gels*: Black pepper, Roman or German chamomile, Clary sage, Eucalyptus globulus, Ginger, Helichrysum, Lavender, Sweet marjoram, Peppermint, Rosemary ct. camphor or cineole
Poor Circulation	*Baths, Footbaths, Massage oils, Gels*: Carrot seed, Black pepper, Ginger, Juniper berry, Laurel, Lemon, Lemongrass, Scots pine, Rosemary ct. camphor or cineole

Therapeutic Dilution

For aging and elderly clients, we generally recommend a 1.5 to 2.5 percent dilution or 9 to 15 drops of essential oil per ounce of carrier oil or lotion. You may want to use a 3 percent dilution, 18 to 20 drops of essential oil per ounce of massage oil, gel, or salve for a limited application to localized areas such as hands, feet, or painful joints. Try 3 to 5 drops of essential oil per cup of hot or cold water when preparing a compress or 3 to 8 drops in a full bathtub of water; making certain the oils are well mixed or blended into an emulsifier such as milk before entering the tub.

Aromatic application ideas:

- ▶ lotions, oils, or gels for massaging sore or fatigued muscles
- ▶ massage gel or salve for painful joints
- ▶ Aloe gel for application on bedsores/ulcers
- ▶ diffuser, nebulizer, cotton pads, aromatic spritzer, or steam to treat the air, relieve sinus congestion, aid sleep, or clear the environment of unwanted odors
- ▶ moisturizing cream or rich massage oil to replenish and restore elasticity to dry skin
- ▶ reflexology combined with essential oils to aid digestion and peristalsis
- ▶ warm or cool compresses for stiff or sore joints and muscles
- ▶ leftover aromatic massage oil or lotion to take home for self-care treatments elicit scent memories to recall the positive emotional and physiological response to touch therapies

Precautions and Special Considerations

Aging clients come in all shapes and sizes, in varying degrees of wellness. For the healthy senior, you will be able to utilize various techniques and essential oils just as you would with younger clients. However, for more frail clients, a caring light touch with lower dilutions of essential oils may be what is called for. It is always important to conduct a thorough interview with special populations so you can be well aware of existing medical conditions and medications the client may be on. This helps in deciding if contraindications may exist.

While some elderly clients are extra-sensitive to aromas or topical applications, others have a diminished sense of smell or sensation with which to give you feedback, so adjust your aromatic blends and pressure accordingly. Keep in mind that elderly clients may bruise easily or have brittle bones. Use great care, monitor the amount of pressure being used, and offer to help your clients to get on, off, or repositioned on the treatment table or chair.

Palliative, Hospice, and End-of-Life Care

Massage and bodywork therapists are playing a growing role in palliative, hospice, and end-of-life care. According to The National Council for Palliative Care (2005), palliative and/or hospice care can be defined as "the active holistic care of patients with advanced progressive illness. Management of pain and other symptoms and provision of psychological, social and spiritual support is paramount. The goal of palliative care is achievement of the best quality of life for patients and their families." Palliative care can be offered at any time during the stages of terminal illness.

End-of-life care, on the other hand, tends to imply that an individual is nearing close to the end of their life. Hospice of Ohio (n/d) summarizes the benefits of massage and hospice care as follows:

Massage can:

- ▶ address feelings of isolation, loneliness, fear, and boredom
- ▶ help to restore feelings of self-acceptance and self-esteem
- ▶ comfort while actively dying
- ▶ provide nurturance and loving care
- ▶ facilitate emotional release
- ▶ provide an opportunity for relationship building
- ▶ enhance memories of positive touch experiences, thus providing peace, joy, and love
- ▶ assist in providing care to family members (excellent stress reliever)

Palliative and hospice services provide physical, social, emotional, and spiritual comfort for the patient, family members, and caregivers as they move through the process of terminal illness and dying. Whatever your chosen modality, bodywork sessions with this population should be gentle, caring, and at times shorter in duration. Aim to incorporate aromatherapy in your massage blends to be comforting, pleasing, refreshing, and nurturing. Always take into account personal preferences, fond memories, and experiences when creating the blends that may comfort your client and those closely involved. Buckle (2003) comments that "Aromatherapy can aid the management of pain and nausea in a complementary way, but perhaps aromatherapy's greatest strength in palliative care lies in its ability to facilitate communication at an emotional and spiritual level, giving feelings of comfort and pleasure" (p. 305). Table 11.6 covers some common conditions, methods of application, and essential oils for hospice and end-of-life care.

TABLE 11.6 Common Conditions, Methods of Application, and Essential Oils for Hospice and End-of-Life Care	
Condition	**Method of Application: Essential Oils**
Appetite Changes	*Inhalation, Massage Oil, Diffusion*: Angelica root, Basil ct. linalol, Black pepper, Cardamom, Carrot seed, Fennel, Lemon
Depression	*Inhalations, Baths, Massage oil, Diffusion*: Bergamot, Clary sage, Frankincense, Jasmine, Lavender, Sweet orange, Mandarin/Tangerine, Rose, Ylang ylang
Fear and/or Anxiety	*Inhalation, Baths, Massage oil, Diffusion*: Angelica root, Bergamot, German chamomile, Roman chamomile, Frankincense, Lavender, Mandarin, Sweet marjoram, Melissa, Neroli, Sweet orange, Petitgrain, Rose, Sandalwood, Vetiver, Ylang ylang
Pain	*Massage oil, Compress, Footbaths*: Black pepper, Birch, Cinnamon leaf, Clove bud, Eucalyptus globulus, Ginger, Lemongrass, Sweet marjoram, Myrrh, Peppermint, Rosemary ct. camphor and cineole
Sleeplessness/Insomnia	*Inhalations, Baths, Massage oil, Diffusion*: German chamomile, Roman chamomile, Lavender, Sweet marjoram
Spiritual Oils for End-of-Life Care	*Diffusion, Massage oil, cream*: Frankincense, Myrrh, Rose, Sandalwood

Therapeutic Dilution

For terminally ill or hospice clients, we generally recommend a .5 to 2.5 percent dilution, that is 3 to 15 drops of essential oil per ounce of carrier oil or lotion. This dilution rate is highly variable based on who you are working with. Terminally ill children and adults or the extremely sensitive or frail may require a lower dilution, although some may desire slightly higher dilutions. You may also need to vary your rate of dilution based on where your client is in their process; outside factors, such as new medications or procedures, sudden physical or emotional decline, or new sensitivities, may be present and may affect the rate of dilution. Try 1 to 3 drops of essential oil per cup of hot or cold water when preparing a compress or 3 to 6 drops per quart of water for a hand or footbath.

Aromatic application ideas:

- ▶ lotions, oils, or gels for offering comfort massage
- ▶ diffuser, nebulizer, cotton pads, aromatic spritzer, or steam to treat the air, relieve sinus congestion, aid sleep, or clear the environment of unwanted odors
- ▶ Use a small amount of moisturizing cream or rich massage oil to replenish dry feet or hands. Show family members or caregivers how to do a gentle hand or foot massage with the aromatherapy blend.
- ▶ light touch reflexology combined with essential oils to help relieve discomfort
- ▶ warm or cool compresses and foot or hand baths
- ▶ Don't forget to offer a tired caregiver or weary family member an aromatic bath blend (or shower gel as they may not have time for a bath), a sachet to tuck in their pillow, or a spritzer to help recharge and revitalize their spirits as well.

HOSPICE BLENDS

Aromatic Comfort Blend 1oz. / 1.5 percent dilution

Roman chamomile	2 drops
Lavender	4 drops
Mandarin	3 drops

Base Oil: 50 percent apricot kernel and 50 percent sunflower oil

Breathe Easy Blend 1oz. / 2.5 percent dilution

Eucalyptus radiata	5 drops
Rosemary	5 drops
Lemon	2 drops
Peppermint	3 drops

Anxiety and Depression Blend 1oz. / 2 percent dilution

Neroli	4 drops
Mandarin	8 drops

Base Oil: 50 percent apricot kernel and 50 percent sunflower oil

Family Support Spritzer 20 drops in 4 oz. bottle of 75 percent distilled water / 25 percent lavender hydrosol

Rose	3 drops
Lavender	7 drops
Mandarin	10 drops

IN PRACTICE

Case Study 11.1

Hospice Care

Jack was a sixty-six-year-old male suffering from stage 4 melanoma, a very aggressive type of cancer. I went out on an aromatherapy consultation. When I arrived he was very sleepy; he had been sleeping for thirteen hours. We weren't sure if he was sleepy from the pain medication or if he was beginning his transition. I talked to him briefly; he suggested that his wife and I make up an aromatherapy blend for him. His wife expressed to me that she would like a blend to address the anxiety he was experiencing and also a blend that would help to open him up spiritually. Together we chose the following oils:

Jack's Spiritual/Anxiety Synergy

Rosa damascena (rose) helps to comfort and release grief. *Cedrus atlantica* (cedar wood) strengthens our connection with the divine. *Boswellia carterii* (frankincense) connects us to our higher self, helps to let go of earthly attachments. *Lavandula angustifolia* (lavender) helps with acceptance; is very comforting and useful with emotional balance. Lavender is also extremely helpful in reducing anxiety. This blend was delivered by means of inhalation (2 drops on a tissue or a cotton ball). We also used a cream base and made a 1 percent dilution to be massaged on his hands and feet two or three times a day to enhance relaxation and also help open him up spiritually.

Results

I made my aromatherapy visit on Tuesday morning. Wednesday afternoon his wife massaged his feet and hands with the aromatherapy cream blend. He died a few hours later. The chaplain came, and they did an anointing with the aromatic synergy. They also rubbed the aroma cream blend on his body. What a wonderful way to transition. Jack's wife also found the synergistic blend to be very comforting after the loss of her loved one.

This case study has been kindly provided by Michelle Thibert, LMT, Seattle, WA.

Precautions and Special Considerations

When working with this population, remember to go slow and easy with whatever modality you use, including aromatherapy. It is always important to conduct a thorough interview with your clients, but especially so with special populations so you can be well aware of any and all conditions they may be suffering and medications they may be taking, in order for you to work (or not work) with any resulting contraindications. While some terminally ill clients are extra-sensitive to aromas or topical applications, others have a diminished sense of smell or sensation or are unable to give you feedback, so keep your aromatic blends light in dilution and be aware of any reactions that may appear. Seek the proper training in your particular bodywork modality in order to work safely and effectively with this special population.

Therapist Self-Care

Although not technically a special population like the ones listed above, we thought it important to mention. As therapists we often wear many hats and fulfill multiple roles. If you are in practice for yourself, you probably do everything from answer the phone, to washing linens, bookkeeping, marketing, and finally working with your clients. If you are an employed therapist, you too most likely have multiple responsibilities and potentially serve a high number of clients each shift. In addition to being therapists or bodyworkers, we may also be parents, spouses, volunteers, friends, or active members of an extended family or community. With so much on our plates, self-care begs to become a priority.

Self-care for massage therapists and other healthcare providers is becoming a hot topic these days. Why? Because all too often the caregiver forgets that they too are in much need of care or that it is important to take time out for self-rejuvenation and nurturing. The nature of bodywork and massage therapy can be extremely taxing physically and emotionally. Some therapists end up leaving the profession after a few years due to physical exhaustion, carpal tunnel, or other repetitive strain injuries. Caring for yourself as a massage therapist is a commitment that can be quite empowering. According to Korn (2003), "self-care may seem like a luxury, but it's not. One of the principles of self-care demands that you deliberately choose to care for yourself."

Some beneficial ways that you can begin to care for yourself: get a massage, take an aromatherapy bath, or get an aromatherapy massage! How often does a massage therapist tell others about the benefits of massage and that they should have one on a regular basis? Well, this holds true for massage therapists and bodyworkers as well. One of the great benefits of being in the field is to connect with other therapists and offer to do trades. Other aspects of self-care include: ensuring that you have great body mechanics while working (this can reduce stress on your body); exercising and stretching regularly to keep your body flexible and strong; drinking plenty of water, to stay hydrated and ensure good circulation; and finally, adding aromatherapy into your life. Aromatherapy can be easily integrated into your home self-care program. Table 11.7 provides some basic ideas on incorporating essential oils for self-care.

Therapeutic Dilution

2.5 to 5 percent dilution, or 15 to 30 drops of essential oil per ounce of carrier. For all over aches and emotional cleansing, try an Epsom or sea salt bath of 3 cups with a strong dilution (10 to 20 drops of essential oil, depending on the oil) added to a full bathtub of water.

Aromatic application ideas:

- ▶ lotions, oils, or gels for massaging sore or fatigued muscles
- ▶ massage gel or salve for painful joints, stressed or strained tissue
- ▶ aromatic spritzer or hydrosol to refresh and revitalize energy
- ▶ warm or cool compresses for stiff or sore joints and muscles
- ▶ cool submersion bath for hands and forearms (between clients)
- ▶ warm Epsom salt/aromatherapy baths for full-body relief and to soothe emotions

TABLE 11.7

Aromatic Self-Care for the Massage Therapist

Condition	Method of Application: Essential Oils
Muscular Aches and Pains	*Baths, Massage oil, Salves, Gels*: Black pepper, Roman or German chamomile, Clary sage, Eucalyptus globulus, Ginger, Helichrysum, Lavender, Sweet marjoram, Peppermint, Rosemary ct. camphor or cineole
Grounding/Centering	*Baths, Inhalation, Massage Oil, Diffusion*: Angelica root, Sandalwood, Vetiver
Release/Detox	*Baths (with salts), Inhalation, Massage Oil, Diffusion*: Grapefruit, Juniper berry, Lemon
Self-Nurture	*Baths, Massage oil, Diffusion*: Rose, Tangerine, Sandalwood, Ylang ylang

AROMATHERAPY FOR THE THERAPIST

Revitalize the Therapist Blend: 1. oz. / 3 percent dilution

Rosemary	6 drops
Peppermint	3 drops
Ginger	5 drops
Clary sage	4 drops

Base Oil: 50 percent apricot kernel and 50 percent sunflower oil

Stress Relief Full-Body Bath Blend: 1 oz. / 2.5 percent dilution

Lavender	8 drops
Roman chamomile	3 drops
Vetiver	4 drops

Base Oil: apricot kernel *or* milk *or* Epsom and/or sea salts

Nurturing the Nurturer: 1 oz. / 2 percent dilution

Rose	3 drops
Vetiver	3 drops
Tangerine	6 drops

Base Oil: 50 percent apricot kernel and 50 percent sunflower oil or lotion

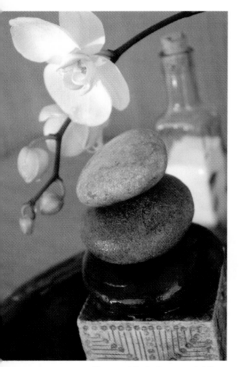

Figure 11-4 Spa orchid
Source: © iStockPhoto.com/elenaray

Precautions and Special Considerations

Be sure to make time for self-care techniques and schedule yourself for regular body-work sessions. Don't work until you are overly fatigued or injured. Each of us is responsible for our own wellness, and bodyworkers are no exception. Be aware of diet, exercise, rest, and body mechanics at all times. Use essential oils and self-care techniques to facilitate your own health and wellness. Be aware of any aromatherapy safety precautions or contraindications that may pertain to your individual situation.

AROMATHERAPY AND PRACTICE SETTINGS

Massage and bodywork practices have made their way into a variety of settings from individual practices to on-site locations. With a little creativity and careful planning, it is possible to offer the benefits of essential oils and/or aromatherapy to whatever and wherever your client base may be. Here we look at some of the challenges and advantages of providing aromatherapy in various treatment settings.

Single Practitioner and Group Settings

Many massage therapists and bodyworkers choose to be self-employed or to work in a small clinic or cooperative practice with other complementary therapists. This type of setting is great for its versatility and flexibility. Obviously if you are on your own and working with aromatherapy in your practice, you need only be concerned about the preferences of your clients in terms of essential oils and the environment.

If, however, you are part of a group practice, you will need to be considerate of other therapists and the reactions *their* clients may have to aromatherapy. In both cases, especially the latter, it is best to remember the importance of adequate ventilation for your treatment area. Also, the use of synthetic or poor-quality essential oils will more readily produce a negative response in sensitive individuals. Explore the tips mentioned in the In Practice 11.1 box for successfully incorporating essential oils in a single therapist practice or group setting.

Destination and Day Spas

There are so many environments for therapists to work in these days that there should be no reason to get bored with the profession. If spa work is your preferred path, congratulations! You are in for a wonderfully diverse experience, most likely working with a variety of body treatments and modalities and an even broader array of clientele. And you're not alone, according to the 2005 ABMP member survey summary; approximately 33 percent of responding ABMP massage therapists work at least part-time in a spa setting.

From world-renowned destination resorts to locally operated day spas, salons, and now more recently, medical spas that are cropping up across the country, Americans are flocking to these retreats for the varied health, wellness, and esthetic services that promise rest, relaxation, and self-improvement. Most spas have a line of products that they work with (Figure 11-4). Often this includes pre-blended aromatherapy products. If this is the case, then you can do either one of two things: become educated on the product line you will be using, understand the essential oils in each product, their therapeutic benefits and potential contraindications; or you can offer to create customized massage blends for the clients you see. For some basic ideas on incorporating aromatherapy into spas, see the In Practice 11.2 box.

The On-Site Environment

As the awareness and acceptance of massage and bodywork grows among the general population, many are experiencing firsthand the amazing health benefits of these complementary therapies. Specialty retailers, shopping malls, and department stores are beginning to offer short chair massages, often in the privacy of small kiosks, to their staff and customers. Employers recognize the importance of a healthy workforce and see on-site massage as a way to reduce stress in their employees, relieve pain-related symptoms, help prevent overuse injuries, improve morale, attention to detail, and overall performance, while at the same time limiting the expense of on-the-job injuries, missed days, and employee turnover.

Even small organizations, special event planners, and individuals are hiring therapists to perform services at various functions, family reunions, parties, and promotions. It is possible to incorporate the use of essential oils in on-site environments, but you need to check with the facility or planner first to determine if there are any policies banning the use of aromas/scents, as some facilities do. Since most on-site massage doesn't include the use of a lubricant, consider other, more subtle methods, such as misting the face cradle with an aromatic spritzer or using a small diffuser if you are working in a private office or kiosk.

Inpatient Hospital or Hospice Setting

As our current model of traditional healthcare continues to grow and evolve, complementary therapies are becoming more and more accepted among doctors, nurses, therapists, and staff. Massage, bodywork, acupuncture, and even aromatherapy

IN PRACTICE 11.1

Aromatherapy in Private Practice, Clinic, or Spa Setting

- Take the time to collect and verify your client's health information. If this is not customary in your facility, be sure to at least ask the basic, necessary questions regarding general health, stress level, and potential allergies before using essential oils in your treatments.

- Never assume that your clients want or even like aromatic oils. Always ask first and be prepared with unscented materials as well.

- For clients who report being very sensitive or not wanting any scent in their treatments, it is especially important to explain the difference between perfume and scented products versus the use of pure essential oils at the proper dilution. Sometimes if they understand the difference they are more apt to want to try a gentle blend with their treatment.

- Insist on using only high-quality, pure, authentic essential oils in your facility.

- Prepare an unscented supply of base oils, lotions, gels, body scrubs, and so forth, then add essential oils to individual portions just prior to each session.

- For common concerns, such as sore muscles, stress, or emotional upsets, make up pre-blended synergies consisting of two or three essential oils each. Then when blending for a specific client, add one or two additional oils based on their personal needs. This saves time, yet it can still become an individualized aromatherapy treatment.

- Have a small variety of basic massage blends, such as "revitalizing," "relaxing," or "harmony" available, then let your client choose.

- Ensure that you have adequate ventilation from a window, air return, or fan.

- If using various essential oils on multiple clients in a given treatment area throughout the day, don't add diffusion or environmental applications on top of it.

- If you use your office or treatment space for creating product, making multiple blends, or a quantity of aromatic treatment materials, try to plan production on days when clients aren't scheduled or after the last appointment of the day.

are cropping up within healthcare institutions around the country. Complementary therapies are often offered in an adjacent building or on the campuses of hospitals or health centers and can also be integrated as a significant part of the inpatient model of care.

If you work in a hospital facility and are a contract or staff employee, you may be given strict guidelines on established policies, such as using only plastic bottles with pump tops, types of lotions or oils that may be used, or permission to access patient chart notes, for example. It is important to discuss your desire to use aromatherapy with massage with the facility first. This may actually take some dedication on your behalf since many in the medical profession still do not understand what holistic aromatherapy is. So be prepared to educate!

Utilizing essential oils in a hospital, hospice, or clinical setting:

▶ Always check with the attending nurse or doctor regarding the current condition of the patient, contraindications, and any site, duration, pressure, or positioning limitations.

▶ Avoid irritating or sensitizing essential oils and steer clear of broken skin or incision sites. Refer to Chapter 3 for safety precautions regarding essential oil use.

▶ Be aware of the increased possibility for deep vein thrombosis (DVT) among individuals with limited activity (e.g., bed bound) and postoperative patients.

▶ Check in with the patient regarding any sensitivities, allergies, or aversions to different aromas.

▶ Use lower dilution rates with special populations and sensitive individuals.

▶ Use caution in a non-private environment so as not to adversely affect neighboring patients with aromas or essential oils. Make sure adequate ventilation is available.

▶ If applying massage oils or lotions to feet, be sure to wipe off excess and replace nonslip socks or slippers on patient before leaving the room.

▶ When working with patients on a hospital bed, raise the bed so as not to place unnecessary strain on your body. Be sure to lower the bed when finished or before leaving the room.

▶ Provide Material Safety Data Sheets (MSDS) on all essential oils being used in a hospital or clinical setting. See Appendix 2.

SUMMARY

▪ To work effectively with a special population clientele, it is important to seek proper training and continued education.

▪ Aromatherapy and prenatal/pregnancy massage can be helpful in alleviating many of the symptoms that accompany pregnancy, including aches and pains, nausea, poor circulation, digestion, insomnia, anxiety, and backache.

▪ When incorporating aromatherapy into prenatal massage, it is recommended that you wait until the pregnancy is well established, usually by the twelfth week.

▪ Infants and children respond quite well to gentle essential oils at low dilutions for a variety of common conditions from sleeplessness to growing pains.

▪ Aromatic massage and bodywork can be pivotal in countering many of the physical and emotional aspects of aging and can be used to positively affect quality of life.

▪ Massage, bodywork, and aromatherapy have a growing role to play in palliative, hospice, and end-of-life care. By maintaining a holistic philosophy and approach, these therapies can positively affect the emotional, spiritual, physical, and social life of the individual whom they work with.

▪ Self-care is a crucial part of being a massage and bodywork therapist, for without it a therapist may experience early burnout or potentially physical and emotional exhaustion.

▪ Massage and bodywork practitioners have a variety of settings in which they are able to practice. The integration of aromatherapy into these different settings can sometimes be challenging but with knowledge, awareness, and careful planning, these obstacles can be easily overcome.

NEW TERMINOLOGY

This chapter does not contain new terminology.

REFERENCES

Associated Bodywork and Massage Professionals (ABMP). (2006). ABMP Member Survey Summary. *Different Strokes, 21* (1).

Buckle, J. (2003). *Clinical Aromatherapy*. New York: Churchill Livingstone.

Field, T. (2001). *Touch*. Boston: First MIT Press.

Field, T., Hernandez-Reif, M., Hart, S., Theakson, H., Seharberg, S., Kuhn, C., and Burman, I. (1998). Pregnant women benefit from massage therapy.

Harris, R. (2005). The use of essential oils in child care. *International Journal of Clinical Aromatherapy*, 2.2, 27–34.

Hospice of Ohio. (n/d). *Massage therapy*. Retrieved on June 20, 2006, from http://www.hospiceohio.org/massage_therapy.asp.

Korn, C. (2003). Taking Care. *Massage Today*, 3 (7).

National Council for Palliative Care. (2005). *Palliative Care Explained*. Retrieved on June 20, 2006, from http://www.ncpc.org.uk/palliative_care.html.

Nelson, D. (2001). Growing Old with Massage in Facility Care. *Massage and Bodywork Magazine*, February/March 2001.

Additional support

England, A. (1994). *Aromatherapy for Mother and Baby*. Rochester, VT: Healing Arts Press.

Fawcett, M. (1993). *Aromatherapy for Pregnancy and Childbirth*. Boston: Element Books, Inc.

Tappan, F., and Benjamin, P. (1998). *Tappan's Handbook of Healing Massage Techniques*. Stamford, CT: Appleton and Lange.

Worwood, V. (1991). *The Complete Book of Essential Oils and Aromatherapy*. Navato, CA: New World Library.

WORKSHEET

Aromatherapy in Practice

Name: _____   Date: _____

Working with Special Populations

1) With your partner, take turns explaining areas in which aromatherapy can benefit at least two of the following special populations:

   - Prenatal and Postpartum Clients
   - Infants and Children
   - Aging and Elderly Clients
   - Terminally Ill and Dying Clients
   - Therapists and Self-Care

2) List four essential oils that you would *not* use on a prenatal client:

   1. _____   3. _____
   2. _____   4. _____

3) List two ways in which you plan to implement self-care techniques over the next week.

   a) _____

   b) _____

4) Create a blend for use with your self-care plan or techniques. 1 oz./ _____ dilution.

   Base: _____ *Total Essential Oil:* _____ drops

Essential Oil—Common Name	Essential Oil—*Latin Name*	Drops	Why Chosen?

5) Design a massage oil blend that could be used for the special population of: _____ 1 oz./ _____ dilution

   Base Oil(s): _____ *Total Essential Oil:* _____ drops

Essential Oil—Common Name	Essential Oil—*Latin Name*	Drops	Why Chosen?

CHAPTER TEST

1. To work with special populations you should:

   a. get started

   b. get the proper training

   c. get better quality essential oils

   d. get another license

2. During pregnancy, women should avoid the following group of essential oils:

   a. lavender and tangerine

   b. frankincense and sandalwood

   c. neroli and Roman chamomile

   d. pennyroyal and wormwood

3. Massage and aromatherapy can help in countering many of the physical and emotional aspects of aging and can enhance quality of life, provide comfort care, and promote healthy aging.

   _____ True_____ False

4. Aging and elderly clients generally:

   a. enjoy bodywork and human touch

   b. don't like to be touched

   c. have too many health problems for massage

   d. have skin that is too thin for aromatherapy

5. Terminally ill and dying clients should be treated:

   a. exactly the same as your other clients

   b. gently and with care

   c. only with lavender

   d. independent of their family or caregiver

6. It is perfectly safe to use just about any essential oil with infants under 6 months of age.

   _____ True_____ False

7. The safest group of essential oils for infants includes:

   a. peppermint and rosemary

   b. thuja and thyme

   c. lemongrass and peppermint

   d. tangerine and lavender

8. List five common prenatal/pregnancy conditions that would benefit from aromatherapy and massage.

   1.

   2.

   3.

   4.

   5.

9. Aromatherapy is meant to be used as a primary treatment for terminal illness.

   _____ True   _____ False

10. Massage therapists and bodyworkers:

    a. need to learn self-care

    b. only need treatments for themselves on special occasions

    c. get enough healing energy from doing the work

    d. should work until they are exhausted

REVIEW QUESTIONS

1. Discuss the special populations you might be interested in working with and where you could get the proper training.

2. What type of practice and location would you like to work in and why?

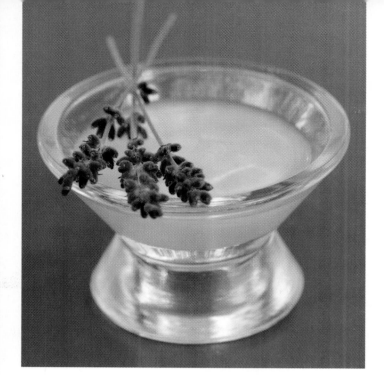

The Business of Aromatherapy

→ LEARNING OBJECTIVES

After reading this chapter, you will be able to

1. Choose a basic set of essential oils to begin your practice with.
2. Choose a basic set of base carriers to begin your practice with.
3. Cost out your essential oils, base materials, and bottles.
4. Discuss basic equipment needs in an aromatherapy practice.
5. Describe general storage needs.
6. Discuss the need for insurance specifically for aromatherapy.
7. List and describe various methods for marketing your aromatherapy business.

INTRODUCTION

As you begin your journey utilizing aromatherapy as a complement to your massage or bodywork practice, you will need to decide upon a number of important issues, such as how will you integrate aromatherapy into your practice; will you customize blends or have a number of pre-blended or generalized blends to work with; how will you charge for aromatherapy; will you provide your client with aromatherapy product to use at home; will you sell aromatherapy product; how will you market your aromatherapy practice; and what type of insurance do you need. This chapter is designed to provide you with some basics about the business of aromatherapy, including necessary supplies, cost accounting, and some marketing tips.

NOTE

Instead of the standard chapter ending like the other chapters in this text, this chapter ends with a series of worksheets to support your introduction of aromatherapy into your practice. Use Appendix 3 and 4 as resources.

⌐▶ AROMATHERAPY SUPPLIES

Throughout this textbook you have learned about forty eight essential oils, a variety of vegetable and specialty oils, as well as other carriers such as creams, lotions, and gels. You have also learned about various equipments that could be used in practice, such as a footbath and hot towel cabinet. Deciding which ones to have in your practice depends upon the goals you have as a practitioner, what type of massage or bodywork you practice, who your clientele is, and what services you would like to offer.

Essential Oils

Beginning your practice in aromatherapy may seem like quite an expensive endeavor; the key is to narrow your potential selection of essential oils to about ten to twenty of the most important essential oils for your type of bodywork or massage technique. If you have decided your practice will be geared mostly toward relaxation massage, then Table 12.1 outlines core essential oils you may want to consider for your practice. If, however, you do mostly treatment work, then Table 12.2 outlines slightly different essential oils to consider. Regardless of what type of massage or bodywork you do, some "must have" essential oils that cover a wide range of therapeutic potential are listed in Table 12.3. It is always wise to start off with essential oils that you enjoy working with and those that are a little more affordable to purchase. Ultimately the choice of essential oils you begin using in your practice is entirely up to you.

Once you have decided on which essential oils you would like to have for your practice, it is a good idea to think about which oils you should have in larger quantities. For instance, lavender can be one of the most used essential oils, and hence it makes sense to purchase 2 to 4 ounces at a time. Neroli, on the other hand, tends to be used less frequently due to cost, and hence it can be purchased in smaller quantities, such as 2 to 5 milliliters.

Vegetable and Specialty Oils and Other Carriers

Like essential oils, which vegetable or specialty oils you choose to incorporate into your practice is entirely up to you. If you don't know what you will be using already, then we suggest you experiment with different oils and other carriers first.

TABLE 12.1

Fifteen Core Essential Oils to Have for Relaxation Bodywork

Essential Oil	Latin Name
Roman chamomile	*Chamaemelum nobile*
Clary sage	*Salvia sclarea*
Frankincense	*Boswellia carterii*
Geranium	*Pelargonium graveolens*
Ginger	*Zingiber officinale*
Lavender	*Lavandula angustifolia*
Mandarin	*Citrus reticulata*
Sweet orange	*Citrus sinensis*
Rose	*Rosa damascena*
Vetiver	*Vetiveria zizanioides*
Ylang ylang	*Cananga odorata*
Bergamot	*Citrus bergamia*
Jasmine	*Jasminum grandiflorum*
Neroli	*Citrus aurantium* var *amara*
Sandalwood	*Santalum album* or *S. spicatum*

TABLE 12.2

Fifteen Core Essential Oils to Have for Treatment Bodywork

Essential Oil	Latin Name
Black pepper	*Piper nigrum*
German chamomile	*Matricaria recutita*
Clary sage	*Salvia sclarea*
Eucalyptus	*Eucalyptus globulus*
Ginger	*Zingiber officinale*
Helichrysum	*Helichrysum italicum*
Juniper	*Juniperus communis*
Lavender	*Lavandula angustifolia*
Lemon	*Citrus limon*
Peppermint	*Mentha* x *piperita*
Rosemary ct. camphor and ct. cineole	*Rosmarinus officinalis*
Birch	*Betula lenta* or *B. alleghaniensis*
Clove bud	*Syzygium aromaticum*
Laurel	*Laurus nobilis*
Scots pine	*Pinus sylvestris*

TABLE 12.3
Fifteen Core Essential Oils for Mixed Practice

Essential Oil	Latin Name
Roman chamomile	*Chamaemelum nobile*
Clary sage	*Salvia sclarea*
Eucalyptus	*Eucalyptus globulus*
Fennel	*Foeniculum vulgare*
Frankincense	*Boswellia carterii*
Geranium	*Pelargonium graveolens*
Ginger	*Zingiber officinale*
Lavender	*Lavandula angustifolia*
Peppermint	*Mentha x piperita*
Rosemary ct. camphor and ct. cineole	*Rosmarinus officinalis*
Tea tree	*Melaleuca alternifolia*
Vetiver	*Vetiveria zizanioides*
Ylang ylang	*Cananga odorata*
And at least two citrus oils: Grapefruit (*Citrus paradisi*),**Lemon** (*Citrus limon*), **Mandarin** (*Citrus reticulata*), **Sweet Orange** (*Citrus sinensis*),or **Bergamot** (*Citrus bergamia*)	

You can usually purchase a small quantity for this purpose. That way you don't waste any oil or money. One of my favorite blends of vegetable oil is 50 percent apricot kernel, 40 percent organic sunflower, and 10 percent organic jojoba. Most massage therapists and bodyworkers will utilize a wide range of bases, including oils, creams, lotions, and gels.

Bottles and Jars

When purchasing bottles (Figure 12-1), it is best to order in large quantities if possible. If you can, find someone to go in on an order with you. The more bottles you buy the less they will cost.

Standard bottles for an aromatherapy massage practice include:

1 or 2 oz. amber glass or PET plastic bottles

1 or 2 oz. amber glass or PET plastic jars

8 oz. PET plastic bottles with pumps to fit in a holster (optional for larger amounts of day-to-day pre-blended massage lotions)

2 or 4 oz. amber or blue cobalt glass bottles with spray tops for aromatic spritzers or hydrosols

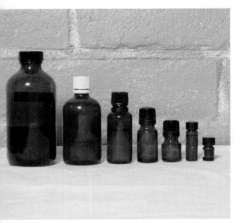

Figure 12-1 Glass essential oil bottles
Source: © Dennis Gallaher

↳ COSTING OUT YOUR PRODUCTS

One of the most important items in the development of an aromatherapy practice is pricing your services and products properly to ensure you are covering your cost and making a profit. When practioners first start selling essential oils, many often forget to add shipping costs to the end price and quickly discover that they are losing money. This can be costly for any practice, so here are a few useful tips on costing your products for aromatherapy.

Basic Cost Accounting: How Much Did It Really Cost You?

When costing out essential oils, or any other product you plan to utilize or carry, it is important to know what items should be included in your costing, such as shipping cost and possible spillage. If you bought your essential oils from a supplier who shipped them to you, then you will have incurred shipping costs or if you bought them from a local shop by driving there, then most likely you spent money on gas. Depending on how many oils you bought and their sizes, you need to add in additional cost for shipping or gas. For instance, let's say you placed the following order from a supplier who shipped them to you. The invoice looked like this:

1 oz Roman Chamomile	$ 49.00
4 oz Eucalyptus	$ 15.00
2 ml Neroli	$ 32.00
10 ml Ginger	$ 12.00
8 oz Lavender	$ 75.00
Shipping cost:	$ 15.00
Total Cost:	$198.00

To figure out the cost for each essential oil:

Step 1: Attach additional cost for shipping to each essential oil by dividing the total shipping cost by the total number of essential oils purchased.

1 oz Roman Chamomile	$ 49.00 + 3. = 52.00
4 oz Eucalyptus	$ 15.00 + 3. = 18.00
2 ml Neroli	$ 32.00 + 3. = 35.00
10 ml Ginger	$ 12.00 + 3. = 15.00
8 oz Lavender	$ 75.00 + 3. = 78.00

Step 2: Figure out how much each drop and milliliter cost. Remember there are approximately 20 drops per milliliter and 30 milliliters per ounce. Also, because there is a possibility of spillage or some loss of essential oil from pipettes, you can reduce your total drops by at least 5 to 10 drops to make up for this loss.

30 mls Roman Chamomile 52 ÷ 30 ml = 1.73 per ml

If there are 20 drops per ml, then there would be 600 drops in a 1 oz. bottle less spillage. This would be 600 − 10 = 590 drops.

4 oz Eucalyptus	18/120 ml = 0.15 per ml
120 mls × 20 drops = 240 drops	
less spillage (10 drops)	18/230 = 0.08 per ml

Step 3: If you are selling essential oils as synergies, single notes, or in a blend for clients to take home, you also need to factor in the cost of the bottle or jar and label. There are wholesale bottle distributors listed in Appendix 3. Decide how much each bottle costs you with shipping, then add it in the next step.

Step 4: Decide how much you are going to charge per drop or ml to earn a profit. Typically a markup of at least 100 percent is done to make a profit, which means you would double the cost.

Roman chamomile   Cost 1.73 per ml × 2 = 3.46 per ml
                              Cost .09 per drop × 2 = .18 per drop

This is great for determining how much it is costing you to include aromatherapy in your treatments. If, however, this is part of a blend or take-home synergy, also add:

Base Material (lotion, oil, gel, etc.) Cost .45 per oz. × 1 oz.
                                        (or number of ounces used)
Bottle and Label   Cost .25
Essential Oils   Cost .72 (total cost based on per drop
                                        of each oil used)
                    Total Cost: $1.42 for a 1 oz. lotions
                                        × 2 =
                    Total Retail Cost: $2.84 for a 1 oz. lotion

Step 5: Write up a sheet that details pricing for each essential oil you will be using in your practice, as well as basic carrier materials, bottles, and labels. Keep on hand for figuring out the total cost of treatments and products.

IN PRACTICE 12.1

Pricing Exercise

On a separate sheet of paper, figure out the cost of neroli, ginger, and lavender.

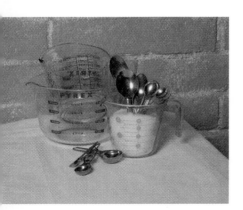

Figure 12-2 Measuring equipment
Source: © Dennis Gallaher

⤷ OTHER EQUIPMENT

There are so many great tools and products on the market today that are designed to supplement a massage therapist's practice. In the interest of starting out with a few key pieces of equipment at a minimal investment, here are a few to consider when incorporating aromatherapy in your practice.

The Basics

▶ glass measuring cups in a few sizes, including an extra-large 8-cup Pyrex for mixing bath salts, larger batches of scrubs, etc.
▶ smaller cups for blending lesser amounts of messy creams and such
▶ good set of stainless measuring spoons

▶ bowls ranging in size from tiny to medium, in glazed ceramic or glass, for holding aromatic materials during treatments (Figure 12-3)

▶ plastic spatula and larger serving spoon for scooping

▶ Stir sticks: Glass rods can be obtained from a science supply shop, but wood sticks can work too; just don't leave the end of the wood sitting in the blend during your treatment or for an extended period as it will absorb the oils.

▶ An electric blender with a glass pitcher for making creams, lotions, and larger batches of product. An electric hand mixer is also a very beneficial tool, as it tends to prevent hand and wrist stirring exhaustion.

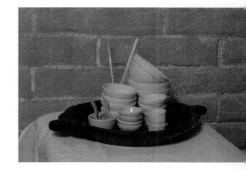

Figure 12-3 Mixing bowls
Source: © Dennis Gallaher

Footbaths

You can purchase a whirlpool-type model that is made of sturdy plastic, plugs into the wall, and will create bubbles and a vibratory action on the feet. Some of the fancier models even add heat and colored light therapy! The downside to these units is that they can be noisy and cumbersome at best, difficult to clean at worse. Large, flat-bottomed ceramic bowls are quiet, beautifully elegant, easy to clean, and relatively affordable if you can scout one out at an antique store or market. This piece is a must-have, as aromatic footbaths go a long way in creating an aromatherapy-based practice.

Hot Towel Cabinet

A hot towel cabinet is an effective way to heat a large number of towels for use throughout the day, but it can be somewhat costly for an initial purchase. The hot towel cabinet also requires you to use several more towels per client because the towels need to be placed back into the cabinet within a few minutes of being applied to client, in order to be reheated. A Crock-Pot or large stainless steel cooking pot on an electric burner, on the other hand, can be a wonderful tool at a minimum investment. This way you can use fewer towels or clothes and return them to the pot for reheating throughout the course of the massage or treatment. Plus, wringing them out each time creates a lovely sound of trickling water that is very relaxing during a session. If it's large enough, you can also use this same piece of equipment for heating larger linens for wraps, for example. The drawback here is that you either have to have several pots or time to wash it out thoroughly between clients. You also have to become very good at getting the temperature just right so you don't burn yourself or your client, whereas the hot towel cabinets stay pretty well regulated in temperature.

Diffuser

What respectable aromatherapist would be without their diffuser? Purchase an electronic nebulizer that will actually suspend essential oil molecules in the environment or an electric or candle version that simply heats a small dish of water to which you've added a few drops of essential oil. Either way, this tool will help you to create an aromatic experience from the moment someone enters your space.

Clean Up

Use rubbing alcohol in a spray bottle and wipe bottles and equipment to remove essential oil and carrier oil residue. Plenty of hot soapy water is also required. Have lots of paper towels on hand and protect wood counters or work surfaces from essential oil damage. Consider wearing an apron to further protect clothing from oil stains. Reusing lotion bottles or jars for repackaging fresh goods is not recommended unless you have the equipment and knowledge of proper sterilization techniques.

STORAGE NEEDS

Considering that essential oils prefer to be stored in a cool, dark place, you wouldn't want to leave them out on a windowsill or shelf that receives sunlight during the day. That being said, just about any little box or cabinet in a cool room will suffice. If possible, store your essential oils in a carrying box and place in a refrigerator either at work or at home.

Labeling your essential oil bottles on the top can be incredibly helpful in finding each oil without having to pick up the whole bottle. Attach a small round sticker with the name to the top of each bottle cap. However you decide to set up, just make sure you have plenty of space in your treatment area to have the minimum supplies required close at hand, as well as a sturdy work surface for blending.

INSURANCE COVERAGE

Each therapist should check with their professional liability policy to ensure that the use of essential oils is covered as part of their regular coverage as a licensed massage therapist. Each company handles things, such as the addition of aromatherapy or other modalities, slightly differently. Some will even insure the products you blend and sell up to a certain quantity, so long as it doesn't become disproportionate to your primary therapy business. If you intend to produce and sell larger amounts of aromatherapy products in your business, then you may need to investigate other insurance policies that further cover product liability. You can contact the Indie Beauty Network (www.indiebeauty.com).

MARKETING AROMATHERAPY IN YOUR SETTING

Some practitioners choose to charge extra for using essential oils in a treatment, while others include it as part of their session to help set their services apart. Still others prefer a combination approach: offering a basic, pre-blended aromatic experience as part of their standard session and customized, true aromatherapy blends upon request and at an additional charge. How you set this up as a therapist is truly based on personal preference and sound business strategy. However you do it, just make sure you're taking into account the cost of base materials and essential oils for each treatment and covering your expenses one way or another. Additional tips on integrating and marketing aromatherapy in your practice:

■ Educate the clients and staff. Education is key to properly using and understanding essential oils. Explain what true aromatherapy is and be clear about the nature and benefits of the services you offer.

■ Create your own informational brochure or purchase preprinted materials that clients can take home that further explains aromatherapy and the healing properties of essential oils.

■ Decide how you want to incorporate aromatherapy into your practice, then get it on your regular menu of services. Let your clients know how excited you are about aromatherapy and the benefits of essential oils. Make sure they know you're dedicated to using only quality oils and skilled techniques. You can include aromatherapy in many of the existing treatments or modalities you currently offer or create new treatments specifically designed as either an aromatic experience or a true aromatherapy session.

■ Develop seasonal specials that center around a particular blend or "scent," such as a spice-scented body mask for fall or a citrus salt glow for summer. Create multiple treatments and even products that can be purchased and used at home, all in the same blend. Market the special like crazy, tell everyone you meet how wonderful it is, print flyers or postcards, and make signs for in your waiting area. Be sure to include an end date for the promotion as this will serve as a call to action for some clients. Use a little of the product on everyone who comes in or have a sample available for them to try, even if they're not there for the seasonal special on that particular visit. Once they try a little of your special blend, they'll book a session and return for it!

■ Host an educational event, such as a tea or short class, where you can introduce prospective and existing clients to aromatherapy and specific essential oils as well as the types of bodywork services you offer. Answer questions and consider doing brief demonstrations or giving out free samples. Make it fun and keep it light, but peak their interest.

■ Make sure to use an aromatic spritzer on the face cradle cover or maybe as a finishing touch to mist your clients at the end of each session. Also, keep a spritzer, lotion, hand-wash, and other samples in the restrooms for clients to try.

■ Occasionally, if a client has had a particularly rough time and you think it helpful, you might make up a 1 oz. custom blend while they get on the table. Use it in the session and send them home with the rest. Let them know it's on the house; you are acknowledging them, you care about their feelings and current state or situation.

■ If you want to entice new customers by running a sale or promotion, it is usually better to offer a free aromatic gift when they purchase a service rather than offering money off the regular session price. If done properly, this will be a great perceived value to your customers, and you will earn more money on each transaction, as it should cost less for you to make a product than give money away. Plus, more clients will experience your aromatic blends, which may lead to more aromatherapy treatments and additional product sales in the future.

■ Remember, you are your best advertising. Use the essential oils in your own day-to-day life. Find out what works well and share your experiences with clients, friends, and family. Let people know how excited you are to have found such a wonderful, helpful gift of nature. Share your knowledge and love of aromatherapy with everyone you meet and let them know where your office is located and what services your provide.

IN PRACTICE 12.2

Sharing Aromatherapy

I like to pour dram-size bottles of various essential oils to take with me on long trips. This way I have the oils with me should I need them for any unexpected occurrence, such as sunburn, dry skin, motion sickness, constipation, or sleeplessness.

But what I like to do most is give them to people I meet along the way, one oil at a time. One of my favorite parts of travel is meeting and talking with people from different parts of the world. Oftentimes during a conversation I'll pick up on subtle (or sometimes not so subtle) hints as to which oil I should leave in their keeping. I enjoy the opportunity to share, however briefly, some of the benefits of aromatherapy. I also mention basic safety precautions when giving an undiluted essential oil away.

↪ CONTINUING YOUR EDUCATION

One of the best things about massage and bodywork is that once you've learned what you need to earn your license, you've basically earned a license to keep on learning. There are so many specialties to master and paths one can travel in this work. Aromatherapy is much the same way. It is not only a modality or technique, but for many it is a way of life.

All knowledge is yours for the taking, and once you've got it no one can take it from you! Developing a specialty or niche that sets you apart from so many other therapists out there will not only make you very good at what you do, but also create a differential advantage to your business or marketability as a therapist.

Now that you have the basics, feel free to play, to experiment, and to practice. Like most things in life, there's always more to learn. So if you are inclined, please seek out additional training on the subject. Educational resources are provided in Appendix 4.

Aromatherapy in Practice (Part I)

Marketing Aromatherapy

1) In the space below, outline a 4" × 6" postcard design (front and back) promoting something special about aromatherapy that you would want your clients to know about.

Front

Back

Aromatherapy in Practice (Part II)

Based on the 48 essential oils covered in this textbook, choose fifteen essential oils you would like to have in your practice, decide what sizes you would like to purchase, and research aromatherapy companies to purchase from. Once you have the necessary information, figure out how much each essential oil will cost you by the milliliter and by the drop (remember to add in shipping charges, gas, and possible spillage). Use the chart below to fill in information.

Essential Oil	Size	Total Cost to Purchase	Cost per ml	Cost per Drop

Aromatherapy in Practice (Part III)

Throughout this textbook and within this chapter you have learned about various supplies you may want to have in your practice. In the table below, fill in each section with the items you would like to have in practice and then spend time researching how much it will cost you to get these supplies into your business.

General Groups	Specific Needs	Cost of Product
Base Oils and Other Carriers	e.g., Apricot Kernel	$25.00 per gallon
Bottles	e.g., 1 oz. amber bottles	$75.00 for case of 250 bottles
Equipment	Foot bath	$25.00 for electric bath
Other Supplies	e.g., table for working on	$50.00

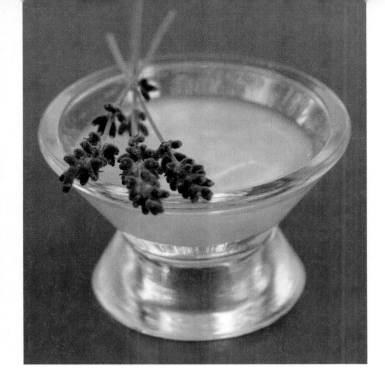

Exploring 48 Essential Oils

24 Essential Oils: In Depth
24 Essential Oils: The Basics

⟶ LEARNING OBJECTIVES

After careful study of this chapter, for each essential oil you will be able to

1. Recognize and state the common and Latin name
2. Identify the botanical family
3. Identify key odor characteristics
4. Identify the blending factor number
5. Describe two therapeutic properties
6. Describe five core aromatic applications
7. Discuss and apply knowledge of safety data
8. Identify the chemical feature/s

INTRODUCTION

This section will explore twenty-four essential oils in depth and an additional twenty-four essential oils in short that can be safely and effectively integrated into a massage therapy or bodywork practice. Each data sheet provides the most current and up-to-date information available on each essential oil. There is a limitless array of clinical trials along with a growing history of empirical uses for each essential oil, and an attempt has been made to focus on each oil's core properties along with other identifying features. The essential oil data sheets provide information on the common and Latin names, botany and history, blending data, chemical information, therapeutic activity, and core aromatic applications for each essential oil. An additional twenty-four essential oils have been covered with the basics, focusing on their therapeutic applications and safety information.

↳ READING AN ESSENTIAL OIL DATA SHEET

Common Name and Latin Name

▪ **Common name:** The common name is provided on the top of each data sheet. When plants have additional common names (synonyms) used in different parts of the world or names that have a historical use, these are placed under the botany section as Other common names.

▪ **Latin binomial:** The Latin binomial is next to the common name and designates the exact genus and species of the essential oil to be portrayed. The data sheets utilize the correct botanical format of Genus, Species, Botanist. The botanist who is attributed with having named the species is noted by an initial or shortened format of his/her last name, for instance, *Lavandula* (genus) *angustifolia* (species) L. (Linnaeus: botanist to name this plant). Occasionally a plant has more than one botanical name, which is represented with the word syn or synonym that means "the same as." Throughout the book, the use of the essential oil Latin binomial will lack the inclusion of the botanist name or initial. It is included here for accuracy.

> **NOTE**
>
> All Latin names have been verified by using Germplasm Resources Information Network and the United States Department of Agriculture, Natural Resources Conservation Service.

Botany and History Information

▪ **Botanical family:** Each essential oil-bearing plant belongs to a specific botanical family. Often a group of plants within one given botanical family will have common characteristics, whether chemically or in therapeutic action. Occasionally there are two names, one followed by the word "syn," meaning "the same as." The first name is the most current and accepted name while the second one is its formerly accepted name. This can be helpful in researching an essential oil as information will be listed under both the older and modern names.

▪ **Botany:** This section provides a basic description of the plant from which the essential oil is derived.

■ **History and myth:** This section contains historical/mythical information on the essential oil.

Extraction Information

■ **Country of origin:** The country of origin reflects the country where the essential oil is either indigenous or where it is cultivated or harvested in the wild and distilled. The country of origin can have an effect on the quality of the oil produced. For instance, many aromatherapists believe Bulgarian rose (*Rosa damascena*) to be far superior to Turkish rose of the same species and Lavender (*Lavandula angustifolia*) from the high altitudes of France to be superior to the Tasmanian, Croatian, or American essential oil from the same species.

■ **Part of plant used:** This is the part of the plant distilled to obtain the essential oil. Please note: The term "flowering tops" means that the flowers and top leaves are distilled.

■ **Extraction method:** The most common method of extraction is provided.

■ **Oil yield:** The oil yield reflects the amount of essential oil found within the plant material.

■ **Color of oil:** A description of the color of the individual essential oil is provided.

Blending Information

■ **Odor description:** The general description of the aroma of the individual essential oil is provided.

■ **Blending factor:** The blending factor is a means to measure the aromatic strength of an essential oil. It is described more completely in Chapter 5.

Safety Information

This section lists the current safety data for the essential oil.

Chemical Feature

Each essential oil has what are considered to be active or major chemical constituents that are thought to influence their therapeutic activity. For instance, an essential oil rich in esters is considered to be generally calming to the nervous system whereas an essential oil rich in phenols will be highly effective as an antimicrobial agent. The chemical feature section is a summary of these key chemical constituents found within the given essential oil. See Chapter 4 for further details.

Chemical Profile

This section lists a small sample of general chemical constituents found within the specified essential oil, listing percentages for major components.

Therapeutic Actions

This section details the known pharmacological activity of the essential oil. The actions listed are those that have either empirical acceptance or can be supported by research. The core actions for which the oil is most used and known for are highlighted in bold text.

Keywords: A small collection of core attributes are expressed as keywords. These are words that may first arise when considering the application of the oil.

Core Aromatic Applications

This section is designed to list the most common and traditional uses of the essential oil. Like the therapeutic actions section, these applications are those with either strong empirical acceptance or those that can be supported by research. It is common in the majority of aromatherapy books to have somewhat of an exhaustive list of potential actions and applications; however, this can be overwhelming and at times inaccurate or misleading. The core aromatic applications section attempts to provide a more focused presentation of therapeutic potentials of the specified essential oil, as supported by empirical acceptance or clinical research.

In Practice: Sample Blends

This section will provide two sample blends for each essential oil.

↪ ESSENTIAL OIL DATA SHEETS

Black Pepper / *Piper nigrum* L.

Botany and History Information

Botanical family: Piperaceae

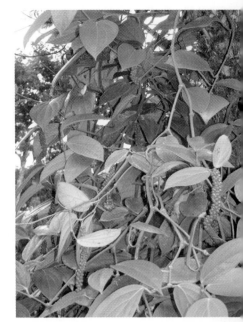

Figure 13-1 Black pepper
Source: Reprinted by permission of David Monniaux

Botany: Black pepper is native to the hills of western India. *Piper nigrum* is a tropical, perennial, woody climber to 20 feet, sometimes taller. Several Piper species have variable physical characteristics. Cultivars are generally hermaphrodite. The leaves are heart-shaped and of a dark green color. The black, white, and green peppercorns are products of the same plant. The green pepper is the whole fresh berry and when dried in the sun becomes black. White peppercorns come from the mature berry that has the skin removed and is then dried. The vines are found in moist soil, particularly in the low-lying forests of monsoon Asia.

History and myth: Black pepper has been used in Ayurvedic medicine for thousands of years. It was an important spice in early East-West trading. Pepper is mentioned in the writings of the early Romans. According to Grieve (1982), Attila the Hun is known to have demanded 3,000 pounds of pepper in ransom for the city of Rome (p. 627). During the time of Hippocrates pepper was used as both a spice for food and as a medicine. It has been employed for treatments of the stomach, for excess gas, and in fever preparations. The Asian world has long considered black pepper to be an important spice for detoxifying and as an antiaging compound.

Extraction Information

Countries of origin:	Indonesia, Malaysia, Madagascar, China, India
Part of plant used:	berries (peppercorns), unripe dried fruit
Extraction method:	steam distillation
Oil content:	1.0 to 4.0 percent
Color of oil:	clear to pale yellow/green

Blending Information

Odor description:	pungent, peppery, spicy, warming
Blending factor:	3 to 4

Safety information:

▶ undiluted application can irritate the skin
▶ avoid use on facial skin
▶ avoid use on infants and young children

Chemical Feature

Rich in monoterpenes supported by sesquiterpenes.

Chemical Profile

Monoterpenes (70 to 90%): limonene (up to 20%), β-pinene (up to 25%), p-cymene (up to 28%), β-phellandrene (up to 20%).

Sesquiterpenes: β-caryophyllene (9 to 33%)

Therapeutic Actions

Analgesic, antibacterial, antimicrobial, antiseptic, antispasmodic, **antiviral**, aphrodisiac, **carminative**, detoxicant, diaphoretic, **digestive**, diuretic, febrifuge, **rubefacient**, **stimulant** (**digestive and circulatory**), stomachic, tonic to nervous system.

Keywords: stimulating, warming, strengthening to the will, empowering

Core Aromatic Applications

Circulatory system: sluggish circulation, chilblains, Raynaud's syndrome, sensitivity to cold

Digestive system: indigestion, encourages peristaltic movement, flatulence, sluggish digestion, may stimulate appetite

Musculoskeletal system: muscular aches and pains, sciatica, pain relief, rheumatism, muscle stiffness, arthritic pain relief

Nervous system: neuritis, peripheral neuropathy, fatigue

Respiratory system: colds, flu, bronchitis, chills, catarrh, smoking cessation aid (Rose and Behm, 1994)

Psyche and emotion: general fatigue, emotional coldness, apathy, low endurance, nervousness, weakness of will, fragile nerves, loss of motivation, mental and emotional exhaustion, insecure with self or others

Subtle/energetic aromatherapy: Represents strength, courage, and strong conviction; can be used to strengthen an individual's intention; can help with motivation, endurance, and stamina; can be employed for emotional blockages, indecision, emotional coldness, apathy, and mental fatigue (Worwood, 1996). Mojay (1997) writes: "Black pepper oil can help to restore a sense of determination—an unwavering single-mindedness that stems from an inner connection with one's *Hara* or *Tanden*, the key vital centre that is situated below the navel."

In Practice: Sample Recipes Using Black Pepper

Muscular Aches and Pains with Spasms	Digestive Tonic
Black pepper	Black pepper
Peppermint	Ginger
Lavender	Lemon

German Chamomile / *Matricaria recutita* L. syn. *Chamomilla recutita* L. syn. *Matricaria chamomilla* L.

Botany and History Information

Other common names: Hungarian Chamomile, Wild Chamomile

Botanical family: Asteraceae syn. Compositae

Botany: German chamomile is an annual herbaceous plant growing to 1 to 2 feet. The daisylike white flowers and yellow center are strongly aromatic. Unlike Roman chamomile, whose leaves and flowers are strongly aromatic, only the flowers of German chamomile yield its beautiful aroma. German chamomile blooms during the late spring to early summer. It does not like the heat of the middle and the end of summer. It is a native of parts of Europe and Asia.

History and myth: German chamomile has been an important medicinal plant since ancient times and was highly prized by the Egyptians, Greeks, and Romans. Its name is derived from the Greek *chamos* (ground) and *melos* (apple), referring to its manner of growth as well as its sweet applelike aroma. Hippocrates, Dioscorides, and Galen are all known to have employed German chamomile in medicinal preparations.

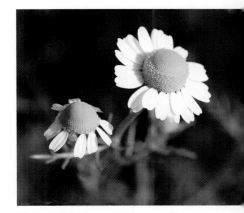

Figure 13-2 German chamomile
Source: Reprinted by permission of Peter Firus

Extraction Information

Countries of origin:	Hungary, Eastern Europe, North America, Australia
Part of plant used:	flowers
Extraction method:	distillation
Oil content:	0.4 to 1.0 percent
Color of oil:	Dark blue. This essential oil is known to oxidize rapidly, turning the color from blue to green and then to brown. Once the essential oil has oxidized it should not be used, as it is no longer of therapeutic value.

Blending Information

Odor description:	sweet, strong, similar to hay, herby aroma
Blending factor:	1

Safety information:

▶ patch test individuals prone to hypersensitivities, particularly to ragweed, which is in the same botanical family

Chemical Feature

Rich in sesquiterpenes, chamazulene, and the sesquiterpene alcohol, (-)-α-bis-abolol.

Chemical Profile

> **Sesquiterpenes: chamazulene** (up to 36%), trans-α-farnesene (up to 25%)
> **Alcohols: (-)-α-bisabolol** (up to 67%)

Therapeutic Actions

Analgesic, antiallergenic, antibacterial, antifungal, **anti-inflammatory**, antirheumatic, antiseptic, **antispasmodic**, carminative, digestive, **muscle relaxant**, **nervine**, **sedative**, stomachic, sudorific, vulnerary.

Keywords: anti-inflammatory, sedative, stress and anxiety relieving, wound/skin healer

Core Aromatic Applications

> **Digestive system:** stress-related digestive upset, general digestive complaints, gastrointestinal spasms, hemorrhoids, colic, swollen gums
>
> **Lymph and immune system:** fever
>
> **Musculoskeletal system:** fibromyalgia, shin splints, spasm, cramps, plantar fasciitis, tendinitis, carpal tunnel syndrome, aches and pains, rheumatism, pain or swelling in joints, bursitis
>
> **Nervous system:** nervous irritability, mild sleep disorders, headaches
>
> **Reproductive/endocrine system:** menstrual cramps or pain, PMS, cracked nipples, postpartum anxiety, dysmenorrhea, emotions associated with menopause
>
> **Respiratory system:** inflammation and irritation of the upper respiratory tract
>
> **Skin:** inflammatory dermatosis and eczema (Blumenthal et al., 1998), acne, inflamed skin conditions, burns, dry itchy skin, wounds, cuts and scrapes, dermabrasion from tattoos; reduces weeping and supports tissue healing (Blumenthal et al., 1998), bacterial skin diseases, broken capillaries, burns including radiation burns, slow-healing wounds, diaper rash, postpartum perineal healing, bedsores
>
> **Psyche and emotion:** agitation, anger, fits, hyperactivity in children, stress-related conditions, anxiety, challenging behavior, self-injury, head banging (w/mentally challenged and autistic children)
>
> **Subtle/energetic aromatherapy:** Has a calm, peaceful, and healing presence; eases the tension of excessive ego-desire and the frustration, resentment, and depression that frequently follow; in TCM, the chamomiles smooth the flow of the body's *Qi-energy*. (Mojay, 1997); helps one to communicate without anger, harmful ego, or animosity and can assist in lessening emotional tension (Leigh, 2001). Leigh recommends German chamomile for the throat chakra.

In Practice: Sample Recipes Using German Chamomile

Anti-Inflammatory Blend	Stress Relief Blend
German chamomile	German chamomile
Helichrysum	Mandarin
Lavender	Patchouli

Roman Chamomile / *Chamaemelum nobile* L. All. syn *Anthemis nobilis* L.

Botany and History Information

Other common names: English Chamomile

Botanical family: Asteraceae syn. Compositae

Botany: A compact, low-growing perennial found in Europe, particularly the Mediterranean region. Roman chamomile has feathery leaves and is a great ground cover. It is strongly aromatic throughout the leaves and flowers. From late spring to early fall, the plant sends out numerous small daisylike flowers.

History and myth: Roman chamomile has been used medicinally since ancient times. During Saxon times, Roman chamomile was known as maythen and was considered to be a sacred herb. During Tudor times, chamomile was used to create aromatic lawns and was often found growing under swings and around benches. The Greeks referred to Roman chamomile as "kamai melon" or ground-apple as its aroma was reminiscent of ripening apples. This characteristic was also noted by the Spaniards who called it "Manzanilla" or "little apple." Throughout the Middle Ages it was a common strewing herb to clean and purify the air as well as to impart its aroma.

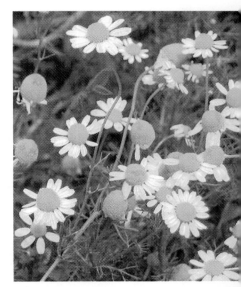

Figure 13-3 Roman chamomile

Extraction Information

Countries of origin:	Italy, France, United States
Part of plant used:	flowers
Extraction method:	distillation
Oil content:	0.4 to 1.0 percent
Color of oil:	yellow, pale yellow to clear

Blending Information

Odor description:	sweet, fruity, applelike, strong
Blending factor:	1

Safety information:

▶ patch test individuals prone to hypersensitivities, particularly to ragweed, which is in the same botanical family

Chemical Feature

Rich in esters (approximately 80%)

Chemical Profile

Sesquiterpenes: sabinene (0 to 10%), caryophyllene (0 to 10%), chamazulene

Aldehydes: myrtenal (0 to 10%)

Esters (75 to 80%): isobutyl angelate (13.1%), propyl angelate (9 to 12%), isobutyl butyrate (15 to 25%), 3-methylpentyl angelate (16%)

Therapeutic Actions

Mild analgesic, antidiuretic, antifungal, **anti-inflammatory**, **antimicrobial**, **antispasmodic**, digestive, febrifuge, **nervine**, **sedative**, **vulnerary**.

Keywords: soothing, anti-inflammatory, anger, temper tantrums (children), wound healing, powerful antispasmodic

Core Aromatic Applications

Head: abscess, conjunctivitis (use Roman chamomile floral water), earache, toothache and teething pain

Digestive system: indigestion, colic, stress-related digestive upsets, hemorrhoids

Musculoskeletal system: spasm, cramps, plantar fasciitis, tendonitis, fibromyalgia, carpal tunnel syndrome, bursitis

Nervous system: headache, insomnia, migraine, hyperactivity in children

Lymph and immune system: fever, chronic fatigue syndrome (symptomatic relief and increase quality of life)

Reproductive/endocrine system: dysmenorrhea, cramps, PMS, irregular periods, sore breasts, postpartum perineal healing

Respiratory system: could be helpful for hayfever, coughs

Skin: dermatitis, eczema, psoriasis, broken capillaries, hives, acne, fungal infections, skin ulcers, slow-healing wounds

Psyche and emotion: anxiety, overactive mind, anger, sensitive people who feel misunderstood or badly hurt, frustration, agitation, nervous stress, anger fits, hyperactivity in children, stress-related conditions, challenging behavior, self-injury/mutilation

Subtle/energetic aromatherapy: For TCM work, Roman chamomile smoothes the flow of the body's *Qi-energy* and regulates the movement of vital energy to relax the nerves, relieve spasm, and ease pain (Mojay, 1997). Leigh (2001) recommends Roman chamomile for healing on the highest spiritual levels as it can assist in seeking higher spiritual truths and channeling information into awareness. Leigh also says that, Roman chamomile can be used for crown chakra work.

Research Notes and Additional Information

According to *PDR for Herbal Medicine* (2000), "The essential oil of Roman chamomile has been found to be active against gram-positive bacteria and dermatomyces. The drug is also cytostatic and acts on the central nervous system, causing a reduction of aggressive behavior in animal tests" (p. 270).

In Practice: Sample Recipes Using Roman Chamomile

Plantar Fasciitis	Sleepy-Time Support
Roman chamomile	Roman chamomile
Lavender	Geranium
Clary sage	Mandarin
Peppermint	Lavender

Clary Sage / *Salvia sclarea* L.

Botany and History Information

Other common names: Clear eye, See bright, Eyebright (Simon et al., 1984), Europe sage, Clarywort

Botanical family: Lamiaceae syn. Labiatae

Botany: *Salvia sclarea* is a medium-sized perennial or biennial, which can grow up to 2 to 3 feet. It is native to Mediterranean countries. Clary sage has an abundance of small blue to purple and white flowers that grow out of large pinky/purple bracts. The leaves are medium-sized heart- or oblong-shaped and are slightly wrinkled. It grows well in loose dry soil. It is cultivated in Central Europe, England, Morocco, the United States and parts of the former Soviet Republic.

History and myth: The English name Clary is derived from the Latin name *sclarea*, a word derived from *clarus* meaning clear. Clary sage has been called "Clear eye" due to the effects the infused seeds have for clearing the eyes from any irritation or infection. Grieve (1982) points out that "Clary sage was listed in the herbals of Hellenic and Roman times, and it has a long history of use in both official Greek/Western medicine and in the unofficial, unwritten tradition of European wise woman healers" (p. 203). Clary sage has been used to make beer in the U.K. and was considered to be quite intoxicating and exhilarating. A wine has also been made with the herb. It was employed during the Middle Ages for its medicinal benefits. Clary sage seems to have fallen into disuse over the years although it continues to be employed in perfumes for its fixative properties and by tobacco companies for its relaxing effect on the nervous system.

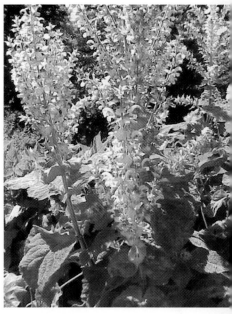

Figure 13-4 Clary sage
Source: Reprinted by permission of Kurt Stueber

Extraction Information

Countries of origin:	France, Germany, Russia
Part of plant used:	Flowering tops
Extraction method:	Distillation
Oil content:	0.12 to 0.15 percent
Color of oil:	Colorless to pale yellow

Blending Information

Odor description:	sweet, nutty, floral, earthy
Blending factor:	2 to 3

Safety information:

▶ nonirritating, nonsensitizing
▶ may increase the effects of alcohol and pain medications
▶ may be prudent to avoid overuse or high dosages during the first trimester or with a woman in unstable pregnancy

Chemical Feature

Major components include sedative alcohol, linalol (up to 20%), and up to 75 percent esters, specifically linalyl acetate.

Chemical Profile

Alcohols: linalol (8.88 to 8.48%), citronellol, nerol, geraniol, borneol, terpinen-4-ol, α bisabol, sclareol (0.2 to 2%)

Esters: linalyl acetate (49 to 74.18%), citronellyl acetate, geranyl acetate, neryl acetate

Therapeutic Actions

Anticonvulsive, **antidepressant**, **antispasmodic**, **aphrodisiac**, balsamic, carminative, deodorant, emmenagogue, **euphoric**, **harmone balance** hypotensive, muscle relaxant, nervine, **parturient**, sedative, stomachic, **uterine relaxant**.

Keywords: feminine (hormone balancer), euphoric, aphrodisiac, antidepressant, antispasmodic, central nervous system relaxant

Core Aromatic Applications

Circulatory system: varicose veins, hemorrhoids, broken capillaries

Musculoskeletal system: aches and pains, arthritis, rheumatism, powerful muscle relaxant, shin splints, spasms, cramps, sciatica, carpal tunnel syndrome, plantar fasciitis

Nervous system: sedative, nerve tonic especially when nervous system is exhausted, anxiety, tension, migraine, headaches, debility, convalescence, insomnia

Reproductive/endocrine system: menstrual cycle irregularities, PMS and related upsets, cramps, menopause, childbirth/labor, impotence, dysmenorrhea, hot flashes, night sweats, hormonal irritability and imbalance, amenorrhea

Respiratory system: asthma attack (reduces spasms in the bronchial tubes), sore dry throats, laryngitis, bronchitis

Skin: eczema caused by stress or anxiety, inflamed skin conditions, mature skin, wrinkles, excessive sebum production, dry itchy skin

Psyche and emotion: irritation, anger, mental fatigue, frigidity, nervous anxiety, insomnia, depression, postnatal depression, exhaustion from overwork, sexual problems, hyperactivity, imbalanced emotional states, and stress

Subtle/energetic aromatherapy: For TCM work, clary sage both strengthens *Qi-energy* that is depleted and relaxes and circulates *Qi-energy* that is "stuck." It can smooth the flow of *Qi-energy* in the stomach and intestines (Mojay, 1997). Leigh (2001) calls clary sage the feminine balancer and recommends it for third eye or vision work. Clary sage quickly dispels shallow feelings and emotional posturing and can give wings to true feelings, heightening them to euphoria (Holmes, 1993). Ultimately, clary sage achieves a harmonizing effect between earth and fire, between our physical body, our feelings, and our aspirations (Holmes, 1993).

In Practice: Sample Recipes Using Clary Sage

Antispasmodic Blend	Pain Relief
Clary sage	Clary sage
Peppermint	Black pepper
Cypress	Lavender

Cypress / *Cupressus sempervirens* L.

Botany and History Information

Other common names: Italian cypress, Mediterranean cypress, Common cypress

Botanical family: Cupressaceae

Botany: *Cupressus sempervirens* L. is a tree that grows 40 to 60 feet high or higher. It has branches either spreading horizontally or narrowly upright; the bark is thin, smooth, grayish-brown, and somewhat fissured. The leaves are a dull dark green. The flowers are small and white and bear round, brownish-grey cones or nuts. The tree is indigenous to the mountains of northern Iran, Asia Minor, Crete, and Cyprus. Cypress was introduced into Italy in ancient times and is now naturalized in many countries, including England, France, Italy, Spain, and Portugal.

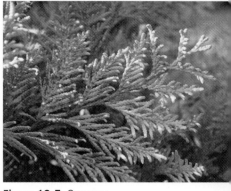

Figure 13-5 Cypress

History and myth: The name sempervirens can be translated to mean "evergreen" or ever-living. The ancient Greeks dedicated this tree to Pluto, god of the underworld. Hippocrates recommended cypress for the treatment of hemorrhoids with bleeding and conditions of excess fluid loss, such as perspiration or menstrual flow. The Chinese have employed cypress for profuse sweating and for its benefits on the respiratory system. Some have said that cypress is superior in its astringent action.

Extraction Information

Countries of origin:	France, Italy
Part of plant used:	leaves, twigs, cones
Extraction method:	distillation
Oil content:	unknown by author
Color of oil:	pale yellow

Blending Information

Odor description:	piney, woody, refreshing
Blending factor:	5

Safety information:

▶ avoid prolonged exposure, particularly with allergy-sensitive individuals
▶ nonirritant, nonsensitizing, non-phototoxic

Chemical Feature

Rich in monoterpenes (up to 45%).

Chemical Profile

Monoterpenes: α-pinene (35 to 40.9%), β-pinene, Δ-camphene, limonene, terpinolene, myrcene, ρ-cymene, sabinene, γ-terpinene

Alcohols: cedrol (5.3 to 7%, α-terpineol, borneol)

Esters: α-terpenyl acetate (4 to 5%)

Therapeutic Actions

Antiperspirant, antirheumatic, **antiseptic**. antispasmodic, anti-sudorific, **antitussive**, **astringent**, decongestant, deodorant, **detoxifier**, diuretic, febrifuge, insecticide, nervine, restorative, sedative, styptic, **vasoconstrictor**, vulnerary.

Keywords: astringent, excessive perspiration, toning effect on veins

Core Aromatic Applications

Circulatory system: varicose veins, nosebleeds, pyorrhea (bleeding gums), chilblains, cellulite, bruises, edema

Digestive system: diarrhea, hemorrhoids

Lymphatic system: congestion in lymph system

Reproductive/endocrine system: excess blood flow during menstruation (menorrhagia), dysmenorrhea, cramps

Respiratory system: infection of the throat, nose, or bronchi in early phase (Schnaubelt, 1995), coughs particularly spasmodic coughs, bronchitis, asthma, flu, sore throat

Skin: oily, sweaty skin and feet, broken capillaries, bruises, cellulite, supportive wound healer

Psyche and emotion: constrictive feelings, overwhelmed, helpful during times of transition and bereavement, anxiety, excessive talking, excessive thinking

Subtle/energetic aromatherapy: Cypress essential oil has a wonderful energy of pulling things together, including thoughts and overwhelming emotions; a useful oil for concentration and to help refocus; used in TCM to enliven and regulate the flow of blood by offering a restorative and toning effect on veins (Mojay, 1997); can be used to purify physical and energetic space and is recommended for the heart chakra to provide comfort and strength to an individual who has experienced the loss of someone close (Leigh, 2001).

In Practice: Sample Recipes Using Cypress

Varicose Veins Blend	Spasmodic Conditions Blend
Cypress	Cypress
Lemon	Clary sage
Geranium	Lavender

Eucalyptus / *Eucalyptus globulus* Labill.

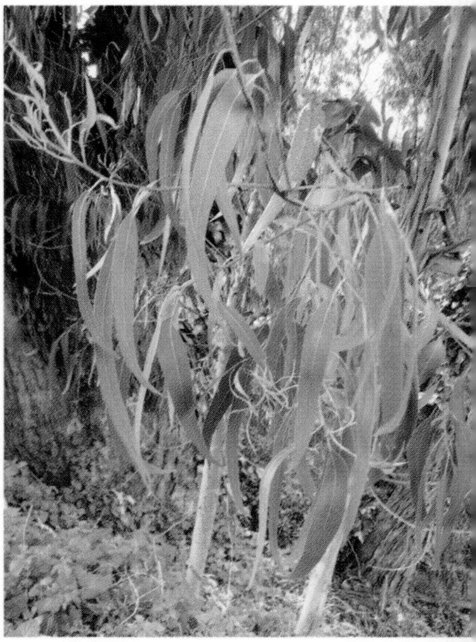

Botany and History Information

Other common names: Blue gum Eucalyptus, Australian fever tree leaf, fever tree leaf, Tasmanian blue gum leaf

Botanical family: Myrtaceae

Botany: *Eucalyptus globulus* is a medium-sized evergreen woodland tree that can grow up to 60m. It is native to Australia. Mature woodland trees usually have extensive roots that are frequently deeply penetrating, but in plantations the roots are often more shallow. There is usually a single trunk, much branched. The lower bark is rough, grayish or brownish, the upper bark smooth, pale, and often with a bluish tinge, decorticating in long strips. The mature leaves are dark glossy green and firm. It bears fragrant white flowers as it matures.

History and myth: Eucalyptus species have a history of traditional use by the Australian aboriginal people who refer to it as "*malee*." According to Grieve (1996): "The genus name *Eucalyptus* comes from Greek *eucalyptos*, meaning 'well-covered,' and refers to its flowers that, in bud, are covered with a cup-like membrane which is thrown off when the flower expands" (p. 287). Eucalyptus has been integrated into traditional medicine systems of the Chinese, Indian Ayurvedic, and Greco-European.

Figure 13-6 Eucalyptus
Source: Reprinted by permission of David Monniaux

Extraction Information

Countries of origin:	Australia, Spain
Part of plant used:	leaves and mature branches
Extraction method:	distillation
Oil content:	1 to 3 percent
Color of oil:	pale yellow to clear

Blending Information

Odor description:	strong, camphorlike, balsamic, fresh
Blending factor:	1

Safety information:

▶ may antidote homeopathic remedies, generally safe to use
▶ avoid applying near the nostrils of infants due to the risk of spasm of the glottis and the cooling effect on the respiratory system; use Eucalyptus smithii or radiata with children
▶ keep essential oil out of reach of children. Ingestion of the oil is toxic and can affect the central nervous, gastrointestinal, and respiratory systems (Blumenthal et al., 1996)

Chemical Feature

Rich in the oxide 1,8 cineole syn eucalyptol and monoterpenes.

Chemical Profile

Monoterpenes (20 to 25%): α-pinene (10.2 to 27%), ρ-cymene, limonene, camphene, β-pinene

Oxides: 1,8 cineole (58.6 to 85%), α-pinene epoxide

Therapeutic Actions

Analgesic (Silva et al., 2003), **antibacterial**, anti-inflammatory, antirheumatic, antiseptic, antispasmodic, antitussive, **antiviral**, balsamic, **decongestant**, depurative, diuretic, **expectorant**, febrifuge, insecticide, rubefacient, stimulant, vermifuge, vulnerary.

Keywords: cooling, stimulating, clearing, antibacterial, expectorant

Core Aromatic Applications

Circulatory system: stimulating, good support oil for the stimulating properties of black pepper or juniper, can support detoxification programs

Digestive system: diarrhea (caused by viral infection), intestinal parasites, candida albicans

Musculoskeletal system: muscular aches and pains, arthritis, rheumatism, plantar fasciitis, sprains

Nervous system: neuralgia, headaches, migraines

Respiratory system: chronic bronchitis (Lu X Q et al., 2004), acute bronchitis, sinusitis, asthma, antiseptic qualities good for sore throat and infections, laryngitis, clears the head especially when used with rosemary and peppermint, nasal congestion

Skin: herpes simplex, shingles, chickenpox, measles, acne, ulcers, wounds, boils, burns, cuts

Psyche and emotion: exhaustion, energy imbalance, negative energies such as present after an argument

Subtle/energetic aromatherapy: Unparalleled in its ability to clear *Lung-Phlegm* for TCM work and as a general tonic to *Lung-Qi* (Mojay, 1997); is suited to the individual who feels emotionally "hemmed-in" or constricted by their surroundings and can help to provide "room to breathe" (Mojay, 1997); can be used as an emotional and energy balancer and is useful for individuals who lack concentration or have cluttered or irrational thoughts (Worwood, 1996); can clear negativity and is recommended for use with the first or base chakra, according to Leigh (2001).

In Practice: Sample Recipes Using Eucalyptus

Respiratory Blend	Breathing Space Blend
Eucalyptus	Eucalyptus
Rosemary ct. cineole or camphor	Lemon
Peppermint	
Tea tree	

Fennel / *Foeniculum vulgare* P. Mill. var. *dulce*

Botany and History Information

Other common names: Fenkel, Wild Fennel, Sweet Fennel

Botanical family: Apiaceae syn. Umbelliferae

Botany: Fennel is a tall perennial that can grow up to 6 feet when flowering. It has hollow yet upright stems and feathery leaves that give rise to beautiful umbels of tiny, vibrant yellow flowers in the summer. The yellow flowers mature into brownish, strongly aromatic seeds. Sweet fennel is most commonly found growing in southern Europe.

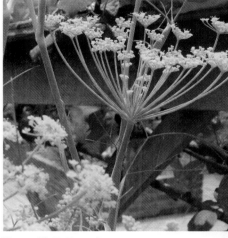

Figure 13-7 Fennel

History and myth: It was the Romans who gave fennel its name "Foeniculum" from the Latin word *foenum* meaning hay. According to Grieve (1996), the name was corrupted in the Middle Ages to *Fanculum*, which gave rise to its more popular name, fenkel. Fennel, together with St. John's wort, is used to protect against evil spirits and witchcraft. Fennel has been well known and well loved since ancient times and has been used to improve vision, lose weight, and promote longevity. It has also been used to provide strength and courage.

Extraction Information

Countries of origin:	France, Spain, Germany
Part of plant used:	seeds
Extraction method:	distillation of crushed seeds
Oil content:	1 to 4 percent
Color of oil:	pale yellow, clear

Blending Information

Odor description:	aniseedy, spicy, warm, sweet, like licorice
Blending factor:	3

Safety information:

▶ bitter fennel essential oil rich in estragole should be avoided

Chemical Feature

Rich in phenylpropanoids, trans-anethole, and monoterpenes.

Chemical Profile

Monoterpenes: α-pinene (1.4 to 10%), limonene (1.4 to 17%), camphene, β-pinene, sabinene, myrcene, β-phellandrene, γ-terpinene (10.5%), cis-ocimene (12%), terpinolene

Phenylpropanoids: methyl chavicol (2 to 10%), cis-anethole, **trans-anethole** (50 to 90%)

Therapeutic Actions

Anti-inflammatory, antimicrobial, **antispasmodic**, bronchodilator, **carminative**, **detoxifier**, estrogenic, emmenagogue, expectorant, **digestive,** galactogogue, **promotes gastrointestinal motility**, **stomachic**.

Keywords: digestive system, menstrual disorders, stimulating

Core Aromatic Applications

Digestive system: colic, indigestion, excess gas, constipation, irritable bowel syndrome, nausea, lack of or decreased appetite, abdominal pain, indigestion, nonspecific colitis (Mills and Bone, 2000)

Musculoskeletal system: muscle spasms or cramps, general muscular aches and pains

Reproductive/endocrine system: balancing to hormones, PMS, dysmenorrhea (Harris, 2001), amenorrhea, lack of or reduced sexual drive, lack of or reduced milk flow in lactating woman, cramps

Respiratory system: bronchitis, coughs, flu

Skin: sluggish circulation, congested or smoker's skin (can be beneficial for stimulating microcirculation and detoxification), fennel hydrosol may be utilized in compresses for conjunctivitis

Psyche and emotion: feelings of being stuck, unexpressed thoughts or emotions, tension, fear or inhibition of expressing self, creative blocks

Subtle/energetic aromatherapy: As a seed oil, fennel contains the energy of potential and creativity. In TCM, fennel regulates the action of *Qi-energy* in the stomach and intestines and is invigorating to *Qi-energy* in the kidneys and spleen (Mojay, 1997). Worwood (1996) recommends fennel for emotional and mental blocks, inability to adjust, and feelings of boredom. She comments that fennel can be useful for enlivening, motivating, and fortifying as well as enhancing confidence and assertiveness. Leigh (2001) recommends fennel for the third or solar plexus chakra and says that fennel helps to give strength and courage when needed.

In Practice: Sample Recipes Using Fennel

Digestive Tonic	Hormonal Imbalance
Fennel	Fennel
Grapefruit	Clary sage
Ginger	Geranium

Frankincense / *Boswellia carterii* Birdw. syn. *Boswellia sacra* Flueckiger

Botany and History Information

Other common names: Pure Incense, Olibanum

Botanical family: Burseraceae

Botany: *Boswellia carterii* is one of approximately five different species of frankincense. It is a deciduous, shrubby, small, much-branched tree that can grow up to 25 feet. It is considered to be highly aromatic due to the resin contained throughout. The resin is extracted by a deep incision into the trunk of the tree. Frankincense grows in desert areas such as Somalia and the Arabia Peninsula.

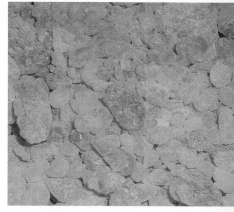

Figure 13-8 Frankincense

History and myth: The name *frankincense* is derived from old French, meaning pure incense. It has been revered by almost all Western religions including Judaism and Christianity. Hindus and Buddhists have employed frankincense as incense for daily ritual and offerings. In Japan it has been incorporated into Shinto meditation and ritual. Frankincense has been highly prized and was one of the three gifts brought to Jesus upon his birth. Frankincense was once considered more valuable than gold. An extensive trade utilizing camels to transport it was carried out along the Frankincense Trail and the Silk Road. The ancient Egyptians used frankincense to make *kohl*, the black powder used by Egyptian women to paint their eyelids black. Modern use of frankincense continues; in Saudi Arabia it is chewed as gum, used as a mouthwash, and is the main ingredient of incense used at births, marriages, deaths, and daily prayer calls. Frankincense was used throughout the ancient world for embalming and as incense for religious ceremonies. In Chinese medicine, frankincense is used in applications for tissue trauma, for pain relief, to increase immunity, to support the respiratory system via its expectorant action, and to act as an antidepressant. Queen Cleopatra's extravagant use of frankincense is legend. Frankincense is also referred to as Olibanum oil from the Latin, Oil of Lebanon.

Extraction Information

Countries of origin:	Somalia, India, North Africa, Oman
Part of plant used:	trunk of tree
Extraction method:	steam distilled gum, white resin
Oil content:	3 to 9 percent
Color of oil:	pale yellow, clear

Blending Information

Odor description:	clean, fresh, earthy, woody
Blending factor:	3 to 4

Safety information:

▶ considered nontoxic, non-photosensitizing, and nonsensitizing

Chemical Feature

Rich in terpenes and esters. The CO_2 extract is rich in terpenes, sesquiterpenes, and sesquiterpene alcohols (Haas, 2004).

Chemical Profile

Monoterpenes: α-pinene, limonene

Sesquiterpenes: α-gurjunene (Haas, 2004)

Esters: octyl acetate (13.4 to 50%), octyl formate (1.4%)

Therapeutic Actions

Antidepressant, **anti-inflammatory**, **antiseptic**, astringent, **balsamic**, carminative, expectorant, **immune enhancer**, **nervine**, sedative, **vulnerary**.

Keywords: wound healing, all around healer, calming, meditation

Core Aromatic Applications

Lymph and immune system: reduced or compromised immunity (Schnaubelt, 1995)

Musculoskeletal system: swollen joints, muscular aches and pains, arthritis

Respiratory system: bronchitis, sinus congestion, asthma

Skin: mature skin, wrinkles, scar tissue, postoperative wound healing (once sutures are removed), eczema, acne, inflamed skin conditions, blackheads, hives, soothing to dry irritated skin

Psyche and emotion: anxiety, tension, inability to focus, frustration, disconnection with self, spiritual unrest

Subtle/energetic aromatherapy: Frankincense has been historically utilized for its powerful and profound effects on the psychological and spiritual well-being of those who use it for meditation, contemplation, and prayer. In TCM, frankincense can smooth the flow of stagnant *Qi-energy* (Mojay, 1997). Worwood (1996) recommends frankincense as an oil to help alleviate feelings of worthlessness, self-destruction, anxiety, and despair. Frankincense is useful for elevating an individual to a more spiritual, meditative place. Leigh (2001) believes frankincense can assist one in connecting to the divinity inside the self as well as to connect to the great divinity of the Divine. She recommends frankincense for the seventh or crown chakra.

Research Notes and Additional Information

According to research by Mikaeil et al. (2003), "Frankincense oil has exhibited a strong immunostimulant activity (90% lymphocyte transformation) when assessed by a lymphocyte proliferation assay."

In Practice: Sample Recipes Using Frankincense

Dry/Irritated Skin Blend	Immune Enhancer
Frankincense	Frankincense
German chamomile	Lemon
Lavender	

Geranium / *Pelargonium graveolens* L'Hér. ex Ait. var. *roseum*, syn. *Pelargonium capitatum* (L.) L'Hér. ex Ait. and *Pelargonium asperum* Willd.

Botany and History Information

Other common names: Sweet scented geranium, Rose geranium.

Botanical family: Geraniaceae

Botany: Lis-Balchin (1996) reports: "The scented *Pelargonium* cultivars used in the production of geranium oil are large bush-like plants with a rosy inflorescence and pinnate, rounded to pointed scented leaves approximately 5cm long. The leaves are fragrantly mint or rose-scented, and a dull green color. There are over 250 natural species of Pelargonium, hundreds of hybrids and thousands of cultivars."

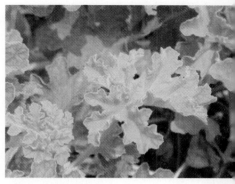

Figure 13-9 Geranium

History and myth: Research on the historical uses of geranium is scarce. According to Kerr (2001), commercial and folk use seems to have appeared sometime in the early 1800s (p. 9).

Extraction Information

Countries of origin:	Reunion Islands, Egypt, Madagascar, China
Part of plant used:	leaves and stems
Extraction method:	distillation
Oil content:	.30 to .45 percent
Color of oil:	pale yellowish, green

Blending Information

Odor description:	fresh, strong, green, feminine
Blending factor:	3

Safety information:

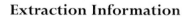

▶ nonirritating, non-phototoxic

Chemical Feature

Rich in alcohols and esters.

Chemical Profile

Alcohols: citronellol (20.89 to 40.23%), **geraniol** (8.7 to 24.97%), linalool (1.89 to 12.9%), nerol, α-terpineol, eugenol (17.3%)

Esters: citronellyl formates (8 to 18%), geranyl formates, citronellyl proprionates, geranyl proprionates, geranyl acetate, citronellyl butyrate

Therapeutic Actions

Analgesic, anticoagulant, antidepressant, **antimicrobial**, antiseptic, **astringent**, deodorant, diuretic, emmenagogue, **hormone balancer**, insecticide, styptic, tonic, vasoconstrictor, vulnerary.

Keywords: balancing (particularly to hormones), harmonizing, uplifting, relaxing, refreshing, cleansing

Core Aromatic Applications

General properties: very useful in treating jet lag or imbalances brought on by travel

Circulatory system: poor circulation, edema, broken capillaries

Digestive system: diarrhea, stomach upsets caused by nerves, hemorrhoids

Lymph and immune system: poor circulation of lymph, lymphatic drainage

Musculoskeletal system: muscle spasms

Reproductive/endocrine system: hormonal imbalance during menstruation, menopause, and puberty, can reduce symptoms of PMS and menopausal experiences of fever and hot flashes, supports the adrenal cortex to help balance hormones

Skin: eczema, psoriasis, dermatitis, itching, acne, sluggish smoker's skin, aids detoxing, ringworm, head lice, dandruff, mouth ulcers, thrush (oral), gum infection, wound healing, abscesses, cellulite

Psyche and emotion: depression, agitation, general fatigue, frustration, anxiety, mood swings, rigidity, unbalanced life, challenging decision-making, mood swings, emotional or physical stress

Subtle/energetic aromatherapy: Mojay (1997) writes: "Geranium has a way of conveying a feeling of calm strength and security, and is therefore beneficial for both chronic and acute anxiety, particularly where there is nervous exhaustion due to stress and overwork. The oil helps us reconnect with our feeling-life—to our emotional sensitivity, relaxed spontaneity, and health thirst for pleasure and enjoyment" (p. 76–77). Leigh (2001) describes geranium as an essential oil that helps to imbue a sense of grace, beauty, and balance. She believes it is beneficial for the fourth or heart chakra. In TCM, geranium clears heat and inflammation due to its cool, moist energy. It can also strengthen *Qi-energy* and encourage the circulation of *Qi* and blood (Mojay, 1997).

In Practice: Sample Recipes Using Geranium

Calming	PMS
Geranium	Geranium
Roman chamomile	Clary sage
Lavender	Lavender
	Sweet orange

Ginger / *Zingiber officinale* Roscoe

Botany and History Information

Other common names: Garden ginger

Botanical family: Zingiberaceae

Botany: *Zingiber officinale* is an erect, leafy perennial that grows to about 1m and is usually cultivated as an annual. It has green reedlike stalks with narrow spear-shaped leaves, white, yellow, or purple orchid-like flowers, and a robust branched rhizome growing horizontally near the soil's surface. The rhizome is firm and can grow to 6 to 20cm depending on the cultivar. The skin color varies from buff to very dark brown (almost black), and the flesh color from pale yellow to deep orange-red. Ginger likes water, humidity, and heat and is grown commercially in many tropical climates. It is native to India and China.

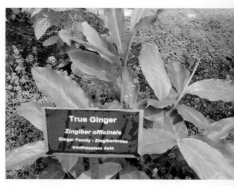

Figure 13-10 Ginger

History and myth: Ginger has been highly prized for its medicinal properties since ancient times. The Greeks, Romans, and Arabs have all utilized ginger for medicinal purposes. For thousands of years, traditional Chinese medicine has employed fresh and dried ginger for the treatment of fevers, cough, and nausea. Ginger spread to Europe during the Middle Ages and is said to have been used to combat the Black Death due to its ability to make a person sweat.

Extraction Information

Countries of origin:	Sri Lanka, China, India, Nigeria
Part of plant used:	rhizome; unpeeled rhizome will result in higher oil yield
Extraction method:	distillation
Oil content:	1.5 to 3 percent
Color of oil:	clear to light amber; oils become thicker with age and exposure to air

Blending Information

Odor description:	warming, spicy
Blending factor:	4

Safety information:

▶ possible irritant to sensitive skin
▶ possible cross-allergic reactions in individuals sensitive to Peru balsam

Chemical Feature

Rich in sesquiterpenes with support from monoterpenes and nonirritant aldehydes.

Chemical Profile

Sesquiterpenes: zingiberene (20 to 50.9%), β-sesquiphellandrene (1.6 to 9%), ar.-curcumene (8 to 19%), β-farnesese (19.8%), β-bisabolene (0.2 to 12%)
Aldehydes: geranial (3 to 20%)
Oxides: 1,8 cineole (4.1 to 13%)

Therapeutic Actions

Analgesic, antibacterial, **antiemetic**, **antispasmodic**, aperitif. **aphrodisiac**, **carminative**, **digestive**, expectorant, febrifuge, rubefacient, stimulant, **stomachic**, sudorific.

Keywords: analgesic, warming, digestive

Core Aromatic Applications

> **Circulatory system:** poor circulation, cold hands or feet
>
> **Digestive system:** stomachache, nausea, vomiting, morning sickness, excess gas, constipation or diarrhea, postoperative or drug-induced nausea (Mills and Bone, 2000, p. 394), loss of appetite
>
> **Lymph/immune systems:** fever (tincture or CO_2 extract)
>
> **Musculoskeletal system:** muscular aches and pains, arthritis, sprains, rheumatism, joint pain and stiffness
>
> **Nervous system:** nervous exhaustion, debility, neuralgia
>
> **Reproductive/endocrine system:** lack of or reduced sex drive, impotence, menstrual cramps and pain, pregnancy nausea (inhalation), amenorrhea and dysmenorrhea (Mills and Bone, 2000, p. 394)
>
> **Respiratory system:** catarrh, bronchitis, congestion, sinusitis, sinus headaches, sore throat, fevers, common cold
>
> **Psyche and emotion:** indecisions, confusion, feeling of being ungrounded, loss or reduced sense of will, loss of motivation, psychic burnout caused by chronic stress
>
> **Subtle/energetic aromatherapy:** Ginger can be used as an emotionally warming oil and is indicated for sexual anxieties, lack of direction, lack of focus, apathy, loneliness, and resignation (Worwood, 1996). In TCM, ginger stimulates and tonifies the *yang* energy of the spleen, stomach, heart, lung, and kidneys (Mojay, 1997). According to Leigh (2001), ginger stimulates the physical body to be open to intimacy and assists an individual in attracting abundance. She recommends it for the eighth or etheric body chakra.

Research Notes and Additional Information

Holmes (1996) confirms that "Ginger has a long history of use for making an individual sweat. The pungent constituents are considered to be responsible for this action. Ginger essential oil does not contain the pungent constituents and hence is not used as a diaphoretic. Ginger tincture and the CO_2 extraction do contain these principles and can be employed as diaphoretics" (p. 18). According to Buckle (2003), "inhaled essential oil is a very effective remedy for nausea and is particularly suitable for pregnancy. (p. 210)"

In Practice: Sample Recipes Using Ginger

Warming/Comfort Blend	Respiratory Blend
Ginger	Ginger
Black pepper	Eucalyptus
	Frankincense

Helichrysum / *Helichrysum italicum* (Roth) G.Don

Botany and History Information

Other common names: Everlasting, Immortelle

Botanical family: Asteraceae syn. Compositae

Botany: This strongly aromatic herb grows up to 20 inches high. The flowers are a cluster of golden-yellow ball-shaped blossoms, the leaves are delicate and oblong and release a distinct aroma when crushed. Helichrysum thrives in sunshine and in the most deprived soil; this is why you can see it growing in many waste places where other plants cannot survive. The name Immortelle or Everlasting comes about because this plant retains its yellow color even when dried.

History and myth: Helichrysum has been praised in aromatherapy as the chosen essential oil for bruises and wound healing. There appears to be very little information available on the traditional uses of this plant.

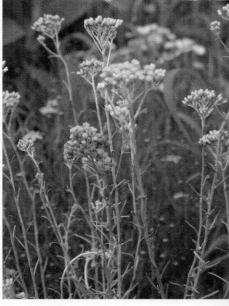

Figure 13-11 Helichrysum

Extraction Information

Countries of origin:	Italy, France, Yugoslavia
Part of plant used:	flowers and flowering tops
Oil content:	unknown
Extraction method:	steam distillation
Color of oil:	yellowish to reddish color

Blending Information

Odor description:	woody, spicy, warm, and herbaceous
Blending factor:	5

Safety information:

▶ considered to be safe when applied diluted or undiluted (Haas, 2004)

Chemical Feature

Rich in esters, supported by 6 percent diketones: italidione (Haas, 2004, p. 36).

Chemical Profile

Monoterpenes:	pinene
Alcohols:	nerol, geraniol, linalol
Esters (30 to 50%):	neryl acetate, geranyl acetate
Ketones:	italidione

Therapeutic Actions

Anti-inflammatory, mucolytic, vulnerary.

Keywords: bruises, skin conditions, anti-inflammatory

Core Aromatic Applications

Circulatory system: varicose veins, bruises, broken capillaries

Musculoskeletal system: gout, arthritis

Nervous system: neuralgia, Herpes Zoster, pain

Respiratory system: bronchitis, common cold, sinus infections

Skin: acne, chronic dermatitis, eczema, scar tissue, burns, dermal inflammation, cuts and wounds, bruises, radiation burns, Herpes simplex

Psyche and emotion: grief and bereavement, inability to heal or overcome adversity

Subtle/energetic aromatherapy: Helichrysum helps to regulate the flow of *Qi-energy* and the blood. It is also useful to clear heat and reduce inflammation (Mojay, 1997). According to Mojay (1997), helichrysum has the power to break through the deepest, most "stuck" of negative emotions and can restore compassion not only for others but for oneself. According to Leigh (2001), helichrysum promotes longevity and can enhance intuition, creativity, and feelings of compassion. She recommends it for personal growth and for application to the third eye chakra.

In Practice: Sample Recipes Using Helichrysum

Wound Healing/Bruises	Emotional Healing
Helichrysum	Helichrysum
Lavendin	Rose
Rosemary ct. verbenon	Mandarin
Carrot seed	

Juniper / *Juniperus communis* L.

Botany and History Information

Other common names: Common juniper, dwarf juniper, genévrier commun (French)

Botanical family: Cupressaceae

Botany: *Juniperus communis* is a coniferous evergreen treelike shrub that grows to a height of about 6 feet, although it can reach upwards of 25 feet. Juniper has spreading branches and densely crowded, needlelike leaves. The tree bears berrylike seed cones. Juniper likes to grow in dry, rocky hillsides or plateaus. The berries can take up to two to three years to ripen.

History and myth: Juniper berries have been historically used in the making of gin. The Dutch word for juniper is "genever," which refers to its most common use as a liqueur. This liqueur was used by Europeans as a tonic and restorative drink. In traditional medicine, juniper berries have been used for digestive upsets as well as for joint and muscle pain. Native American Indians utilized juniper for treating colds, flu, arthritis, and muscle aches.

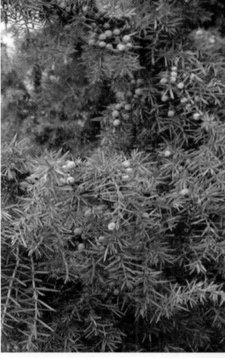

Figure 13-12 Juniper

Extraction Information

Country of origin:	Balkans
Part of plant used:	berries
Extraction method:	distillation
Oil content:	0.5 to 1.5 percent
Color of oil:	pale yellow

Blending Information

Odor description:	fresh, piney, fruity
Blending factor:	4

Safety information:

▶ avoid internal use if kidney inflammation or irritation is present (Blumenthal, 1998)

Chemical Feature

Rich in monoterpenes supported by alcohols and esters.

Chemical Profile

Monoterpenes (60 to 80%): α-**pinene** (26.5 to 70.82%), β-pinene (1.7 to 13.67%), **limonene** (0.68 to 40%), δ-3-carene (0.03 to 20.2%)

Alcohols: terpinen-4-ol, α-terpineol, borneol, geraniol, elemol, α-eudesmol, -cadinol

Esters: bornyl acetate, terpinyl acetate

Therapeutic Actions

Anti-inflammatory, **antirheumatic**, antiseptic, antispasmodic, antiviral, depurative, **detoxifier**, digestive, **diuretic**, stimulant.

Keywords: detoxifying, clearing, stimulating, strengthening, cleansing

Core Aromatic Applications

Circulatory system: poor circulation

Digestive system: poor appetite, flatulence/gas, dyspepsia, lack of appetite

Musculoskeletal system: muscular aches and pains, rheumatism, cellulite, joint pain and stiffness, strains and sprains, carpal tunnel syndrome, sciatica, spasms, shin splints

Skin: poor elimination from skin, slow-healing sores

Psyche and emotion: low energy level, worry, cold, fear, trembling, emotionally frozen, feelings of being blocked, lack of motivation

Subtle/energetic aromatherapy: Juniper cleanses, detoxifies, and helps to clear negative energy. It is recommended for the sixth chakra or third eye (Leigh, 2001). According to Mojay (1997), juniper is a powerful tonic of the body's warming and stimulating *yang energy*, especially of the *Kidney-yang*. He states that juniper is useful to break through psychological stagnation and consolidate willpower. Juniper may be beneficial for cleansing, purifying, and for visionary work and is indicated for those suffering from nervous or emotional exhaustion, lack of self-worth, emptiness, and listlessness (Worwood, 1996).

Research Notes and Additional Information

According to Blumenthal et al. (1998), "Junipers therapeutic actions are due primarily to its volatile oil, which contains the constituent terpinen-4-ol. Diuretic actions stimulated by terpinen-4-ol are reportedly aquaretic, meaning that glomerular filtration rates increase, but electrolyte secretion does not." Avoid internal use if kidney inflammation or irritation is present (Blumenthal, 1998). External application is considered safe.

In Practice: Sample Recipes Using Juniper

Lymphatic Tonic	Dysmenorrhea
Juniper	Juniper
Lemon	Clary sage
Rosemary	Peppermint
Grapefruit	Lavender

Lavender / *Lavandula angustifolia* P. Mill. syn. *L. officinalis* Chaix syn. *L. vera* DC.

Botany and History Information

Other common names: Lavander, English lavender, True lavender

Botanical family: Lamiaceae syn. Labiatae

Botany: *Lavandula angustifolia* is a compact, bushy shrub with linear gray-green leaves. In mid to late summer, long unbranched stalks produce fragrant, pale to deep purple flowers in dense spikes. *Lavandula angustifolia* can reach a height of 2 to 3 feet. There are approximately twenty species of lavender with a number of varieties and cultivars as well. All species of lavender flourish in the Mediterranean regions.

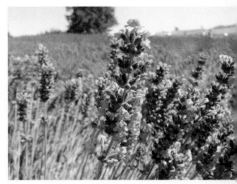

Figure 13-13 Lavender
Source: Reprinted by permission of Kent Goodwin McKay

History and myth: Lavender has been used since ancient times and appears in the writings of the Greek naturalist, Discorides, during the first century. The word lavender is thought to be derived from the medieval Latin "*Lavo*" or "*Lavare*," which means to wash or to bathe. Lavender was used to protect against the plague during the Middle Ages and the Renaissance. The Romans are considered responsible for the introduction of lavender into England. Lavender has some traditional use for being used for headaches, insomnia, and upset stomach due to nerves. Lavender has been traditionally utilized for scenting laundry. According to Hajhashemi et al. (2003), "Extracts obtained from the leaves of *Lavandula angustifolia* are used in Iranian folk medicine as remedies for the treatment of various inflammatory diseases."

Extraction Information

Countries of origin:	France, Bulgaria, England, United States
Part of plant used:	flowering tops
Extraction method:	distillation
Oil content:	0.5 to 3 percent
Color of oil:	clear

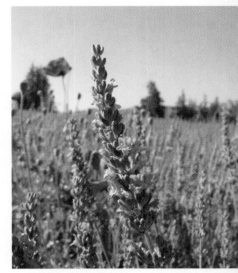

Figure 13-14 Lavendin
Source: Reprinted by permission of Kent Goodwin McKay

Blending Information

Odor description:	fresh, floral, sweet, herbaceous
Blending factor:	7

Safety information:

▶ nonirritant, non-phototoxic, nontoxic

Chemical Feature

Rich in the ester, linalyl acetate, and the sedative alcohol, linalol.

Chemical Profile

Sesquiterpenes: β-caryophyllene (2.6 to 12.37%), β-farnesene
Alcohols: linalol (29.45 to 49.9%), terpinen-4-ol, α-terpineol, borneol, geraniol, lavandulol
Esters: linalyl acetate (46.71 to 53.8%), lavandulyl acetate, terpenyl acetate

Therapeutic Actions

Analgesic, antidepressant, **anti-inflammatory**, antirheumatic, antiseptic, **anti-spasmodic**, antiviral, hypotensive, **nervine**, **sedative**, **vulnerary**.

Keywords: Balancing, extreme changeable emotions, nervous exhaustion, anxiety, wound healing, CNS sedative.

Core Aromatic Applications

Digestive system: stress-related digestive upsets, including irritable bowel syndrome, abdominal cramps, nervous stomach

Musculoskeletal system: muscular aches and pains, arthritis, sprains, strains, muscle spasms, growing pains, plantar faciitis, tendonitis, shin splints, rheumatic conditions, joint pain and stiffness, bursitis

Nervous system: restlessness, insomnia (Blumenthal et al., 1998), stress, shock, headaches, migraines, neuralgia

Reproductive/endocrine system: calms during delivery, can help reduce severity of contractions (use with clary sage), helps in relieving pain, cramps, PMS, perineal discomfort and repair following childbirth (Dale and Cornwell, 1994), postpartum perineal healing

Skin: burns, scrapes, abscesses, acne, athlete's foot, eczema, inflamed skin conditions, psoriasis (as an anti-inflammatory), sunburn, relieves itching, hives, open wounds or sores, poorly healing wounds

Psyche and emotion: depression (including manic), anxiety, hyperactivity, fears and delusions, extreme emotions, panic attacks, hysteria, fainting, self-injury, challenging behavior, limited communication skills, fear of touch, disturbed sleep patterns

Subtle/energetic aromatherapy: In TCM, lavender works to regulate and cool an overheated liver and to soothe and support the *Qi-energy* of the heart (Mojay, 1997). According to Leigh (2001), lavender may assist in bringing the lower and higher chakras into harmony. She recommends it to be used with the fourth or heart chakra to bring about joy. Worwood (1996) states that due to its ability to address a wide range of physical and emotional issues, lavender could be called the mother or grandmother of essential oils. Lavender is beneficial in working with individuals who suffer from or with anxiety, mental exhaustion, insecurity, trauma or emotional violence, conflict, psychosomatic illness, and a multitude of other issues (Worwood, 1996).

Research Notes and Additional Information

There is practically no health condition for which lavender would not provide some kind of relief (Haas, 2004).

In Practice: Sample Recipes Using Lavender

Sleepy-Time Remedy	Relaxation Blend
Lavender	Lavender
Roman chamomile	Marjoram
Mandarin	Clary sage
	Mandarin

Lemon / *Citrus limon* (L.) Burm. f.

Botany and History Information

Botanical family: Rutaceae

Botany: *Citrus limon* has small branches and twigs, pointed, slightly serrate light to mid-green leaves. The flowers are white, the buds pink-tinged. The flowers will occur as single flowers or in small groups. The fruit is light to medium green becoming yellow to bright yellow upon ripening. The peel is relatively thin, smooth, and tight; or rough, thicker, and somewhat loosely attached.

History and myth: The lemon tree, like other citrus trees, appears to have originated in Asia and then was carried over to other continents. Christopher Columbus introduced it into the new world in the late 1400s. During the seventeenth century, lemon was used as a blood cleanser and purifier agent. Lemon juice was once an important remedy for scurvy (long before vitamin C was discovered).

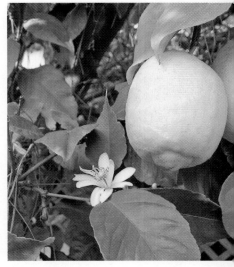

Figure 13-15 Lemon
Source: Reprinted by permission of Ellen Levy Finch

Extraction Information

Countries of origin:	Italy, United States, Argentina, Sicily, Cyprus
Part of plant used:	peel or zest of fruit
Extraction method:	expression
Oil content:	0.5 to 2.5 percent cold pressed .05 to .1 percent distillation of expressed peel
Color of oil:	pale yellow

Blending Information

Odor description:	sharp, citrus, refreshing
Blending factor:	4

Safety information:

▶ patch test for sensitivity
▶ potential photo-sensitization; recommended dosage less than 2 percent
▶ Use less than 7 to 10 drops of citrus oils, combined or singly, in a bath to avoid skin irritation. The use of a dispersant for citrus oils in a bath is highly recommended.

Chemical Feature

Rich in monoterpenes, particularly limonene.

Chemical Profile

Monoterpenes (90 to 95%): limonene (66 to 85%), α-pinene, β-pinene (12.27 to 17.29%), γ-terpinene, sabinene, α-thujene, myrcene, α-phellandrene, β-phellandrene, α-terpinene, ρ-cymene, camphene

Therapeutic Actions

Antacid, antidepressive, **antiseptic**, antispasmodic, **astringent**, carminative, depurative, **detoxifier**, **digestive**, **diuretic**, escharotic, febrifuge, hepatic, hypotensive, **immune enhancer**, laxative, **stomachic**, tonic.

Keywords: cleansing, astringent, antiseptic, uplifting

Core Aromatic Applications

Circulatory system: poor circulation, detoxing

Digestive system: poor or sluggish digestion (Schnaubelt, 1995, p. 76), toxic overload

Lymph/immune system: lymphatic congestion, preventative for contagious illnesses (Schnaubelt, 1995, p. 76)

Musculoskeletal system: muscular or joint aches and pains, arthritis, cellulite, rheumatism, joint swelling, gout

Skin: acne, boils, corns, oily complexions, mouth ulcers, cellulite, varicose veins (can help to prevent and also to prevent them from getting worse), tired, sagging and grayish (smoker's) skin, broken capillaries, ulcers where a large amount of puss or debridement is present: use 1.5 percent dilution in distilled water with lemon and tea tree and apply via a mister to whole area of ulcer at frequent intervals (Barker, 1994, p. 6)

Psyche and emotion: anxiety, depression, dislike of exercise, limited communication skills, inability to let go

Subtle/energetic aromatherapy: In Oriental medicine, lemon essential oil is cool and dry in nature and can be used to clear heat, dampness, and phlegm (Mojay, 1997). Lemon is able to heighten consciousness and is generally activating, stabilizing, and calming during a potential emotional outburst due to its cooling, clearing, and refreshing effect (Gumbel, 1993). Lemon has the ability to dispel sluggishness and can help to clear negative blockages and revitalize energy (Leigh, 2001). Leigh (2001) recommends lemon for the base of the spine chakra.

In Practice: Sample Recipes Using Lemon

Detoxification	Muscular Aches and Pains
Lemon	Lemon
Juniper	Rosemary
Cypress	Peppermint

Mandarin/Tangerine / *Citrus reticulata* Blanco

Botany and History Information

Other common names: Red mandarin, Tangerine (USA)

Botanical family: Rutaceae

Botany: *Citrus reticulata* is normally a small spreading tree that grows to 4 m. It is native to the Far East, particularly southern China. The tree has a core trunk with numerous branches and delicate green leaves. The peel color varies from yellow to deep orange-red when ripe and is loose and easily removable. The peel contains oil secreted in the glands of the zest of the fruit. The tree prefers a hot, humid climate (tropical) and rich soil, although trees in a more temperate climate grow more slowly and produce a greater quantity of oil. Semi-ripe fruit has the greatest oil yield.

History and myth: The tangerine tree was originally cultivated in southern China. The fruit was traditionally offered to the rulers or Mandarins as a token of respect. It was introduced to Europe and America in the 1800s.

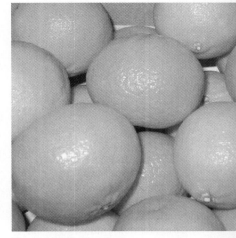

Figure 13-16 Mandarin

Extraction Information

Countries of origin:	Italy, Argentina
Part of plant used:	peel or zest of fruit
Extraction method:	expression or steam distilled
Oil content:	17 to 22 percent
Color of oil:	yellowy, green

Blending Information

Odor description:	sweet, fresh, citrus
Blending factor:	7

Safety information:

▶ one of the safest oils to use with everyone (with proper dilution)
▶ nonirritating, nonsensitizing, nontoxic
▶ Use less than 7 to 10 drops of citrus oils, combined or singly, in a bath to avoid skin irritation. Dilute citrus oils into a dispersant prior to adding to the bath to reduce potential skin irritation.

Chemical Feature

Rich in monoterpenes supported by aldehydes.

Chemical Profile

Monoterpenes: limonene (65 to 95%), α-pinene, β-pinene, myrcene, **γ-terpinene** (13.7 to 21.02%), camphene, ρ-cymene, α-phellandrene, sabinene, terpinolene

Aldehydes: hexanol, decanal (0.05 to 24%), dodecanal (13.5%), α-sinensal, perillaldehyde, octanal, neral (5%), geranial (5.7%), nonanal, citronellal

Therapeutic Actions

Antidepressant, antiseptic, antispasmodic, cholagogue, digestive, **nervine**, sedative

Keywords: calming yet uplifting, soothing, gentle

Core Aromatic Applications

Circulatory system: improves general circulation, aids excess fluid elimination

Digestive system: stress-related digestive upset, said to stimulate appetite (especially after illness or depression)

Nervous system: nervous tension, insomnia (use with lavender), nervous disorders, headaches

Reproductive/endocrine system: PMS, hormonal imbalance, birth and labor stress

Skin: detoxing to congested skin, oily skin

Psyche and emotion: temper tantrums, depression, anxiety, disturbed eating patterns, fear of physical contact, dislike of exercise, limited communication skills, hyperactivity in children

Subtle/energetic aromatherapy: Mandarin speaks to the child within and assists an individual in clearing out clogged ideas (Leigh, 2001). Leigh recommends the use of mandarin for the eighth chakra or etheric body. Mandarin regulates *Liver-Qi* and can ease depressive stress (Mojay, 1997).

In Practice: Sample Recipes Using Mandarin

Hormonal Balancer	Meditation Blend
Mandarin	Mandarin
Clary sage	Frankincense
Geranium	Rose
Lavender	

> **NOTE**
> **The Difference between Mandarin and Tangerine**
>
> According to Arctander (1994), tangerine and mandarin are from two trees, both of which are botanically *Citrus reticulata*, however they are varieties of this species. The mandarin originated in China and is cultivated in Europe. It is considered to have a superior aroma to U.S. tangerine, which is derived from the variety *Citrus reticulata* Blanco var. *deliciosa*. Arctander (1994) comments that the U.S. tangerine is much larger than the mandarin and has a different aroma; it should not be used as a replacement for mandarin oil.

Sweet Marjoram / *Origanum marjorana* L.

Botany and History Information

Botanical family: Lamiaceae syn. Labiatae

Botany: *Origanum marjorana* is a dainty, low, shrubby plant with woody stems, hairy, delicate, oval, opposite leaves, and white or pink flowers. It can grow up to 20 inches and is native to Portugal. It can be either a perennial or annual and prefers to grow in the light warm soil of a garden, rather than in high altitude. It grows in abundance in Tunisia, carpeting the fields between almond trees. Although much of the oil is obtained from Europe, there are varieties: sweet or knotted marjoram, pot marjoram, and wild Spanish marjoram, which is not a true marjoram (it is of the same family but is of inferior quality).

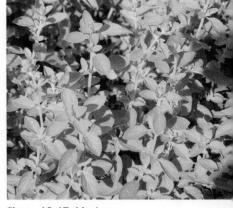

Figure 13-17 Marjoram

History and myth: Originating in Asia, it was considered a sacred plant to Osiris in Egypt, Vishnu in India, and Venus by the Romans. The Greeks and Romans would weave crowns for the newly married, a symbol of love and honor known by the Greeks as "joy of the mountain"; Aphrodite was known to have used it to heal her son Aeneas' wounds. The Greeks also planted marjoram in grave sites to bring peace to the departed spirit. It was used both as a digestive herb and also for spasms, cold and rheumatic pain, chest infections, dropsy, and narcotic poisoning. It is also used in liquors, foods, and perfumeries.

Extraction Information

Countries of origin:	France, Germany, Egypt
Part of plant used:	flowering tops
Extraction method:	distillation
Oil content:	unknown
Color of oil:	pale yellow

Blending Information

Odor description:	spicy, herbaceous
Blending factor:	3

Safety information:

▶ not recommended for individuals with asthma (Haas, 2004)
▶ nonirritating and nonsensitizing

Chemical Feature

Rich in monoterpenes and alcohols.

Chemical Profile

Monoterpenes (40%): sabinene, myrcene, ρ-cymene, terpinolene, α-pinene, β-pinene, ocimene, cadinene, 3-carene, α-terpinene, α-phellandrene, β-phellandrene, myrcene, limonene

Alcohols (50%): terpinen-1-ol-4 (14 to 20%), cis-thujanol-4 (4 to 13%), linalol, α-terpineol (7 to 27%), piperitol

Therapeutic Actions

Analgesic, anaphrodisiac, **antiseptic**, **antispasmodic**, carminative, digestive, emmenagogue, expectorant, hypotensive, **nervine**, **sedative**, vulnerary.

Keywords: warming, antispasmodic, comforting, calming

Core aromatic applications

Circulatory system: poor circulation, chilblains, Raynaud's syndrome, bruises, can reduce blood pressure (Haas, 2004)

Digestive system: stress-related digestive upset, tonic to digestive processes

Musculoskeletal system: muscular or joint aches and pains, rheumatic aches and pains, joint swelling, muscle spasms, growing pains (adolescents), cramps, sciatica, carpal tunnel syndrome, plantar fasciitis

Nervous system: headaches, insomnia, stress reliever, lethargy, nervous exhaustion

Respiratory system: spasmodic coughs, bronchitis

Reproductive system: dysmenorrhea, menstrual cramps

Psyche and emotion: may have a "deadening effect" on emotions when overused or with prolonged use, anxiety, over-thinking, obsessive thinking (Mojay, 1997), grief

Subtle/energetic aromatherapy: In TCM, marjoram tonifies and circulates *Qi-energy*, clears cold phlegm, and calms the mind (Mojay, 1997). According to Leigh (2001), marjoram offers protection on a vibrational level from grief, anxiety, and irritability and could be used for the second or sacral chakra. Marjoram offers comfort, strength and warmth during times of anguish, mental strain, and irritability (Worwood, 1996).

In Practice: Sample Recipes Using Marjoram

Muscular Cramps	Centering
Marjoram	Marjoram
Clary sage	Lavender
Peppermint	Cypress

Sweet Orange / *Citrus sinensis* (L.) Osbeck syn. *Citrus aurantium* var. *sinensis* (L.)

Botany and History Information

Other common names: Orange

Botanical family: Rutaceae

Botany: *Citrus sinensis* is a medium-sized tree that can reach between 8 to 15 m. The tree normally has a single trunk with many branches and leaves that are dark green above and slightly lighter underneath. The flowers are fragrant and white. The peel is orange when ripe with a smooth, somewhat wrinkled texture.

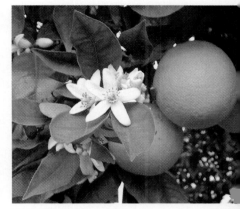

Figure 13-18 Sweet Orange
Source: Reprinted by permission of Ellen Levy Finch

History and myth: The English word for the color orange is derived from the Arabic name of the fruit. Simpson and Ogorzaly (1995) share the following story: "Oranges were considered by some to be the 'golden apples' of Greek mythology that the goddess of fertility gave to Hera when she married Zeus" (p. 121). It is believed that the Moors brought the orange to Spain, and the Spanish and Portuguese introduced them to the new world in the 1500s. The orange grows well in cooler climates, which promote the formation of carotene. Through the eighteenth and nineteenth centuries, sweet oranges were considered to be a delicacy for the wealthy.

Extraction Information

Countries of origin:	Israel, United States, Spain, Italy
Part of plant used:	peel or zest of fruit
Extraction method:	expression
Oil content:	0.5 to 3.5 percent
Color of oil:	clear to light yellow

Blending Information

Odor description:	refreshing, citrusy, orange
Blending factor:	7

Safety information:

▶ nonirritant, nonsensitizing

▶ Use less than 7 to 10 drops of citrus oils, combined or singly, in a bath to avoid skin irritation. Dilute citrus oils into a dispersant prior to adding to the bath to reduce potential skin irritation.

Chemical Feature

Rich in monoterpenes.

Chemical Profile

Monoterpenes: limonene (94.87 to 95.37%), α-pinene, β-pinene, sabinene, myrcene, β-farnesene, valencene

Therapeutic Actions

Antidepressant, antiseptic, antispasmodic, aperitive, carminative, digestive, febrifuge, **nervine**, **uplifting**.

Keywords: uplifting, refreshing, warming, happy, cheerful, digestive

Core Aromatic Applications

Digestive system: indigestion, nervous stomach

Nervous system: insomnia, anxiety, depression, agitation

Psyche and emotion: depression, challenging behavior, limited communication skills, disturbed eating patterns

Subtle/energetic aromatherapy: Sweet orange is a happy, uplifting essential oil that can bring the sunshine into an individual's life. Leigh (2001) says that orange allows one to expel any sour feeling in the heart and soul as well as attracts good fortune and luck. In TCM, orange unblocks and circulates stagnant *Qi-energy*, mainly when it accumulates in the liver, stomach, and intestines (Mojay, 1997).

In Practice: Sample Recipes Using Sweet Orange

Emotional Balancer	Uplifting
Sweet orange	Sweet orange
Geranium	Lavender
Patchouli	Ylang ylang

Patchouli / *Pogostemon cablin* (Blanco) Benth.

Botany and History Information

Botanical family: Lamiaceae syn. Labiatae

Botany: Patchouli is a perennial herb that can grow up to 2 feet tall. It has dark green leaves and, at times, small pale-pink tubular flowers. The leaves are very aromatic.

History and myth: According to Bown (2001), "In India, dried patchouli leaves were traditionally placed among clothes and their lingering scent in imported shawls entranced the Victorians; in the 1860s patchouli was the height of fashion" (p. 118). It was used by individuals in the 1960s and 70s in the United States to serve as a masking agent for the scent of marijuana. Patchouli remains fashionable in perfumes as a fixative and base note. According to Holmes (1997), patchouli is used in all three major world medical systems, traditional Chinese, Ayurvedic, and Greek medicine, for both topical and internal applications (p. 18).

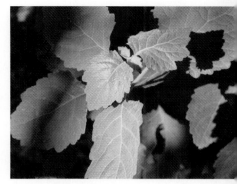

Figure 13-19 Patchouli
Source: Reprinted by permission of Kent Goodwin McKay

Extraction Information

Countries of origin:	Indonesia, India, China, Brazil
Part of plant used:	dried leaves
Extraction method:	distillation
Oil content:	0.25 to 0.75 percent fresh leaves 1.8 to 5 percent dried leaves
Color of oil:	red/brown to clear

Blending Information

Odor description:	strong, musty, hot, earthy, dry
Blending factor:	5

Safety information:

▶ nontoxic, nonirritant

Chemical Feature

Rich in sesquiterpenes and alcohols.

Chemical Profile

Sesquiterpenes (40 to 50%): α-bulnesene (10 to 25%), β-bulnesene (14 to 17.2%), α-guaiene (6 to 15%), β-guaiene, α-patchoulene, β-patchoulene, seychellene, cyclo-seychellene, β-caryophyllene, Δ-cadinene, aromadendrene (10 to 20%).

Alcohols (23 to 55%): patchoulol (32 to 46%), pogostol, bulnesol, nor-patchoulenol, patchoulic alcohol

Therapeutic Actions

Antibacterial, **antidepressant, antifungal, anti-inflammatory**, antiseptic, aphrodisiac, **astringent**, insect repellant, sedative, vulnerary.

Keywords: grounding, centering, meditative, calming, skin care

Core Aromatic Applications

Circulatory system: varicose veins

Reproductive/endocrine system: frigidity, menstrual cramps, reduced or lack of sex drive

Skin: astringent, useful in treating aging, sagging skin, itchy or inflamed skin conditions (Van Wyk and Wink, 2004, p. 249), acne, athlete's foot, cracked or chapped skin, eczema (weeping), fungal infections, wrinkles, irritated skin conditions, sores, fissures, scar tissue, fungal or parasitic skin infections (Holmes, 1997), soothing

Psyche and emotion: anxiety, confusion, poor concentration, mood swings, challenging behavior, hyperactivity, very relaxing, anxiety, feelings of being overwhelmed, depression, lacking connection with body

Subtle/energetic aromatherapy: Patchouli has a gentle yet persistent sensualizing nature that seduces us into accepting our body needs (Holmes, 1997). It can be used for individuals who are experiencing sexual frigidity or detachment. Patchouli can also benefit those who seek to develop or enhance intuitive and empathetic abilities. According to Holmes (1997), patchouli helps us become more integrated in our immediate environment. As a more viscous earthy aroma, patchouli is grounding and soothing for those who are feeling depressed, anxious, stressed out, or tense. Leigh (2001) writes that patchouli is very grounding and helps to root or maintain connection with the physical body. She recommends it for the second or sacral chakra.

In Practice: Sample Recipes Using Patchouli

Antidepressant	Oily Skin
Patchouli	Patchouli
Mandarin	Lemon
Ylang ylang	Geranium

Peppermint / *Mentha* x *piperita* L. (pro sp.)

Botany and History Information

Botanical family: Lamiaceae syn. Labiatae

Botany: There are approximately twenty true species of *Mentha, all of which readily hybridize with other Lamiaceae/Labiatae* species. There are thousands of known variations of the *Mentha* species, and *Mentha* x *piperita* is one of them. Considered a cross between *Mentha spicata* and *Mentha aquatica*, peppermint is a perennial that can grow up to 3 feet tall. It likes to spread and sends out its root system quite extensively. The leaves are dark green, purple-tinged, oval, and sharply toothed. In the summer the plant produces small lilac-pink flowers.

History and myth: According to Pliny, peppermint was popular both for adornment and flavoring in classical times, after which its only mention for many centuries was in a thirteenth-century Icelandic pharmacopoeia (Bown, 2001, p. 170). The name comes from the myth of the nymph Menthe. Pluto fell in love with her, and when his infuriated wife, Persephone, discovered them, she pursued Menthe and trod her ferociously into the ground. Pluto then turned Menthe into a wonderful healing plant (Grieve, 1996, p. 534). Today peppermint is widely used in commercial flavoring for such items as candy, toothpaste, jelly, muscle pain medicine, chewing gum, and mouthwash. Washington, Oregon, and Indiana are large producers of peppermint for the herb and essential oil. The United States is the world's largest producer of peppermint and spearmint oil, producing more than 80 percent of the world's supply (Foster, 1993, p. 150).

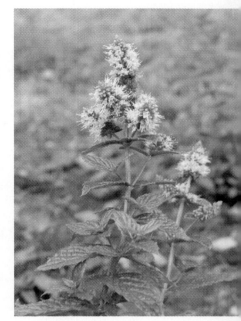

Figure 13-20 Peppermint
Source: Reprinted by permission of Kent Goodwin McKay

Extraction Information

Countries of origin:	France, England, United States
Part of plant used:	leaves and flowering tops
Extraction method:	distillation
Oil content:	0.9 to 3 percent
Color of oil:	pale yellow, clear

Blending Information

Odor description:	fresh, menthol, clean, cool, strong
Blending factor:	1 to 2

Safety information:

▶ Menthol is an irritant in high concentration, especially if evaporation from the skin is prevented. Peppermint oil should not be applied over large areas of skin because of its freezing effect (Schnaubelt, 2004).

▶ Peppermint oil should not be applied to the facial region or near the nose of infants or small children due to the risk of spasm and respiratory arrest (Van Wyk and Wink, 2004, p. 206), nor should it be applied to infants or children under the age of thirty months (Schnaubelt, 2004).

▶ Avoid undiluted application to open wounds and sensitive skin.

▶ Peppermint is a potent essential oil and can have differing effects depending on concentration used. Reactions to peppermint range from mildly heating or cooling to burning.

Chemical Feature

Rich in the alcohol, menthol, and the ketone, menthone.

Chemical Profile

Alcohols (50%): menthol (38 to 46.2%), isomenthol, neo-menthol, piperitol, piperitenol, isopiperitenol, α-terpineol, linalol (<1%), terpinen-4-ol, viridiflorol, myrtenol, nerolidol (trace)

Ketones: menthone (16 to 25%), iso-menthone, neomenthone, piperitone, caryophyllene oxide, pulegone

Therapeutic Actions

Analgesic, antiemetic, anti-inflammatory, antiseptic, **antispasmodic**, antitussive, **carminative**, cephalic, decongestant, **expectorant**, febrifuge, insecticidal, stimulant, **stomachic**, sudorific.

Keywords: refreshing, cooling/warming, stimulating, digestive, pain relieving

Core Aromatic Applications

Circulatory system: sluggish circulation (use with rosemary or black pepper), varicose veins, Raynaud's syndrome

Digestive system: travel sickness, stomach upsets, colic, cramping, dyspepsia, excess gas, nausea, stomach cramps, irritable bowel syndrome (Foster, 1993), spastic colon, postsurgical nausea

Lymph/immune system: supports lymphatic drainage massage, chronic fatigue syndrome

Musculoskeletal system: muscular stiffness, aches and pains, tight muscles, rheumatism, pain, fibromyalgia, sprains, strains, plantar fasciitis, carpal tunnel syndrome, sciatica, bursitis, bruises, can reduce swelling and pain (Haas, 2004)

Nervous system: mental fatigue, headache (Gobel et al., 1994), migraine, neuralgia

Reproductive/endocrine system: dysmenorrhea, painful cramps

Respiratory system: bronchitis, halitosis, spasmodic cough, head cold, common cold, congestion, sinusitis, flu

Psyche and emotion: dislike of exercise, limited communication skills, mental fatigue, low energy, lack of clarity

Subtle/energetic aromatherapy: Peppermint is an invigorating and consciousness-expanding essential oil. In TCM, peppermint is energetically cool and dry and helps to circulate *Qi-energy*, clear hot phlegm, and stimulates the nerves and brain (Mojay, 1997). Peppermint can be used to facilitate the digestion of new ideas and impressions (Mojay, 1997). Peppermint can help to clarify and refresh the emotional state of the individual. According to Leigh (2001), peppermint can assist in overcoming feelings of inferiority and is used for the third or solar plexus chakra.

> **NOTE**
> Buckle (2003) reports that peppermint is routinely offered in many chemotherapy units in the United States and England to prevent and relieve nausea. Inhalation is recommended at a low dosage: 2 to 3 drops on a cotton swab.

In Practice: Sample Recipes Using Peppermint

Muscular Aches and Pains	Headaches/Migraines
Peppermint	Peppermint
Eucalyptus	Lavender
Lemon	
Rosemary ct. camphor	

Rose / *Rosa* x *damascena* P. Mill.

Botany and History Information

Other common names: Damask rose

Botanical family: Rosaceae

Botany: There are over 250 different species and many thousands more hybrids and varieties. *Rosa damascena* and *Rosa centifolia* are the most commonly used rose species for extracting the essential oil and absolute. *Rosa centifolia* has also been called Cabbage Rose due to its highly aromatic small pink flowers. It can grow up to 6 feet tall. *Rosa damascena*, commonly referred to as the Damask rose, bears pink to red flowers. All rose species have flowers with five petals.

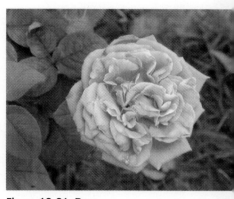

Figure 13-21 Rose

History and myth: Rose petals, fruits, leaves, and roots have been utilized throughout the ages for their medicine and perfume. The rose finds a place among the medicine of the Chinese, Persians, Indians, Arabs, Romans, and Greeks. The rose has been given the power of healing and beauty as well as for soothing the heart. According to Grieve (1996), "The word *rosa* comes from the Greek word *rodon* (red), and the rose of the Ancients was of a deep crimson color, which probably suggested the fable of its springing from the blood of Adonis" (p. 684). During the Middle Ages, the rose was commonly found in monastery gardens and used for medicinal purposes. The rose was called the "Queen of Flowers" in 600 BC by the famed poet, Sappho. Throughout its history the rose has been a symbol of beauty, love, joy, perfection, and even immortality. The Romans were probably the most lavish in their use of roses for they used them extensively in celebrations, feasts, weddings, and funerals. The Romans would also place rose petals in their wine during the winter months and wore rose garlands to ward off the hangover during festivals. The first rose distillation for the rose water is believed to have been accomplished by Avicenna during the tenth century. According to Grieve (1996), rose oil was accidentally discovered during the wedding feast of Princess Nour-Djihan and the Emperor Djihanguyr. A canal that circled their garden was filled with rose water. Due to the heat of the sun, the essential oil of rose separated from the water, floated to the top, and was observed by all who smelled its captivating aroma (p. 684).

Extraction Information

Countries of origin:	Bulgaria, Turkey, India
Part of plant used:	petals
Extraction method:	distillation produces Rose otto also known as rose essential oil solvent extraction produces Rose absolute
Oil content:	1kg oil per 2000 to 4000 kilograms of rose petals
Color of oil:	Rose otto: clear to pale yellow; Rose absolute: dark yellow/orange to clear

Blending Information

Odor description:	floral, rich, warm, fresh, feminine
Blending factor:	1

Safety information:

▶ nonirritant, non-photosensitizing, non-phototoxic

Chemical Feature

Rich in alcohols supported by monoterpenes.

Chemical Profile

Monoterpenes: stearoptene (16 to 22% [Price & Price, 1995]), α-pinene, β-pinene, α-terpinene, limonene, myrcene, ocimene, p-cymene, camphene

Alcohols: geraniol (11.87 to 35%), **citronellol** (33 to 45.04%), ethanol, **nerol** (3.6 to 10%), linalool (less than 1%)

Therapeutic Actions

Antibacterial, **antidepressant**, antifungal, anti-inflammatory, antiseptic, antiviral, aphrodisiac, **astringent**, emmenagogue, **nervine**, sedative, stomachic, **vulnerary (cell regenerative)**.

Keywords: calming, soothing, female disorders, antidepressant

Core Aromatic Applications

Circulatory system: varicose veins, broken capillaries

Reproductive/endocrine system: irregular menstruation, impotence, sterility, frigidity, reduced or low libido, PMS, amenorrhea, dysmenorrhea, menopause, ovary problems, polycystic ovarian disease, postnatal depression

Skin: broken capillaries, conjunctivitis (rose water), oily skin, mature and sensitive skin, aging skin

Psyche and emotion: depression, shock, grief, challenging behavior, fear of physical contact, mood swings, frigidity, heartbreak, anger, frustration, jealousy, resentment, difficulty loving or trusting, lack of creativity, inability to forgive

Subtle/energetic aromatherapy: Rose, the queen of essential oils, represents the feminine water element and is a core essential oil for addressing sexuality, self-nurturing, and self-esteem. It can be used to give comfort in heartbreaks, emotional losses, broken trusts, and violated feelings in general (Holmes, 1994). The oil should be considered for all people in states of emotional disconnection, showing coldness, harshness—an emotional void—toward themselves and others (Holmes, 1994). For TCM, rose is cool and moist in nature, clears heat and inflammation, and helps to restore the body's yin energy (Mojay, 1997).

> **NOTE**
>
> True rose essential oil is one of the most expensive oils on the market. The average cost of 1 ml is $27 to $39, which means that each drop can cost up to $2 to $4. One ounce of true rose essential oil can cost well over $400. Many companies will sell rose essential oil either by the drop or ml or as a 5 to 10 percent dilution in Jojoba oil. True rose essential oil is commonly adulterated to bring the cost down, so beware. A true rose essential oil will be solid at cool room temperatures. Rose absolute (solvent extracted) is less expensive and averages $30 for 2 ml or $15 for 1 ml. Some retailers may be selling rose absolute as rose essential oil, so beware of low-priced true rose essential oil. Although the absolute is beautiful and has many similar uses as rose essential oil, it does not replace it nor is it the same.

In Practice: Sample Recipes Using Rose

Soothing the Heart Blend	Skin Care Blend (Oily Skin)
Rose	Rose
Tangerine	Patchouli
Ylang ylang	

Rosemary / *Rosmarinus officinalis* L. ct. camphor

Botany and History Information

Botanical family: Lamiaceae syn. Labiatae

Botany: *Rosmarinus officinalis* is an aromatic, evergreen, flowering shrub that grows from 3 to 6 feet tall. The numerous branches have an ash-colored, scaly bark and bear opposite, leathery, thick leaves that are lustrous, linear, dark yet bright green above and downy white underneath. The pale blue/lilac flowers grow in short racemes, and both the leaves and flowers are highly aromatic. The shrub is native to the Mediterranean region where it grows along the seashore, hence its Latin name which means "Dew of the sea."

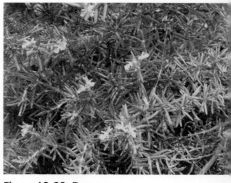

Figure 13-22 Rosemary

History and myth: Rosemary has been associated with memory and fidelity since the famed times of the Egyptians. It has been used at funerals, religious ceremonies, weddings, and as an emblem for fidelity. Shakespeare's Ophelia echoed these associations when she said, "There's rosemary, that's for remembrance; pray, love, remember." The word *Rosmarinus* can be translated to "dew of the sea," which is reflected by rosemary's attraction to growing along the coastal region. Rosemary and juniper were once utilized in French hospitals to reduce microbes and purify the air. The PDR for Herbal Medicines (2000) reports that "Rosemary is used in folk medicine for digestive symptoms, headaches and migraine, dysmenorrhea, amenorrhea and oligomenorrhea, states of exhaustion, dizziness and poor memory" (p. 645).

Extraction Information

Countries of origin:	Croatia (Haas, 2004), Spain (Bowles, 2003)
Part of plant used:	flowers and leaves
Extraction method:	distillation
Oil content:	1 to 2.5 percent
Color of oil:	clear to pale yellow

Blending Information

Odor description:	fresh, strong, vibrant, herbaceous
Blending factor:	2

Safety information:

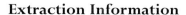

▶ Caution is expressed when using camphor-rich oils on individuals with hypertension or epilepsy. Avoid internal use of the oil. Low dilutions are recommended.

Chemical Feature

Monoterpenes 25 percent, oxides 30 percent, ketones 30 percent (camphor), alcohols (linalol) 8 percent (Haas, 2004).

Chemical Profile

Monoterpenes 25–30%: α-pinene (17.9–25%), β-pinene (3–7%), camphene (8–19%), myrcene (3–5%)

Alcohols: linalool (0.6–4%), α-terpineol (1–5%), borneol (1–3%)

Oxides: 1,8 cineol (15–20%), caryophyllene oxide

Ketones: α-thujone, β-thujone, camphor (6.4-30%)

Therapeutic Actions

Mild analgesic, antirheumatic, antiviral, carminative, **cephalic**, **decongesting**, digestive, **mucolytic**, rubefacient, **stimulant**, vulnerary.

Keywords: stimulating, memory aid, muscular system

Core Aromatic Applications

Circulatory system: poor circulation (Van Wyk and Wink, 2004, p. 276) Lymph

Lymph/immune system: sluggish lymph

Musculoskeletal system: cramps, sprains, swellings, arthritis, stiffness, pain relieving, lack of muscle tone, neuralgic pain, fibromyalgia, rheumatoid arthritis, plantar fasciitis, carpal tunnel syndrome, bursitis, cramping pains in the legs (Barker, 1996), for neuromuscular problems including muscular aches and pains, cramps, spasms, and neuralgic and rheumatic pain (Goeb, 1996)

Nervous system: poor memory, headaches, hypotension, neuralgia, mental fatigue, nervous exhaustion, lack of energy, foggy mind/thinking

Respiratory system: bronchitis, excess mucus, flu, colds, sinus congestion

Skin: varicose veins (Haas, 2004), slow healing wounds, slow hair growth

Psyche and emotion: poor memory, lack of concentration, difficulty studying, exhaustion, lethargy, depression, limited communication skills, dislike of exercise, lack of energy or clarity of thought

Subtle/energetic aromatherapy: According to Mojay (1997), rosemary is one of the most valuable and invigorating of essences and is an excellent tonic of the body's *yang* energy, able in addition to promote the circulation of both *Qi-energy* and blood. Mojay writes that rosemary is suited to the cold, debilitated individual who has a poor sense of self-worth and who lacks a strong, healthy ego. Leigh (2001) believes that rosemary is a psychic protector and helps to promote clear thought, clear sight or vision, and to develop clairvoyance. She therefore recommends it for the sixth or third eye chakra.

In Practice: Sample Recipes Using Rosemary ct. camphor

General Poor Circulation: Tonic	Scalp Tonic
Rosemary ct. camphor	Rosemary ct. camphor
Black pepper	Lemon
Ginger	Peppermint

Tea tree / *Melaleuca alternifolia* Cheel

Botany and History Information

Other common names: T-tree, Ti tree

Botanical family: Myrtaceae

Botany: *Melaleuca alternifolia* is an evergreen tree growing to a height of 15 to 20 feet. The leaves are bluish-green, very narrow, and similar in appearance to cypress leaves. Tea tree produces a small creamy white to purplish flower. The tree thrives in natural swampy conditions and is found in the Bungawalbyn wetlands of New South Wales.

History and myth: Tea tree has a long history of use by the Australian Aborigines who employed it as medicine for a variety of skin disorders (bruises, insect bites, skin infections) and other ailments. It was the famous British explorer, Captain Hook, who gave it its name after his sailors brewed it as tea in hopes of preventing scurvy. Captain Hook pronounced it "Tea Tree" and the name stuck. Tea tree is one of the most thoroughly researched essential oils. It was utilized during World War II by the Royal Australian army and navy as an antiseptic for wounds and for treatment of various skin conditions.

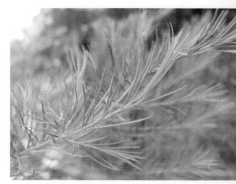

Figure 13-23 Tea tree
Source: Reprinted by permission of Kent Goodwin McKay

Extraction Information

Countries of origin:	Australia, New Zealand
Part of plant used:	leaves
Extraction method:	steam distillation
Oil content:	2.0 to 5.0 percent
Color of oil:	clear to pale yellow

Blending Information

Odor description:	spicy, warm, balsamic
Blending factor:	3

Safety information:

▶ nonirritating, nonsensitizing, non-phototoxic

Chemical Feature

Rich in the oxide, 1,8 cineole, and the alcohol, terpinene-4-ol, and monoterpenes.

Chemical Profile

Monoterpenes (25 to 40%): α-pinene, β-pinene, α-terpinene (4.6 to 13%), γ-terpinene, ρ-cymene (<12%), limonene, terpinolene, α-thujene, sabinene, myrcene, α-phellandrene, β-phellandrene, terpinolene

Alcohols: terpinen-4-ol (1.7 to 52.9%), α-terpineol (5.3 to 11.8%), globulol, viridiflorol, cubenol, linalool

Oxides: 1,8 cineole (10 to 64.1%), 1,4-cineole (trace)

Therapeutic Actions

Antibacterial, antibiotic, **antifungal**, (Riley et al., 2002), anti-inflammatory, **antimicrobial** (Riley, 2005), antiseptic, antispasmodic, **antiviral**, **expectorant**, **immuno-stimulant**, stimulant.

Keywords: antibacterial, antifungal, antiviral, immune enhancing

Core Aromatic Applications

Digestive system: colic, diarrhea, enteritis, intestinal parasites, dental hygiene (Hammer et al., 2002), gum problems, mouth ulcers, oral thrush, *Candida albicans*

Lymph/immune system: lowered or compromised immunity, lymph congestion

Musculoskeletal system: tired, achy muscles and joints, arthritis, rheumatism

Reproductive/endocrine system: leucorrhoea, vaginal candidiasis (Hammer et al., 2002)

Respiratory system: colds, flu, bronchitis, sinus infections or congestion, coughs, sore throat, tonsillitis, ear infections

Skin: acne, nail fungus, oily skins, abscesses, boils, cold sores (Riley, 2005), cuts, dandruff, herpes simplex (Riley, 2005), insect bites, lice, rashes, shingles, infected wounds, varicose ulcers, athlete's foot, ringworm, inflamed skin conditions (Koh et al., 2002)

Subtle/energetic aromatherapy: In TCM, tea tree can tonify *Qi-energy* in cases of chronic lethargy, shallow breathing, palpitations, and poor circulation (Mojay, 1997).

NOTE

The chemistry of tea tree, in particular its 1,8 cineole and terpinen-4-ol content, has been a subject of great debate, mostly for safety considerations. According to Kerr (2000), "the Australian Government has a standard for Tea tree essential oil which states that the 1,8 cineole content should not exceed 15% and the terpinen-4-ol content should be at least 30%" (p. 9). Buckle (2003) says that one should look for Melaleuca alternifolia CT terpineol rather than a tea tree rich in cineol, as cineol can produce discomfort when applied to mucus membranes as well as increase the chance of skin irritation.

However, according to Southwell (n.d.), his research shows that "there are no grounds for promoting low cineole oils other than for avoiding low terpinen-4-ol oils. If all buyers could be convinced of this, more tea tree oil could be offered for sale, providing a yield boost to many producers." Carson (1999) reports "1,8 cineole was regarded as an undesirable constituent in tea tree oil due to its reputation as a skin and mucous membrane irritant. However, the latter 2 case studies (Knight & Hausen, 1994 and Southwell et al., 1997) indicate that this component is not responsible for a large proportion of sensitivity reactions" (p. 9).

In Practice: Sample Recipes Using Tea Tree

Room Cleanser	Skin Antiseptic
Tea tree	Tea tree
Lemon	Lavender
Eucalyptus	Lemon
	Roman chamomile

Vetiver / *Vetiveria zizanioides* (L.) Nash ex Small

Botany and History Information

Other common names: Khas Khas, Khus Khus

Botanical family: Poaceae syn. Gramineae.

Botany: *Vetiveria zizanioides* is a tall, densely tufted perennial scented grass that grows to 3 m. The grass normally develops large clumps with a rhizome and fibrous root system that contains the essential oil. The main rootstock is a stout, branching rhizome that develops an extensive but not deeply penetrating system of aromatic roots. The roots are whitish yellow when young and change to a reddish brown as they mature. The roots yield very little oil, making the oil expensive; this can lead to adulteration with synthetics. The plant is botanically related to lemongrass and citronella.

History and myth: Vetiver has a history of use as an insect repellant. Bundles of vetiver root would be used to infuse wardrobes and rooms with its aroma. The root fibers would be woven into mats and screens. Vetiver has a long traditional use as a fixative or base note in perfumes. The aroma of vetiver has been used to bring about tranquility and protection from evil spirits or influences.

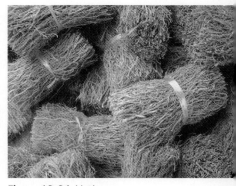

Figure 13-24 Vetiver
Source: Reprinted by permission of David Monniaux

Extraction Information

Countries of origin:	Haiti, Sri Lanka, India
Part of plant used:	roots of grass
Extraction method:	distillation
Oil content:	2 to 3 percent
Color of oil:	golden orange to dark brown, viscous oil

Blending Information

Odor description:	sweet, earthy, warm, woody, deep
Blending factor:	1

Safety information:

▶ non-phototoxic, nonirritant, nonsensitizing

Chemical Feature

Rich in the alcohol, vetiverol.

Chemical Profile

Sesquiterpenes: vetivene, vetivazulene, tricyclovetivene

Alcohols: vetiverol (50 to 70%), bicyclovetiverol (12%), tricyclovetiverol (3 to 4%)

Esters: vetiverol acetate

Ketones: α-vetiverone (3 to 4%), β-vetiverone (3%)

Therapeutic Actions

Anti-inflammatory, antirheumatic, antiseptic, antispasmodic, aphrodisiac, astringent, **nervine**, sedative.

Keywords: calming, grounding, balancing

Core Aromatic Applications

Circulatory system: varicose veins, cold hands and/or cold feet, poor circulation, circulatory tonic

Lymph/immune system: lowered immunity, particularly due to stress

Musculoskeletal system: muscular aches and pains, sprains and stiffness, arthritis, rheumatism

Nervous system: debility, nervous tension, insomnia

Reproductive/endocrine system: menopause, postnatal depression, PMS, reduced or lowered sex drive

Skin: acne, inflamed conditions, oily skin (due to its slight astringent effect), preventative for stretch marks and wrinkles, nourishing and balancing for dry skin, wound care, irritated skin, rashes, and topical bacterial or fungal infections (Kerr, 2003)

Psyche and emotion: anxiety, feelings of being ungrounded, mental burnout, lack of confidence, depression, lack of center/focus, lack of clarity, overwhelming thoughts or feelings

Subtle/energetic aromatherapy: Vetiver is one of the most grounding and centering essential oils available. On the mental level, vetiver can serve to pull together scattered ideas and ground them into more practical concepts. On the feeling level, vetiver cools down emotional flightiness and dizzy passions and grounds them in the reality of true body-centered feelings (Holmes, 1997). Vetiver grounds energy and promotes strength. It is a wonderful essential oil for those who tend to float outside their bodies and yet need to be grounded and centered in life. In TCM, vetiver is cool and moist energy that can be used to clear heat while also nourishing, calming, and uplifting (Mojay, 1997). Leigh (2001) recommends vetiver for balancing the entire chakra/aura system and for protecting the solar plexus chakra from oversensitivity.

In Practice: Sample Recipes Using Vetiver

Heart-Centered Blend	Grounding and Centering Blend
Rose	Vetiver
Vetiver	Patchouli
Mandarin	Mandarin

Ylang ylang / *Cananga odorata* (Lam.) Hook. f. & T. Thomson or *Cananga odorata* var genuina

Botany and History Information

Other common names: ilang ilang

Botanical family: Annonaceae

Botany: Ylang ylang is a tropical aromatic tree that originated in the Philippines and has now spread throughout tropical Asia. The tree can grow up to 100 feet. The leaves are large, oval, and shiny. At first when the flowers appear, they are greenish. Over a period of twenty days, they open and become mainly yellow-green flowers that exude an intense aroma at night. The flowers appear constantly and are more abundant during the rainy season.

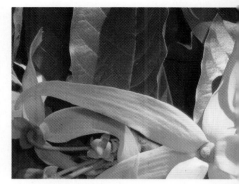

Figure13-25 Ylang ylang
Source: Reprinted by permission of Kent Goodwin McKay

History and myth: The name ylang ylang has been interpreted as "flowers of flowers." It originates from the Malay "ilang-ilang." On the Hawaiian Islands, ylang is mixed with coconut oil to create a mixture known as "borriborri," which is rubbed into the body for its aroma as well as its protective abilities. The women used this mixture to protect their hair from the sea salt, while the flowers were used to adorn their hair. The oil was an ingredient of Macassar oil (hair tonic), hence the use of antimacassars on the backs of chairs to prevent greasy stains. The oil is sometimes called "poorman's Jasmine" and blends well with jasmine, neroli, and sandalwood.

Extraction Information

Countries of origin:	Reunion Islands, Comoros, Madagascar, Costa Rica
Part of plant used:	flowers
Extraction method:	Distillation: fractional distillation (see note at end of profile)
Oil content:	2.0 to 2.5 percent
Color of oil:	clear, pale yellow

Blending Information:

Odor description:	warm, exotic, sweet, heavy, sensual
Blending factor:	4

Safety information:

▶ nontoxic, nonirritant, non-photo toxic

Chemical Feature

Rich sesquiterpenes and supported by alcohols and esters.

Chemical Profile

Sesquiterpenes(28.8 to 54%): α-farnesene (6.5 to 18%), β-caryophyllene (6.8 to 33%), germacrene D (11 to 25%), Δ-cadinene (2 to 5%)

Alcohols: linalool (18.6 to 50%)

Esters (15%): benzyl acetate (3.7 to 17.4%)

Therapeutic Actions

Antidepressant, antiseptic, antispasmodic, **aphrodisiac**, hypotensive, **nervine**

Keywords: Euphoric, aphrodisiac, antidepressant, calming, regulator

Core Aromatic Applications

Circulatory system: high blood pressure, tachycardia, heart palpitations

Reproductive/endocrine system: male impotence, PMS (low self-esteem), dysmenorrhea

Skin: oily/combination skin, aging or stressed skin, scalp tonic (Kerr, 1997)

Psyche and emotion: anxiety, anger, and fright, depression, lack of inner trust, reduced libido, lack of self confidence or trust, grief/bereavement, post-traumatic stress syndrome, nervous tension, frigidity

Subtle/energetic aromatherapy: According to Leigh (2001), ylang ylang helps to dispel anger and negative emotional states and can assist an individual in overcoming sexual dysfunctions or concerns. She recommends its use for the second or sacral charka. For TCM, ylang ylang can help to clear heat from the heart while simultaneously harmonizing the mind (*Shen*) (Mojay, 1997). Ylang ylang has an incredible ability to calm the heart and ease the mind.

Research Notes and Additional Information

In 2005 Bob Harris reported "Ylang ylang was found to be a 'harmonizing'; essential oil during research conducted by a Thai/Austrian study. The results indicated that ylang ylang can reduce pulse rate while at the same time increase alertness and arousal. The reduced level of arousal of the ANS (autonomic nervous system) did not lead to deactivation at the behavioural level; in contrast the subjects reported to feel more attentive and alert" (p. 55–56).

> **NOTE**
>
> Ylang ylang is different from other essential oils as it is not actually a whole essential oil. During the distillation process, various grades or fractions are removed at different time intervals. For instance, after the first hour of distillation the first fraction is removed. This fraction is called "extra" and considered to be superior in aroma to the other fractions. This first fraction also contains higher levels of esters, up to 40 to 50 percent, and hence could be considered more calming. During the next two to three hours of distillation, a second fraction is removed, and this is called "ylang ylang #1" or "complete." The second fraction tends to be rich in sesquiterpenes and esters. Two further fractions are removed at five to six hours (called ylang ylang #3) and then at nine to ten hours. Ylang ylang extra, complete, and #3 are available to the aromatherapy practitioner. Extra and complete will both be more expensive than #3.

In Practice: Sample Recipes Using Ylang Ylang

Aphrodisiac	Uplifting
Ylang ylang	Ylang ylang
Rose	Mandarin
Mandarin	Patchouli

Angelica root / *Angelica archangelica* syn. *officinalis*

Other common names:	Garden angelica, archangel
Botanical family:	Apiaceae syn. Umbelliferae
Countries of origin:	Hungary, Belgium, Germany, England, France
Part of plant used:	roots
Odor description:	sweet, herbaceous, woody
Blending factor:	3
Chemical feature:	Rich in monoterpenes (up to 70%) supported by sesquiterpenes and furanocoumarins.

Safety information: Photosensitizing.

Actions on the body: Antiseptic, **antispasmodic**, aphrodisiac, carminative, depurative, **digestive**, diuretic, emmenagogue, expectorant, febrifuge, **nervine**, sedative, stomachic, tonic.

Keywords: balancing, strengthening, rejuvenating (especially after long illness), grounding

Core aromatic applications:

- ▶ tonic to digestive system: constipation, indigestion, excess gas, poor appetite (may stimulate appetite)
- ▶ nervous tension or upset, irritability, nervous exhaustion, stress, heart palpitations, anxiety, insomnia
- ▶ irregular menstruation, PMS, hormonal imbalance, menopause, frigidity, cramps, supportive to clary sage
- ▶ nervous dispositions, grounding, fortifying, healing during times of great emotions, soothes weaknesses of the nervous system, helps to discover our own stamina, inner strength, provides a connection to our Higher Self and the angelic realms

Bergamot / *Citrus* x *aurantium* ssp. *bergamia* syn. *Citrus bergamia*

Other common names:	Bitter orange, Seville orange tree
Botanical family:	Rutaceae
Countries of origin:	Calabria, Southern Italy, Sicily
Part of plant used:	zest, peel of fruit
Odor description:	rich, exotic, fresh, sweet, sharp, citrus becoming more spicy over time
Blending factor:	7 to 8
Chemical feature:	Up to 60 percent esters (linalyl acetate), monoterpenes (limonene, pinene), furanocoumarin (5 to 10% bergaptene).

Safety information: Strong photosensitizer. •Do not use prior to going into the sun or other similar light. •To overcome problems with phototoxicity, bergamot oil can be vacuum distilled to create a terpeneless and bergaptenless oil. This process will result in an essential oil that has a slightly stronger and finer aroma.

Actions of the body: Analgesic, **antidepressant**, **antiseptic**, antispasmodic, carminative, deodorant, digestive, febrifuge, insecticide, **nervine**, stomachic, tonic, vermifuge, vulnerary.

Keywords: "brings in the sunshine," uplifting, antidepressant, antiseptic, refreshing.

Core aromatic applications:

- ▶ calming yet uplifting, anxiety, nervous tension, insomnia, anger, depression, irritability, frustration, stress-related disorders
- ▶ oily complexions, shingles, acne
- ▶ PMS, hormone-related moodiness or depression, emotional ups and downs during menopause
- ▶ has an ability to relax the nerves and refresh the spirit, indicated for depressive states that stem from stress and pent up feelings, has an ability to harmonize *Liver-Qi* (Mojay, 1997)

Birch / *Betula lenta* (Sweet birch), *Betula alleghaniensis* (Yellow birch), or *Betula nigra* (Black or River birch)

Botanical family:	Betulaceae
Country of origin:	Canada
Part of plant used:	wood/bark
Odor description:	wintergreen-like, minty
Blending factor:	2
Chemical feature:	98 percent methylsalicylate (esters).

Safety information: Avoid use throughout pregnancy and breast-feeding. •Do not use birch or wintergreen on infants, on damaged skin, or with individuals on other salicylate-based medication. •Do not use with individuals who are taking warfarin. •This oil is often adulterated with synthetic methyl salicylate. Please be assured that you are buying the distilled birch extract. •Methyl salicylate can be absorbed through the skin, resulting in human fatalities (Duke, 1983). See chemistry chapter for additional information.

Actions on the body: **Analgesic**, antiseptic, astringent, diuretic, tonic.

Keywords: pain relieving, stimulating, warming yet cooling

Core aromatic applications:

- ▶ muscular aches and pains, sciatica, rheumatism, muscle stiffness or tightness, increase range of motion, joint pain and stiffness, plantar fasciitis, cramps, carpal tunnel syndrome, whiplash, spasms or cramps, sprains or strains, neuralgia, TMJ
- ▶ stimulating, refreshing, energizing aroma

Cardamom / *Elettaria cardamomum*

Botanical family:	Zingiberaceae
Part of plant used:	fruit/seed
Extraction method:	distillation

Countries of origin:	Sri Lanka, Ceylon, Guatemala
Odor description:	spicy, bitter lemon, sweet
Blending factor:	4
Chemical feature:	Oxides (32 to 50% 1,8 cineole) and esters (terpinyl acetate).

Safety information: None known.

Actions on the body: Antibacterial, antiseptic, antispasmodic, aperitive, **aphrodisiac**, **carminative**, cephalic, decongestant, **digestive**, diuretic, **expectorant**, **stimulant**, stomachic, tonic.

Keywords: aphrodisiac, warming, stimulating yet comforting

Core aromatic applications:

- ▸ constipation, excess gas, colic, soothing to stomach upsets caused by emotional upsets or nervous conditions, encourages flow of saliva, soothes nausea, heartburn, indigestion
- ▸ muscular aches and pains, joint pain or stiffness, sports warm-up
- ▸ bronchitis, coughs, warming effect makes it good for a "cold" in the lungs, liquefies dry mucus, asthma
- ▸ emotionally warming, impotence, frigidity, aphrodisiac
- ▸ stimulates the movement of digestive Qi, indicated for poor concentration, over-thinking, worry, nervous exhaustion, can restore an "appetite for life" (Mojay, 1997)

Carrot seed / *Daucus carota*

Other common names:	Bird's neat
Botanical family:	Apiaceae syn. Umbelliferae
Part of plant used:	dried seed
Countries of origin:	France, Holland, Hungary
Odor description:	sweet, fresh, tenacious, slightly spicy, warm-spicy
Blending factor:	6
Chemical feature:	Sesquiterpene alcohols (carotol) and monoterpenes.

Safety information: None known.

Actions on the body: Antiseptic, antispasmodic, **carminative**, **detoxifier**, **digestive**, diuretic, stimulant, stomachic, tonic, **vulnerary**.

Keywords: wound healing, digestive, stimulating

Core aromatic applications:

- ▸ constipation, excess gas, heartburn, indigestion
- ▸ wound healing, eczema, brown spots (Haas, 2004), aging/mature skin, congested skin, postsurgical wound healing, revitalizes dry, pallid skin (Schnaubelt, 1995)
- ▸ edema, sluggish lymph flow

Cedarwood / *Cedrus atlantica*

Other common names: Atlas Cedar, African Cedar, Moroccan Cedarwood

Botanical family: Pinaceae

Place of origin: Atlas Mountains in Morocco and Algeria

Part of plant used: bark, leaves, and twigs

Odor description: fairly viscous with a warm, woody, balsamic fragrance and a camphoraceous top note

Blending factor: 7 to 8

Chemical feature: Sesquiterpenes

Safety information: None known.

Actions on the body: Antifungal, antiseptic, antiviral, aphrodisiac, **astringent**, diuretic, emmenagogue, expectorant, **mucolytic,** sedative (nervous), stimulant (circulatory), tonic.

Keywords: antiseptic, preserving, soothing, spiritual

Core aromatic applications:

▶ oily skin, acne, athlete's foot, blemishes, dandruff, cellulite, varicose veins
▶ bronchitis, coughs, asthma, excess mucus in upper respiratory tract
▶ nervous tension, stress-related conditions, anxiety
▶ fortifying and strengthening, a powerful tonic of the body's *Qi-energy*, use for general lethargy, nervous debility, lower backache, and poor concentration (Mojay, 1997)

Cinnamon leaf / *Cinnamomum zeylanicum* or *Cinnamomum verum*

Botanical family: Lauraceae

Countries of origin: Sri Lanka, Madagascar, East Indies, Jamaica

Part of plant used: leaves

Odor description: warm-woody, spicy, sweet aroma

Blending factor: 3 or 4

Chemical feature: Phenols, up to 70 percent eugenol with phenylpropanoids (cinnamic aldehyde).

Safety information: Avoid undiluted application, strong irritation. • Dermal and mucus membrane irritant. Do not use in the bath. • The oil from the leaf is less irritating than the bark oil. • Sensitizer. Avoid prolonged use.

Actions on the body: Analgesic, **antibacterial, antifungal, antimicrobial,** antiseptic, antispasmodic, **antiviral, aphrodisiac,** astringent, carminative, digestive, emmenagogue, escharotic, stimulant (circulatory, cardiac, respiratory).

Keywords: antimicrobial, antiviral, warming, stimulating, digestive

Core aromatic applications:

- colds, flu, bronchitis
- loss of appetite, diarrhea, dyspepsia, flatulence, intestinal spasm, sluggish digestion, nausea
- debility, nervous exhaustion, neuralgia, chronic fatigue
- rheumatism, muscular spasms, muscular aches and pains, muscle stiffness, sciatica
- painful periods, scanty periods, impotency, frigidity, cramps, PMS

Clove bud / *Syzygium aromaticum* syn. *Eugenia caryophyllata*

Botanical family:	Myrtaceae
Countries of origin:	Madagascar, Indonesia, India
Part of plant used:	bud
Odor description:	spicy clove, warming
Blending factor:	5
Chemical feature:	Phenol (eugenol up to 70%).

Safety information: Skin irritant, always recommended to dilute down Mucous membrane irritant "The authors commented that eugenol progressively destroys the cells of the mucosal epithelium, and causes an acute inflammatory response."[1]

Actions on the body: **Analgesic, a**ntibacterial, **antifungal**, antiseptic, antispasmodic, **antiviral**, **carminative**, rubefacient, stomachic.

Keywords: warming, pain relieving, aphrodisiac

Core aromatic applications:

- muscular aches and pains or stiffness, joint stiffness, sciatica, pain relief, sprains, myalgia, rheumatism, fibromyalgia, plantar fasciitis, carpal tunnel syndrome
- excess gas, sluggish digestion

Grapefruit / *Citrus* x *paradisi*

Botanical family:	Rutaceae
Country of origin:	Israel, United States
Part of plant used:	zest, peel of fruit
Odor description:	fresh-citrusy, sweet
Blending factor:	8
Chemical feature:	Rich in monoterpenes, up to 95 percent.

---

[1] Robert Tisserand and Tony Balacs, *Essential Oil Safety*, Churchill Livingston: New York, 1995, p. 60.

Safety information: Use less than 7 to 10 drops of citrus oils, combined or singly, in bath to avoid skin irritation. Dilute citrus oils into a dispersant prior to adding to the bath to reduce potential skin irritation. A potential mild photosensitizer, avoid direct sun and tanning booths for up to twenty-four hours after application to the skin.

Actions on the body: **Antidepressant**, **antiseptic**, antiviral, astringent, **detoxifier**, disinfectant, diuretic, **stimulant** (lymphatic and digestive), uplifting tonic

Keywords: uplifting, refreshing, cleansing, stimulating, refreshing to air (spritzer or diffuser)

Core aromatic applications:

- ▶ constipation, sluggish digestion, general digestive fatigue, digestion-related migraine
- ▶ sluggish lymph, edema, supportive to detoxification
- ▶ muscular aches and pains, rheumatism, muscle fatigue
- ▶ depression, nervous exhaustion, performance stress
- ▶ uplifting, may help to shift blocked energy, cleansing, agitation, stress-related conditions, anxiety, challenging behavior
- ▶ releases feelings of tension, frustration, irritability, and moodiness (Mojay, 1997)

Jasmine / *Jasminum grandiflorum* syn. *Jasminum officinale* L. var. *grandiflorum*

Other common names:	Poets Jasmine
Botanical family:	Oleaceae
Countries of origin:	France, India, Egypt
Part of plant used:	flowers
Extraction method:	solvent extraction or enfleurage
Color of oil:	dark orange, brown
Odor description:	rich, floral, fruity, heady, exotic
Blending factor:	1
Chemical feature:	Complex composition (Haas, 2004), rich in esters.

Safety information: None known.

Actions on the body: **Antidepressant**, **aphrodisiac**, nervine, parturient, sedative/stimulant.

Keywords: heady, exotic, antidepressant

Core aromatic applications:

- ▶ depression, nervous exhaustion, postpartum depression, calming, lack of confidence, lethargy, anxiety
- ▶ frigidity and impotence, useful during childbirth, uterine spasms

▶ encourages creativity, uplifting the mind (*Shen*) in a gentle and sensuous way, warming, reassuring, relaxes the mind and harmonizes the heart (Mojay, 1997)

Laurel / *Laurus nobilis*

Other common names: Bay laurel, Sweet bay

Botanical family: Lauraceae

Countries of origin: Morocco, France, Croatia

Part of plant used: leaves

Odor description: Christmas-like, cinnamon, spicy, sweet, warm

Blending factor: 2

Chemical feature: Rich in oxide (1,8 cineole up to 40%), linalol (10%).

Safety information: None known, potential skin irritant with prolonged use.

Actions on the body: Analgesic, antibacterial, antimicrobial, antiseptic, **antispasmodic**, astringent, diuretic, **expectorant**, febrifuge, **immune enhancer**, stimulant, tonic.

Keywords: immune supportive (Haas, 2004), stimulates lymphatic flow

Core aromatic applications:

▶ lymphatic congestion, edema
▶ strains, rheumatism, muscle or joint stiffness, excellent in combination with birch and lavender in treating muscular aches and pains, especially after physical exertion, fibromyalgia, plantar fasciitis, carpal tunnel syndrome
▶ fortifying, nervous tension or exhaustion, poor concentration, lack of memory
▶ bronchitis, colds, flu
▶ in TCM, its principal actions are to circulate and regulate *Qi-energy* and to clear cold phlegm (Mojay, 1997)

Lemongrass / *Cymbopogon citratus* syn. *Andropogon citratus*

Other common names: West Indian lemongrass

Botanical family: Poaceae syn. Gramineae

Countries of origin: Nepal, West Indies

Part of plant used: grass

Odor description: lemony, strong

Blending factor: 1

Chemical feature: Rich in the aldehyde, citral, and monoterpenes.

Safety information: A skin irritant when used undiluted on the skin. Avoid undiluted application! Citral is a known sensitizer.

Actions on the body: Analgesic, antibacterial, antidepressant, **antifungal,** anti-inflammatory, **antimicrobial, antiseptic, antiviral,** astringent, carminative, febrifuge, galactogogue, immune stimulant, insecticidal, nervine, peripheral analgesic.

Keywords: antimicrobial, cleanses the air, strengthens connective tissue oil (Gumbel, 1993, p. 204)

Core aromatic applications:

- ▶ poor or sluggish circulation, varicose veins
- ▶ candida (Abe et al., 2003), lowered immune response, compromised immunity, lymph drainage
- ▶ muscular aches and pains, tired and sore muscles, sprains, bruises, weakness of connective tissue (Gumbel, 1993, p. 204), pain in joints
- ▶ nervous exhaustion, fatigue, grieving process, strengthening during weak emotional period, release work
- ▶ sinus congestion, lowered immune response for respiratory illness, respiratory infection (Inouye et al., 2001)
- ▶ acne, oily skin, boils, athlete's foot, herpes simplex (Minami et al., 2003)

Melissa / *Melissa officinalis*

Other common names:	Lemon balm, Sweet balm, Common balm
Botanical family:	Lamiaceae syn. Labiatae
Country of origin:	France
Part of plant used:	fresh leaves and tops
Odor description:	strong, sweet, lemony, earthy
Blending factor:	1
Chemical feature:	Aldehydes

Adulterations: Due to the low oil content of melissa and therefore the high cost of production, melissa is known to be one of the most adulterated oils on the market. Melissa may be adulterated by the addition of lemon oil, lemongrass oil, citronella oil, lemon verbena oil, or other various isolates to increase total yield.

Safety information: Could cause skin irritation; dilute to 1 percent •Due to the difficulty in obtaining *true* melissa oil, this author advises caution in applying melissa oil to the skin.

Actions on the body: Antibacterial, **antidepressant,** anti-inflammatory, antiseptic, antispasmodic, **antiviral,** carminative, febrifuge, hypotensive, **nervine, sedative,** stomachic, sudorific, tonic.

Keywords: calming, soothing, tonic (heart, digestive, and nervous systems), revives and strengthens the spirit

Core aromatic applications:

- ▶ Herpes simplex, shingles
- ▶ sedative to the CNS, nervous tension, anxiety, depression
- ▶ PMS, helps regulate ovulation
- ▶ overactive skins, oily, or sluggish skin, nervous or allergic skin disorders, eczema, bug bites and bee stings
- ▶ energetically, melissa is cool and dry and is indicated for stagnation of *Qi-energy*, for heat in the liver and heart, and for disturbance of the mind (*Shen*) (Mojay, 1997)

Myrrh / *Commiphora molmol*

Botanical family:	Burseraceae
Part of plant used:	resin
Country of origin:	Morocco
Odor description:	musky, smoky
Blending factor:	4 to 5
Chemical feature:	Sesquiterpenes

Safety information: None known.

Actions on the body: Analgesic, antifungal, anti-inflammatory, antimicrobial, antiseptic, **antiviral**, astringent, balsamic, carminative, diuretic, expectorant, stomachic, sudorific, tonic, **vulnerary**.

Keywords: drying, cooling, rejuvenating, astringent

Core aromatic applications:

- nervous tension, anxiety
- bronchitis, asthma, catarrh, coughs, gum infections, mouth ulcers, sore throat, laryngitis
- athlete's foot, chapped, dry, or cracked skin, wound healing (use with lavender), antiseptic, oily skins, soothes inflammations, acne complexions, broken capillaries, aging skin, ulcers, bedsores, weeping wounds, eczema, slow-healing wounds
- calming, centering, relaxing, warming, strengthens base chakra, has a cooling effect on the emotions, gives lift to feelings of weakness, apathy, and lack of incentive, good when feeling stuck either emotionally or spiritually

Neroli / *Citrus aurantium* syn. *Citrus* x *aurantium* ssp. *aurantium*

Other common names:	Bitter orange tree, Seville tree
Botanical family:	Rutaceae
Countries of origin:	Tunisia, France, Spain
Part of plant used:	flower (orange blossoms)
Odor description:	fresh, floral, sweet, light, exotic
Blending factor:	2
Chemical feature:	Alcohols (linalol), esters (linalyl acetate), and monoterpenes.

Safety information: None known.

Actions on the body: Antibacterial, **antidepressant**, anti-inflammatory, antiseptic, **antispasmodic**, antiviral, aphrodisiac, astringent, carminative, deodorant, digestive, hypotensive, **nervine**, sedative, tonic (cardiac, circulatory), **vulnerary**.

Keywords: overwrought, sudden shock and fear, depression, lightly hypnotic, euphoric, aphrodisiac

Core aromatic applications:

> ▶ depression, anxiety, shock, heartache, agitation, tachycardia, insomnia, stress, stress-related conditions, panic attacks
> ▶ colitis (stress-related episodes), chronic diarrhea related to long-standing stress or fear
> ▶ PMS, menopause, pregnancy and labor, calms sexual nerves, frigidity
> ▶ astringent and toning effect on the skin, reduces stretch marks and scars, acne, thread veins, dry, sensitive, and/or mature skin types
> ▶ nourishes the heart, calms the spirit, and relieves anxiety (Holmes, 1995)
> ▶ particularly good for hot, agitated conditions of the heart characterized by restlessness, insomnia, and palpitations and is indicated for hypertension (Mojay, 1997)

Niaouli / *Melaleuca quinquenervia* syn. *viridiflora*

Botanical family:	Myrtaceae
Countries of origin:	Madagascar, New Caledonia, Australia
Part of plant used:	leaves
Odor description:	pungent, bitter, putrid
Blending factor:	2
Chemical feature:	Oxides (up to 60% 1,8 cineole), alcohols.

Safety information: None known.

Actions on the body: Analgesic, **antibacterial**, **antifungal**, antirheumatic, antiseptic, antispasmodic, **antiviral**, decongestant, **expectorant**, febrifuge, **immune enhancer**, stimulant, vermifuge, vulnerary.

Keywords: Antiseptic, stimulating, immune enhancer

Core aromatic applications:

> ▶ respiratory infections, catarrh (excess mucus), coughs, sinusitis, sore throats, laryngitis, bronchitis, colds, flu
> ▶ acne, boils, burns, ulcers, dermatitis, wounds, cuts, aids in healing and firming the tissue, oily skin, insect bites
> ▶ muscular aches and pains, tired and sore muscles, sore joints

Palmarosa / *Cymbopogon martinii*

Botanical family:	Gramineae
Countries of origin:	India, Brazil, Nepal (Haas, 2004)
Part of plant used:	fresh or dried grass
Odor description:	sweet, somewhat rosy aroma
Blending factor:	4
Chemical feature:	Alcohols up to 80 percent (geraniol) supported by esters.

Safety information: None known.

Actions on the body: **Antibacterial**, **antifungal**, anti-inflammatory, **anti-septic**, **antiviral**, digestive, vulnerary.

Keywords: calming yet uplifting, inspiring

Core aromatic applications:

▶ acne, athlete's foot, eczema, slow-healing wounds, bedsores, oily skin, dermatitis, wounds, sores
▶ stress, anxiety, restlessness, nervous exhaustion, tension
▶ neuralgia, sciatica, rheumatic pain (Mojay, 1997)
▶ In TCM, it is cool and moist in energy, able to clear heat and strengthen the *yin-energy*; the oil comforts the heart and mind and can clear away oppression (Mojay, 1997)

Petitgrain / *Citrus x aurantium* ssp. *aurantium*

Botanical family:	Rutaceae
Country of origin:	Italy
Part of plant used:	leaves and green twigs (of bitter orange tree)
Odor description:	woody, dry, floral, light
Blending factor:	6
Chemical feature:	Esters approx 60 to 65% (linalyl acetate 40 to 50%), alcohols 30 to 40%.

Safety information: None known.

Actions on the body: Antibacterial, **antidepressant**, antiseptic, **antispasmodic**, deodorant, digestive, **nervine**, sedative, stomachic.

Keywords: pleasant, earthy, relaxing, soothing, delicate, refreshing

Core aromatic applications:

▶ aids digestion, dyspepsia, calms nervous stomach upsets
▶ anxiety, tension, nervousness, irritation, insomnia, anger, panic attacks, heart palpitations, stress-related conditions
▶ PMS, cramps, hormonal irritability
▶ acne, inflamed skin (supports neroli and lavender), oily skin, excessive perspiration, oily hair
▶ muscular spasms

Scots Pine / *Pinus sylvestris*

Other common names:	Pine
Botanical family:	Pinaceae
Countries of origin:	France, Canada
Part of plant used:	pine needles
Odor description:	balsamic, woody, piney
Blending factor:	6
Chemical feature:	monoterpenes (pinene), Esters (bornyl acetate)

Safety information: None known.

Actions on the body: Anti-inflammatory, antimicrobial, antirheumatic, **antiseptic**, antiviral, balsamic, **decongestant**, disinfectant, diuretic, **expectorant**, insecticide, **restorative**, rubefacient, stimulant (adrenal cortex, circulatory, nervous), tonic, vermifuge.

Keywords: refreshing, antiseptic, energizing, opens up the lungs, breathing space

Core aromatic applications:

▶ muscular aches and pains, arthritis, rheumatism, neuralgia
▶ refreshing, relaxing, evokes deep breathing, uplifting, cleansing, nervous exhaustion, fatigue
▶ asthma, bronchitis, catarrh, coughs, sinusitis, sore throat
▶ restores confidence through its effect on the bodily soul (*P'o*), revives the spirits, dispels the gloom of a negative outlook (Mojay, 1997)

Ravensara / *Ravensara aromatica*

Botanical family:	Lauraceae
Country of origin:	Madagascar
Part of plant used:	leaves
Odor description:	light, fresh
Blending factor:	7
Chemical feature:	Up to 35 to 40 percent monoterpenes (sabinene, limonene), oxides (4 to 5% 1,8 cineole).

Safety information: None known.

Actions on the body: Antibacterial, antiseptic, antispasmodic, **antiviral**, balsamic, **expectorant**, **immune enhancer**, stimulant.

Keywords: immune enhancing, antiviral, opens the lungs

Core aromatic applications:

▶ muscular aches and pains
▶ bronchitis, asthma
▶ refreshing, calming, breathing becomes slower and deeper
▶ herpes simplex, shingles, lowered or poor immunity

Sage / *Salvia officinalis*

Botanical family:	Lamiaceae syn. Labiatae
Country of origin:	France
Part of plant used:	flowering plant/leaves
Odor description:	strong, warm-spicy, herbaceous, and somewhat camphoraceous
Blending factor:	4
Chemical feature:	Ketones (up to 60%), oxides.

Safety information: Avoid use with pregnant women, infants, and young children.

Actions on the body: Analgesic, **antibacterial**, anti-inflammatory, antirheumatic, antiseptic, **antispasmodic**, **antiviral**, astringent, carminative, digestive, emmenagogue, **expectorant**, febrifuge, hypertensive, **mucolytic**, tonic, **vulnerary**.

Keywords: restorative effect on the whole body, female reproductive system

Core aromatic applications:

- ▶ bronchitis, flu, colds
- ▶ slow-healing wounds, wound healing
- ▶ menopause, hot flashes (hydrosol may be used), PMS, painful menstruation, cramps
- ▶ muscular aches and pains, spasms

Sandalwood / *Santalum album* (India) or *Santalum spicatum* (Australia)

Botanical family:	Santalaceae
Countries of origin:	India, New Caledonia, Australia
Part of plant used:	heartwood of tree trunk
Odor description:	soft, woody, balsamic
Blending factor:	6
Chemical feature:	Alcohols

Safety information: None known.

Actions on the body: Antibacterial, antidepressant, **anti-inflammatory,** antiseptic (urinary and pulmonary), antispasmodic, **antiviral**, aphrodisiac, **balsamic**, carminative, diuretic, **emollient**, expectorant, **nervine**, sedative, tonic (adrenals, spleen, reproductive), vulnerary.

Keywords: relaxing, soothing, meditative, dry conditions

Core aromatic applications:

- ▶ insomnia, nervous tension, stress, depression, anger, stress-related conditions, agitation
- ▶ dry nasal conditions, dry irritated throat conditions, bronchitis, laryngitis, sore throat, dry cough
- ▶ acne, dry, cracked, and/or chapped skin, dry eczema, razor/shaving rash, balancing to sebum, itchy or inflamed skin, mature or aging skin, varicose veins, oily skin
- ▶ calming, soothing, balancing, wonderful oil to use during meditation (as it has been historically), inner awareness, indicated for hot, agitated emotional states that lead to headache, insomnia, and nervous exhaustion (Mojay, 1997)

Spearmint / *Mentha spicata* syn. *Mentha viridis*

Botanical family:	Lamiaceae syn. Labiatae
Countries of origin:	Europe, Morocco, United States
Part of plant used:	fresh leaves

Odor description:	herbaceous, minty, refreshing
Blending factor:	2 to 3
Chemical feature:	Ketones (carvone up to 50%), monoterpenes (limonene).

Safety information: None known.

Actions on the body: Antiseptic, antispasmodic, **carminative**, cephalic, emmenagogue, stimulant, **stomachic**.

Core aromatic applications:

- ▶ nausea, indigestion, dyspepsia
- ▶ bronchitis, colds, flu
- ▶ muscular stiffness, aches and pains, tight muscles, rheumatism, pain, fibromyalgia, sprains, strains, plantar fasciitis, carpal tunnel syndrome, sciatica, bursitis.

Thyme / *Thymus vulgaris*

Other common names:	Common thyme
Botanical family:	Lamiaceae syn. Labiatae
Country of origin:	France
Part of plant used:	partially dried herb
Odor description:	strong, spicy, balsamic
Blending factor:	1
Chemical feature:	Phenols (thymol 30 to 50% and carvacrol 1 to 5%), supported by monoterpenes.

Safety information: Dermal irritant.

Actions on the body: **Antibacterial**, **antifungal**, anti-inflammatory, **antimicrobial**, antirheumatic, antiseptic, antispasmodic, antitussive, **antiviral**, carminative, diuretic, emmenagogue, expectorant, hypertensive, **immune enhancer**, insecticide, rubefacient, stimulant, tonic, vermifuge

Keywords: antimicrobial, immune enhancing, strengthening

Core aromatic applications:

- ▶ lowered or poor immunity
- ▶ diarrhea, dyspepsia, flatulence, gastritis, excess gas (flatulence), intestinal parasites
- ▶ arthritis, rheumatism, muscular aches and pains, sprains, strains, sciatica
- ▶ improves concentration and strengthens memory, nerve tonic, mental debility
- ▶ bronchitis, flu, sore throat, colds
- ▶ abscess, acne, bruises, cuts, insect bites, lice, gum infections, general antiseptic (use in .5 to 1% dilutions; may irritate sensitive skins)
- ▶ stimulating, energizing, strengthening, uplifting, used for conscious intellectual thought, promotes bravery to face challenges, especially good during convalescence

⟳→ REFERENCES

Abe, S., et al. (2003). Anti-Candida albicans activity of essential oils including Lemongrass (Cymbopogon citratus) oil and its component, citral. *Nippon Ishinkin Gakkai Zasshi*, *44* (4): 285–291.

Arctander, S. (1994). *Perfume and Flavor Materials of Natural Origin*. Carol Stream, Illinois: Allured Publishing Corp.

Barker, A. (1996). Exploring the Chemotypes of Rosemary. *Aromatherapy Quarterly*, 51, 9.

Barker, A. (1994). Pressure Sores. *Aromatherapy Quarterly*, 41, 5–7.

Blumenthal M., et al., Klein, S., and Rister, R.S. (trans.). (1998). *The Complete German Commission E Monographs: Therapeutic Guide to Herbal Medicines*. Austin: American Botanical Council; Boston: Integrative Medicine Communications. Retrieved on August 10, 2005, from www.herbalgram.org.

Blumenthal, et al. (1998). *Expanded Commission E on Lavender Flower*. Austin: American Botanical Council; Boston: Integrative Medicine Communications. Retrieved on August 10, 2005, from www.herbalgram.org.

Blumenthal, et al. (1998). *Expanded Commission E on Juniperberry*. Austin: American Botanical Council; Boston: Integrative Medicine Communications. Retrieved on August 10, 2005, from www.herbalgram.org.

Blumenthal, et al. (1998). *Expanded Commission E on German chamomile*. Austin: American Botanical Council; Boston: Integrative Medicine Communications. Retrieved on August 10, 2005, from www.herbalgram.org.

Blumenthal, et al. (1996). *Review of Clinical Effects and Management of Eucalyptus Oil Poisoning in Infants and Children*. HerbClip. Retrieved on August 10, 2005, from www.herbalgram.org.

Bowles, E.J. (2003). *The Chemistry of Aromatherapeutic Oils*. Crows Nest, Australia: Allen & Unwin.

Bown, D. (2001). *Herbal*. London: Barnes and Noble.

Buckle, J. (2003). *Clinical Aromatherapy*. Philadelphia: Elsevier Science.

Buckle, J. (1997). *Clinical Aromatherapy in Nursing*. San Diego: Singular Publishing Group.

Carson, C.F. (1999). Tea Tree Essential Oil Fact and Fiction. *Aromatherapy Today*, Vol. 10, June 1999.

Dale, A., and Cornwell, S. (1994). The role of lavender oil in relieving perineal discomfort following childbirth: A blind randomized clinical trial. *J Adv Nurs*. 19 (1): 89–96. PMID: 8138636, Retrieved August 10, 2004, from http://www.ncbi.nlm.nih.gov.

Duke, J. (1983). *Betula lenta*. Handbook of Energy Crops. Unpublished. Retrieved June 14, 2006, from http://www.hort.purdue.edu/newcrop/duke_energy/Betula_lenta.html.

Foster, S. (1993). *Herbal Renaissance*. Layton, Utah: Gibbs Smith.

Goeb, P. (1996). Properties and Indications of Rosmarinus officinalis. *Les Cahiers de lAromatherapie—Aromatherapy Records*, 2, 45–51.

Gobel, H., Schmidt, G., and Soyka, D. (1994). *Effect of peppermint and eucalyptus oil preparations on neurophysiological and experimental algesimetric headache parameters*. *Cephalalgia*, 14 (3): 228–234; discussion 182. PMID: 7954745, Retrieved August 15, 2004, from http://www.ncbi.nlm.nih.gov.

Grieve, M. (1996). *A Modern Herbal*. Kent, U.K.: Barnes and Noble.

Grieve, M. (1982). *A Modern Herbal, Vol. I*. New York: Dover Publications.

Gumbel, D. (1993). *Principles of Holistic Therapy with Herbal Essences*. Brussels: Haug International.

Haas, M. (2004). *Quick Reference Guide for 114 Important Essential Oils*. San Rafael, CA: Linda Scent and Image Books.

Hajhashemi, V., Ghannadi, A., and Sharif, B. (2003). Anti-inflammatory and analgesic properties of the leaf extracts and essential oil of Lavendula angustifolia Mill., *J Ethnopharmacol*, *89* (1): 67–71. PMID: 14522434, Retrieved on August 15, 2004, from http://www.ncbi.nlm.nih.gov.

Hammer, K.A., Carson, C.F., and Riley, T.V. (2002). In vitro activity of Melaleuca alternfolia (tea tree) oil against dermatophytes and other filamentous fungi. *Journal of Antimicrobial Chemotherapy* 50, 195–199.

Harris, B. (2005). Research Reports: Harmonizing Ylang Ylang. *International Journal of Aromatherapy, 15* (1): 55–56.

Harris, B. (2001) Fennel and Dysmenorrhea. *International Journal of Aromatherapy, 11* (4): 225–226.

Holmes, P. (1993). Clary sage. *International Journal of Aromatherapy, 5* (1): 15–17.

Holmes, P. (1994). Rose – The Water Goddess. *International Journal of Aromatherapy, 6* (2): 8–11.

Holmes, P. (1995). Neroli – The lightness of being. *International Journal of Aromatherapy, 7* (2): 14–17.

Holmes, P. (1997). Patchouli—The colours within the darkness. *International Journal of Aromatherapy, 8* (4): 16–19.

Holmes, P. (1997). Vetiver—The power of mother earth. *International Journal of Aromatherapy, 5* (3): 13–15.

Holmes, P. (1996). Ginger. *International Journal of Aromatherapy, 7* (4): 16–19.

Inouye, S., Yamaguchi, H., and Takizawa, T. (2001). Screening of the antibacterial effects of a variety of essential oils on respiratory tract pathogens, using a modified dilution assay method. *J Infect Chemother*, *7* (4): 251–254.

Kerr, J. (2003). Essential Oil Profile: Vetiver. *Aromatherapy Today*, Vol. 28, December 2003.

Kerr, J. (2001). Essential Oil Profile: Geranium. *Aromatherapy Today*, Vol. 20, December 2001.

Kerr, J. (2000). Essential Oil Profile: Tea Tree. *Aromatherapy Today*, Vol. 13, March 2000.

Kerr, J. (1997). Essential Oil Profile: Ylang ylang. *Aromatherapy Today*, Vol. 4, December 1997.

Koh, K.J., Pearce, A.L., Marshman, G., Finlay-Jones, J.J., Hart, and P.H. (2002). *Regulation of Immune Responses in Human Skin by Tea Tree Oil*. Flinders University. Accessed on August 24, 2005, http://www.rirdc.gov.au/comp00/tto1.htm.

Leigh, I. (2001). *Aromatic Alchemy*. Winchester, MA: Mansion Publishing Ltd.

Lis-Balchin, M. (1996). Geranium Oil. *International Journal of Aromatherapy, 7* (3): 16–19.

Lis-Balchin, M. (1995). *The Chemistry and Bioactivity of Essential Oils*. Surrey, England: Amberwood Publishing Ltd.

Lu X.Q, et al. (2004). Effect of Eucalyptus globulus oil on lipopolysaccharide-induced chronic bronchitis and mucin hypersecretion in rats. *Zhongguo Zhong Yao Za Zhi. 29* (2): 168–171. PMID: 15719688, Retrieved August 10, 2004, from http://www.ncbi.nlm.nih.gov.

Mikhaeil, B.R., et al. (2003). Chemistry and immunomodulatory activity of frankincense oil. *Z Naturforsch [C]. 58* (3–4): 230–238. PMID: 12710734, Retrieved August 10, 2004, from http://www.ncbi.nlm.nih.gov.

Mills, S., and Bone, K. (2000). *Principles and Practice of Phytotherapy*. London: Churchill Livingstone.

Minami, M., et al. (2003). The Inhibitory Effect of Essential Oils on Herpes Simplex Virus Type-1 Replication In Vitro. *Microbiol. Immunol.*, *47* (9): 681–684.

Mojay, G. (1997). *Aromatherapy for Healing the Spirit*. Rochester, VT: Healing Arts Press.

PDR for Herbal Medicines. (2000). Montvale, New Jersey: Medical Economics Company, Inc.

Riley, T. (n.d.). *The antimicrobial activity of tea tree oil.* Australian Government, Rural Industries Research and Development, University of Australia. Retrieved on August 24, 2005, from http://www.rirdc.gov.au/comp00/tto1.htm.

Riley, T. (n.d.). *Antimicrobial activity of tea tree oil against oral microorganisms.* Australian Government, Rural Industries Research and Development, University of Australia. Retrieved on August 24, 2005, from WWW.rirdc.gov.au/comp03/tto1#UWA58A.

Riley, T. (n.d.). *Clinical efficacy of tea tree oil for treating coldsores.* Australian Government, Rural Industries Research and Development, University of Australia. Retrieved on August 24, 2005, from WWW.rirdc.gov.au/comp03/tto1#UWA58A.

Riley, T., Hammer, K.A., and Carson, C.F. *The antifungal activity of tea tree oil.* Australian Government, Rural Industries Research and Development, University of Australia, Retrieved on August 24, 2005 from http://www.rirdc.gov.au/comp00/tto1.htm.

Rose, J.E., and Behm, B.M. (1994). Inhalation of vapor from black pepper extract reduces smoking withdrawal symptoms. *Drug Alcohol Depend. 34* (3): 225–229. PMID: 8033760.

Schnaubelt, K. (1995). *Advanced Aromatherapy.* Rochester, Vermont: Healing Arts Press.

Silva, J., Abebe, W., Sousa, S. M., Duarte, V. G., Machado, M. I., and Matos, F. J. (2003). Analgesic and anti-inflammatory effects of essential oils of Eucalyptus. *J Ethnopharmacol. 89* (2–3): 277–283. PMID: 14611892, Retrieved August 10, 2004, from http://www.ncbi.nlm.nih.gov.

Simon, J.E., Chadwick, A.F., and Craker, L.E. (1984). *Herbs: An Indexed Bibliography. 1971–1980. The Scientific Literature on Selected Herbs, and Aromatic and Medicinal Plants of the Temperate Zone.* Hamden, CT: Archon Books. Retrieved on August 24, 2005, from http://www.hort.purdue.edu/newcrop/medaro/factsheets/CLARY_SAGE.html.

Simpson, B., and Ogorzaly, M.C. (1995). *Plants in Our World.* United States: McGraw-Hill, Inc.

Southwell, I. (n.d.). *Significance of cineole for the bioactivity and irritancy of tea tree oil.* Retrieved on January 15, 2006, from http://www.rirdc.gov.au/comp03/tto1.html#DAN104A.

Van Wyk, B., and Wink, M. (2004). *Medicinal Plants of the World.* Portland, Oregon: Timber Press.

Worwood, V. (1996). *The Fragrant Mind.* Novato, CA: New World Library. Plant database: http://plants.usda.gov/.

Therapeutic Activity and Core Essential Oils

Analgesic: a substance that relieves or reduces pain

Black pepper, Birch, Cinnamon leaf, Clove bud, Eucalyptus globulus, Ginger, Lemongrass, Sweet marjoram, Myrrh, Peppermint, Rosemary ct. camphor and cineole

Antibacterial: a substance that destroys bacteria

Cinnamon leaf, Eucalyptus globulus, Lemongrass, Niaouli, Palmarosa, Sage, Tea tree, Thyme

Antidepressant: a substance that relieves depression

Bergamot, Clary sage, Grapefruit, Jasmine, Mandarin, Melissa, Neroli, Orange, Patchouli, Petitgrain, Rose, Ylang ylang

Antiemetic: a substance that prevents vomiting

Ginger, Peppermint

Antifungal: a substance that destroys or inhibits fungal growth

Cinnamon leaf, Clove bud, Lemongrass, Myrrh, Niaouli, Palmarosa, Patchouli, Tea tree, Thyme

Anti-inflammatory: a substance that soothes and reduces inflammations

German chamomile, Frankincense, Helichrysum, Lavender, Myrrh, Patchouli, Sandalwood

Antimicrobial: a substance that destroys or resists pathogenic microorganisms

Roman chamomile, Cinnamon leaf, Clove bud, Eucalyptus, Lemongrass, Tea tree, Thyme

Antirheumatic: a substance that helps to relieve the symptoms of rheumatism

Juniper berry

Antiseptic: a substance that destroys or prevents the growth of microbes

Bergamot, Roman chamomile, Cypress, Frankincense, Grapefruit, Lavender, Lemon, Lemongrass, Sweet marjoram, Scots pine, Tea tree

Antispasmodic: a substance that relieves smooth/skeletal muscle spasms

Angelica root, Bay laurel, German chamomile, Roman chamomile, Clary sage, Cypress, Fennel, Ginger, Lavender, Sweet marjoram, Neroli, Peppermint, Petitgrain, Sage

Antitussive: a substance that helps to relieve coughs

Cypress

Antiviral: a substance that inhibits growth of a virus

Cinnamon leaf, Clove bud, Eucalyptus globulus, Lemongrass, Melissa, Myrrh, Niaouli, Palmarosa, Ravensara, Rosemary ct. cineole, Sandalwood, Thyme ct. thymol

Aphrodisiac: a substance that increases sexual stimulation and excitement

Cardamom, Cinnamon leaf, Clary sage, Ginger, Jasmine, Ylang ylang

Astringent: a substance that causes cells to shrink; contracts, tightens, and binds tissues

Cedarwood, Cypress, Geranium, Lemon, Patchouli, Rose

Balsamic: a substance that soothes the lungs

Frankincense, Sandalwood

Carminative: a substance that relieves flatulence or excess gas in stomach

Black pepper, Cardamom, Carrot seed, Clove bud, Fennel, Ginger, Peppermint, Spearmint

Cephalic: a substance that clears the mind, relating to the head

Rosemary ct. cineole or camphor

Decongestant: a substance that reduces or relieves nasal congestion

Eucalyptus species, Scots pine, Rosemary ct. camphor

Detoxifier: a substance that enhances the removal of toxic substances from the body

Carrot seed, Cypress, Fennel, Grapefruit, Juniper berry, Lemon

Digestive: a substance that aids digestion, tonic

Angelica root, Basil ct. linalol, Black pepper, Cardamom, Carrot seed, Fennel, Lemon

Diuretic: a substance that increases the flow of urine

Juniper berry, Lemon

Emmenagogue: a substance that promotes and helps regulate menstruation

Clary sage, Geranium

Emollient: a substance that softens and soothes the skin, e.g., oils and fats

Sandalwood

Estrogenic: a substance that may act similar to estrogen

Fennel, Lemon, Rose

Expectorant: a substance that aids the removal of phlegm or mucus from the respiratory system

Cardamom, Eucalyptus, Fennel, Bay laurel, Niaouli, Scots pine, Peppermint, Ravensara, Rosemary ct. cineole or camphor, Sage, Tea tree

Hypertensive: a substance that raises blood pressure

Black pepper, Rosemary ct. camphor or cineole, Thyme ct. thymol

Hypotensive: a substance that lowers blood pressure

German chamomile, Clary sage, Lavender, Sweet marjoram, Neroli, Ylang ylang

Immune enhancer: a substance that enhances immunity, either by stimulating the immune system or by destroying microbes

Frankincense, Bay laurel, Lemon, Lemongrass, Niaouli, Ravensara, Tea tree, Thyme

Mucolytic: a substance that dissolves mucus or breaks down mucus. Mucolytics are used to treat chest conditions involving excessive or thickened mucus secretions

Cedarwood, Helichrysum, Rosemary ct. camphor or cineole or verbenon, Sage

Muscle relaxant: a substance that relaxes the muscles

German chamomile, Clary sage, Ginger, Lavender, Peppermint

Nervine: a substance that relaxes the nervous system; can reduce nervous disorders

Angelica root, Bergamot, German chamomile, Roman chamomile, Clary sage, Frankincense, Lavender,

Mandarin, Sweet marjoram, Melissa, Neroli, Sweet orange, Petitgrain, Rose, Sandalwood, Vetiver, Ylang ylang

Parturient: a substance that helps to ease delivery in childbirth

Clary sage, Jasmine, Lavender, Rose

Restorative: a substance that strengthens and revives the body systems

Scots pine

Rubefacient: a substance that causes reddening and warming of the skin

Black pepper, Clove bud, Ginger, Juniper berry, Sweet marjoram, Rosemary ct. camphor, Thyme

Sedative: a substance that has a calming effect, relieving anxiety and tension

German chamomile, Roman chamomile, Clary sage, Lavender, Sweet marjoram, Melissa

Stimulant: a substance that increases body or organ function and activity

Black pepper, Cardamom, Grapefruit, Juniper berry, Rosemary ct. camphor or cineole

Stomachic: digestive aid and tonic, improving appetite

Cardamom, Fennel, Ginger, Lemon, Peppermint, Spearmint

Uterine relaxant: a substance that relaxes the uterus

Clary sage, Jasmine, Rose

Vasoconstrictor: a substance that decreases blood flow by narrowing the blood vessels

Cypress, Lemon, Rose

Vulnerary: a substance that promotes wound healing, particularly skin wounds

Carrot seed, Roman chamomile, Frankincense, Helichrysum, Lavender, Myrrh, Neroli, Rosemary ct. verbenon, Sage, German chamomile, Patchouli

Sample Material Safety Data Sheet

Section I: Identification

Manufacturer Name: Company X

Emergency Telephone Number:

Address:

Chemical Name and Synonyms: Oil of Peppermint

Trade Names and Synonyms: *Mentha* x *piperita*

CAS Number: 8006-90-4

Section II: Fire, Explosion, and Reactivity Data

Flash Point Closed Cup Method: 151 degrees F

Extinguishing Media: FOG CO_2 yes, FOAM yes, DRY CHEMICAL yes

Dot Hazard Classification: Flammable liquid

Special Fire Fighting and Explosion Hazards: Cool containers exposed to flame with water

Hazardous Combustible of Decomposition Products: None. Material is not pyrophoric (does not ignite spontaneously), does not react with water, not an oxygen donor, material is shock stable

Stability: Normally stable

Conditions To Avoid: Excessive heat

Materials To Avoid: Strong oxidizing agents

Hazardous Polymerization Products: None

Section III: Physical Data

Odor, Appearance, and Physical State: Colorless to pale yellow liquid with strong penetrating peppermint odor and pungent taste

Boiling Point: Mixed

Melting Point: Liquid

Specific Gravity (H_2O = 1): 0.90

Vapor Pressure: Not found

Solubility in H_2O: Insoluble

Vapor Density (Air = 1): Greater than air

Section IV: Protection Information

Respiratory: As with all materials, avoid casual breathing of vapors

Ventilation: Local exhaust is recommended to avoid casual breathing of vapors

Eyes: Use OSHA approved safety glasses

Skin: Wear gloves to avoid skin contact

Other Protective Devices or Procedures: Follow good manufacturing practice

Section V: Occupation Exposure Limit

Threshold Limit Value (TLV): None established

OSHA Permissible Exposure Limit: None established

Section VI: Health Hazard Information

Health Hazard Information: Council of Europe evaluation was approval; FEMA evaluation was GRAS (Generally recognized as safe)

Irritation Data: Liquid may be irritating to skin and is irritating to eyes and other mucus membranes

Section VII: Emergency and First Aid Procedures

Inhalation Exposure: Remove person to ventilated area and follow normal first aid procedures

Eyes: Wash eyes by normal first aid procedures. Flush with water and seek medical attention if necessary.

Skin Contact: Wash with soap and water

Other: If ingested, see physician

Section VIII: Spill Leak and Disposal Procedures

Precaution If Material is Spilled or Released:

For small spills, wipe up with paper towels and place contaminated items in closed metal waste container; for large spills, use nonflammable absorbent cloth and dispose in the same manner.

Waste Disposal Methods: Follow local, state, and federal laws

Section IX: Handling and Storage Procedures

Store in cool dry area in closed containers. Do not expose to temperatures over 35 degrees C

Supply Resources

Organic Essential Oils

Essential Aura Aromatherapy
1935 Doran Road
Cobble Hill, BC V0R 1L0
250.758.9464
www.essentialaura.com
www.organicfair.com

Fragrant Earth
www.Fragrant-earth.com

Florihana
Les Grands Prés, 06460 Caussols, France
+33 (0) 493 09 06 09 -
www.florihana.com

Original Swiss Aromatics
P.O. Box 6842
San Rafael, CA 94903
415.459.3998
www.originalswissaromatics.com

Universal Companies
www.universalcompanies.com

Organic Vegetable Oils

The Aroma Tree
139 South Eastbourne Avenue
Tucson, AZ 85716
866.276.6287
520.327.5456
email: info@thearomatree.com

Omega Nutrition
800.661.3529
www.omeganutrition.com

Base Materials

Essential Wholesale
503.722.7557
http://www.essentialwholesale.com

Jedwards International
39 Broad Street
Quincy, MA 02169
617.472.9300
www.bulknaturaloils.com

Massage Warehouse
2775 Pacific Drive
Norcross, GA 30071
800.910.9955
www.massagewarehouse.com

Mountain Rose Herbs
85472 Dilley Lane
Eugene, OR 97405
800.879.3337
www.mountainroseherbs.com

New Life Systems
2853 Hedberg Drive
Minnetonka, MN 55305-3404
800.852.3082
www.newlifesystems.com

Organic Herbal Oils

Blessed Herbs
109 Barre Plains Road
Oakham, MA 01068
800.489.4372
www.blessedherbs.com

Bottles/Packaging

SKS Bottle
2600 7th Avenue, Building 60
West Watervliet, NY 12189
518.880.6980 ph
518.880.6990 fx
www.sks-bottle.com

Specialty Bottle
5215 5th Avenue South
Seattle, WA 98108
206.340.0459 ph
206.903.0785 fx
www.specialtybottle.com

Bags & Bows
33 Union
Sudbury, MA 01776
800.225.8155
www.bagsandbowsonline.com

Packaging Specialties
515 South Michigan
Seattle, WA 98108
206.762.0540 ph
206.762.4413 fx
www.ps-stores.com

Business/Marketing Support

Information for People
P.O. Box 1038
Olympia, WA 98507
800.754.9790 ph
360.754.9799 fx
www.info4people.com

Sharper Communication Tools
110 Pacific Avenue, Suite 850
San Francisco, CA 94111
800.561.6677 ph
888.251.4454 fx
www.sharpercards.com

Sohnen-Moe Associates
3906 West Ina Road
Tucson, AZ 85741
520.743.3936
www.sohnen-moe.com

VistaPrint
800.961.2075
www.vistaprint.com

Indie Beauty Network
(704) 843-9877
www.indiebeauty.com

Diffusors

Leyden House Limited
200 Brattleboro Road
Leyden, MA 01337
413.772.0858 and Toll-Free 800.754.0668
www.leydenhouse.com/

APPENDIX 4

Education, Associations, and Publications

Aromatherapy Education

East-West School for Herbal and Aromatic Studies
Jade Shutes
335 Amber Lane
Willow Spring, NC 27592
919.892.7230
www.TheIDA.com

Zsuzsana Davidson
Zobiana Aromatherapy
7280 Candleshine Court
Columbia MD 21045
443.283.1462
http://www.zobiana.com/

Cheryl's Herbs
Cheryl Hoard
7159 Manchester Road
Maplewood, MO 63143
314.645.2165 or 800.231.5971
http://www.cherylsherbs.com/

Pacific Institute of Aromatherapy
Kurt Schnaubelt
P.O. Box 6723
San Rafael, CA 94903
415.479.9120
www.pacificinstituteofaromatherapy.com

Essential Oil Resource Consultants
Bob and Rhiannon Harris
Au Village
83840 La Martre
Provence, France
http://www.essentialorc.com/

Michelle Thibert
EWSHAS-WA State
Bonney Lake, WA
253.221.7312
www.TheIDA.com

Aromatherapy Associations

USA

National Association for Holistic Aromatherapy
3327 West Indian Trail Road PMB 144
Spokane, WA 99208
509.325.3419 or 888.Ask.NAHA
www.NAHA.org

Canada

Canadian Federation of Aromatherapists (CFA)
#103-1200 Centre Street
Thornhill, ON L4J 3M9
905.886.2567
www.cfacanada.com | www.aromascentsjournal.ca

Massage Therapy Associations

American Massage Therapy Association
500 Davis Street, Suite 900
Evanston, IL 60201-4695
Toll-Free 1.877.905.2700
http://www.amtamassage.org

Associated Bodywork & Massage Professionals
1271 Sugarbush Drive
Evergreen, CO 80439
800.458.2267 or 303.674.8478 ph
800.667.8260 fx
email: expectmore@abmp.com
www.abmp.com

*National Certification Board for Therapeutic Massage
and Bodywork (NCBTMB)*
1901 South Meyers Road, Suite 240
Oakbrook Terrace, IL 60181
www.NCBTMB.com

Aromatherapy Publications

The International Journal for Clinical Aromatherapy
http://www.ijca.net/index.php

Absolutes: an aromatic extract produced via solvent extraction

Acid mantle: the slightly acidic layer on our skin that protects the skin from infection

Active listening: demonstrating that we are energetically engaged in the discussion, not just passive listeners, and that we have brought in our intellect and knowledge, too

Acute stress: the most common form of stress we all experience on a day-to-day basis; is short term

Alcohols: organic compounds that contain a hydroxyl group (–OH) attached to a saturated carbon

Aldehydes: organic compounds that contain the polar carbonyl group (C=O) with the carbonyl group directly attached to at least one hydrogen atom and a second attached directly to a hydrogen or carbon atom

Allelochemics: the chemicals that deter competing growth, e.g., terpenes

Allelopathy: when a plant releases chemicals to prevent competing vegetation from growing within its area or zone

Amenorrhea: a condition in which there is an absence or cessation of menstruation

Amygdala: an almond-shaped mass located deep within the temporal lobes, close to the hypothalamus and adjacent to the hippocampus

Analgesic: a substance that relieves or reduces pain

Anesthetic: a substance that causes loss of feeling or sensation

Angiosperm: flowering plants

Anosmia: total inability to smell any aromatic substance

Anti-allergenic: a substance that reduces symptoms of allergy

Antibacterial: a substance that destroys bacteria

Anticoagulant: a substance that prevents blood from clotting

Anticonvulsive: a substance that prevents or reduces seizures

Antidepressant: a substance that relieves depression

Antidiuretic: a substance that reduces the amount of water your body eliminates

Antiemetic: a substance that prevents vomiting

Antifungal: a substance that destroys or inhibits fungal growth

Anti-inflammatory: a substance that soothes and reduces inflammations

Antimicrobial: a substance that destroys or resists pathogenic microorganisms

Antioxidants: substances that are able to prevent cell damage from the destructive elements of free radicals

Antiperspirant: a substance that reduces excessive sweating

Antirheumatic: a substance that helps to relieve the symptoms of rheumatism

Antiseptic: a substance that destroys or prevents the growth of microbes

Antispasmodic: a substance that relieves smooth/skeletal muscle spasms

Antisudorific: a substance that prevents sweating

Antitussive: a substance that helps to relieve coughs

Antiviral: a substance that inhibits growth of a virus

Aperitive: a substance that stimulates the appetite

Aphrodisiac: a substance that increases sexual stimulation and excitement

Aroma: an odor arising from spices, plants, cooking, etc., especially an agreeable odor

Aromatherapy: the holistic therapeutic application of genuine essential oils for enhancing the physical, emotional, mental, and spiritual health of the individual

Aromatherapy blend: a combination of essential oils within a base or carrier product

Aromatherapy synergy: a combination of essential oils without a base or carrier product, 100 percent essential oils

Aromatic: having an aroma; fragrant or sweet-scented; odoriferous

Aromatic experience: refers to using pre-blended plant-based materials or essential oils to create aromatic or fragrant materials for massage, bodywork, or spa treatments

Aromatic spritzer: the combination of essential oils and water or essential oils, water, and a dispersing agent

Aromaticity: the quality or state of being aromatic

Aromatize: to make aromatic or fragrant

Astringent: a substance that causes cells to shrink; contracts, tightens, and binds tissues

Atopic eczema: often found in people with a family history of allergic reactions, for example, hay fever or asthma

Attending: the manner in which the therapist is present with the client, both physically and psychologically

Balneotherapy: the use of baths for therapeutic purposes, the use of baths which aim to enhance the immune system, stimulate the circulatory process including lymph and blood circulation, accelerate cell activity, by dilating tissue and vessels and activating the self healing potential naturally

Balsamic: a substance that soothes the lungs

Basal cells: found on the underside of the epithelium; are capable of neurogenesis

Batch number: a number used to identify a specific batch or drum of essential oil, from a specific supplier, during a specific year

Biochemical specificity: refers to the identification of a chemotype of a specific essential oil

Biosynthesized: diverse organic compounds that are created or manufactured by a plant

Blends: as a product this term implies the combination of essential oils with a base product, e.g., a vegetable oil or cream base

Blending factor: an aromatic potency scale utilized as a tool for determining the appropriate and specific number of drops for each essential oil within a given blend or synergy

Botanical specificity: refers to the specific Latin binomial of a given essential oil/plant

Bronchodilator: a substance that causes widening of the air passages by relaxing bronchial muscles

Bursitis: inflammation of the bursae; commonly called by such names as "housemaid's knee" and "student's elbow"

Cacosmia: smelling a continuous foul odor

Carcinogenic: a chemical that may give rise to tumor production, which is an unrestrained malignant proliferation of a somatic cell, resulting in a progressively growing mass of abnormal tissue

Carminative: a substance that relieves flatulence or excess gas in the stomach

Carpal tunnel syndrome: irritation of the median nerve in the wrist; can be caused by edema or repetitive movements

Carrier oils: vegetable, nut, or seed oils used to dilute essential oils and carry them onto the skin and into the body

Cephalic: a substance that clears the mind, relating to the head

Chemoreceptors: olfactory receptor neurons that register chemical sensory input

Chemotype: when a plant of a specific genus and species produces a particular chemical in a higher than normal amount because of geographic location, weather, altitude, insect and environmental interactions, and the like

Chronic stress: when acute stress becomes long term

Cilia: fine hairlike projections of olfactory receptor neurons in the olfactory epithelium

CO_2 extraction: a relatively new process used for the extraction of aromatic products. The basic concept is that CO_2 under pressure will turn from a gas into a liquid, which can then be used as an inert liquid solvent.

Cold pressing: a method of extraction specific to citrus essential oils, such as tangerine, lemon, bergamot, sweet orange, and lime

Collagen: a complex, long-chained protein that is tough and does not stretch easily

Concrete: concentrated extract that contains the waxes and/or fats as well as the odoriferous material from the plant

Connective tissue: the type of tissue in the body that gives the skin strength, resiliency, and flexibility

Contact eczema: an allergic reaction to irritating substances, for example, chemicals, rubber, metals, soaps, and washing powders

Contrast therapy: involves the altering of hot and cold applications to the same area of the body

Core essential oil: is chosen based upon your primary purpose/goal and is considered the heart of the synergy

Decongestant: a substance that reduces or relieves nasal congestion

Deodorant: a substance that reduces or removes unpleasant body odor

Depurative: a substance that purifies the blood

Dermal irritant: a substance that produces an immediate effect of irritation on the skin; the reaction, represented on the skin as blotches or redness, can be painful to some individuals

Dermal sensitizer: To initiate this reaction, the substance, such as an essential oil, must enter the skin, bind with the lymphatic tissues, and then cause the T-lymphocytes to become sensitized. Upon further exposure to the same or a chemically related substance, the immune system will react to the substance by perceiving it as an invader, causing a similar reaction to occur as in dermal irritation

Detoxicant: the process whereby toxic substances are removed or toxic effects are neutralized

Detoxifier: a substance that enhances the removal of toxic substances from the body

Diaphoretic: a substance that causes an increase in sweating

Digestive: a substance that aids digestion, tonic

Discoid eczema: scaly, itchy, round-shaped patches found on the limbs

Disinfectant: a substance that destroys or removes bacteria and other microorganisms

Dispersant: a substance used to combine essential oils with water, e.g., polysorbate 20, milk, or honey

Distillation: an extraction technique to produce essential oils and hydrosols

Diuretic: a substance that increases the flow of urine

Dosage/Dilution: the number of drops of essential oil to add to a specified quantity of base material

Dysmenorrhea: the technical term for menstrual pain that is severe enough to interfere with and limit the activities of women of childbearing age

ecuelle a piquer: a process that involves a prodding, pricking, sticking action to release the essential oil

Eczema: an inflammatory skin disorder usually brought on by an outside agent

Edema: the accumulation of fluid between cells; sometimes associated with inflammation or poor circulation

Elastin: a protein component of the fibers that give the skin its elasticity—the ability to stretch and return to its original shape

Electrolytes: salts or substances that conduct an electrical current in solution

Emmenagogue: a substance that promotes and helps regulate menstruation

Emollient: a substance that softens and soothes the skin, e.g., oils and fats

Empathy: involves listening to clients, understanding them and their concerns to the degree that this is possible, and communicating this understanding to them so that they might understand themselves more fully and act on their understanding

Enfleurage: a method of extracting odoriferous substances from flowers which continue giving off their aroma even after harvesting. It is based upon the principles that fat possesses a high *power of absorption*, particularly animal fat and must be relatively stable against rancidity.

Enhancer essential oil: strengthens the core essential oil in its purpose and therapeutic action

Episodic acute stress: when an individual is always in a rush, they take on too much, have too many irons in the fire and seem to always be doing something or going somewhere

Escharotic: caustic agent that dries the skin

Essential oil: a product made by distillation with either water or steam or by mechanical processing of citrus rinds or by dry distillation of natural materials; highly concentrated aromatic extracts that are distilled or expressed from a variety of aromatic plant material, including flowers, flowering tops, fruits/zests, grasses, leaves, needles and twigs, resins, roots, seeds, and woods

Essential oil cells: found within the plant tissue and are unique from other cells in content and size

Esters: organic compounds that result from a chemical reaction that occurs between an alcohol and an organic acid

Estrogenic: a substance that may act similar to estrogen

Euphoric: tending to induce a feeling of happiness, well-being

Expectorant: a substance that aids the removal of phlegm or mucus

Expression: a method of extraction specific to citrus essential oils, such as tangerine, lemon, bergamot, sweet orange, and lime

External secretory structures: essential oil structures found on the surface of the plant

External stressors: include adverse physical conditions (such as pain or hot or cold temperatures) or stressful psychological environments

Febrifuge: a substance that reduces or prevents fever; cools body temperature

Fibromyalgia: a widespread musculoskeletal pain and fatigue disorder; cause is still unknown

Flatulence: the presence of gas or air in the stomach

Fragrance: perfume, cologne, toilet water, or the like; the quality of being fragrant

Fragrant: having a pleasant scent or aroma

Functional group: an atom or group of atoms that imparts specific chemical and physical properties to a molecule

Furanocoumarins: a type of coumarin

Galactogogue: a substance that stimulates the flow of milk or increases milk flow

Gas chromatography: a chemical analysis instrument used to separate and identify individual constituents found within a given essential oil

Genus: a group or category of plants that are similar in botanical structure

Glandular trichomes: external secretory structures in plants

Gymnosperm: plants that lack flowers but produce seeds such as the conifers

Haleakala Red: a medicinal clay that is reddish in color, high in trace minerals and iron-oxide

Hard water: rich in minerals, such as magnesium, iron, sulfur, and/or calcium

Harmonizing essential oil: supports and enhances the vitality and purpose of the overall synergy

Hepatic: relating to the liver

Herbal oils: vegetable oil infusions of herbal medicinal plants

Heterotrophs: humans and other life that depend on the release of oxygen from plants to provide the necessary energy to sustain life

Himalayan Pink: a naturally occurring, pure salt that is hand-mined deep inside the Himalayan Mountains

Hippocampus: curved band of gray matter located inside the temporal lobe (humans have two hippocampi, one in each side of the brain); forms a part of the limbic system and plays a part in learning and memory

Hyaluronic acid: attracts and retains water to maintain moisture and flexibility in the skin

Hybrid: the result of a cross-fertilization between two different plant species and/or two varieties within a species

Hydrocarbons: the simplest organic compounds consisting solely of hydrogen and carbon

Hydrosol: the water by-product of distillation; contains the water soluble principles of the essential oil

Hydrotherapy: the use of water in any form (solid, liquid, vapor) for the treatment of disease or injury as well as for the maintenance of good health

Hyperosmia: extreme sensitivity to aromas

Hypersensitivity: prone to respond abnormally to the presence of a particular antigen; may cause a variety of tissue reactions

Hypertensive: a substance that raises blood pressure

Hyposmia: partial loss of smell

Hypotensive: a substance that lowers blood pressure

Hypothalamus: part of the brain below the thalamus and above the pituitary gland in the heart of the brain; has numerous functions, most importantly serves as a control for the endocrine and autonomic nervous system

Idiosyncratic irritation: an uncharacteristic or unusual reaction to a commonly used essential oil

Immune enhancer: a substance that enhances immunity, either by stimulating the immune system or by destroying microbes

Insecticide: a substance that kills or wards off insects and other threats

Internal secretory structures: essential oil structures found inside the plant material

Internal stressors: can be physical (infections, inflammation) or psychological

Irritable bowel syndrome: a common condition of the digestive system often attributed to prolonged anxiety or stress-related states

Irritant: a substance that produces redness, itching, swelling, or blisters on the skin

Isoprene unit: contains five carbon atoms and eight hydrogen atoms

Ketones: organic compounds that are similar to aldehydes with the exception that only carbons are directly attached to the carbonyl group (C=O)

Langerhans' cells: phagocytic cells (cells that ingest and destroy foreign matter such as microorganisms or debris) that play a role in immunity

Latin binomial: refers to one kind of plant, critically distinguished from all others, and identifies a biological species name consisting of two terms: genus and species

Limbic system: known as the emotional brain; is considered to be one of the oldest parts of the human brain, it includes the amygdala, the anterior thalamus, the nucleus accumbens, the hypothalamus, the septum, and the hippocampus including the cingulate gyrus and parahippocampal gyrus

Lipophilic: substances that are attracted to and soluble in fatty substances

Magnesium: a necessary component in the body's ability to form adequate amounts of serotonin, a chemical within the brain that elicits feelings of well-being and relaxation

Mass spectrometry: a technique that allows for the detection of compounds (chemical constituents) by separating ions by their unique mass

Massage delivery systems: a carrier substance such as vegetable oil, gel, lotion, salves, or creams

Memory-based response: a learned response based upon the experiences and emotions while smelling a specific aroma or combination thereof

Mitosis: cell reproduction

Monoterpenes: compounds formed from the joining of two isoprene units; have ten carbon atoms and sixteen hydrogen atoms ($C_{10}H_{16}$)

Morphological structures: parts of a plant, such as the leaf, seed, and root, or the flower and leaf

MSDS: Material Safety Data Sheet

Mucolytic: a substance that dissolves mucus or breaks down mucus; used to treat chest conditions involving excessive or thickened mucus secretions

Mucous membrane irritant: a substance that will produce a heating or drying effect on the mucous membranes of the mouth, nose, and reproductive organs

Muscle relaxant: a substance that relaxes the muscles

"Neat" application: the undiluted or direct application of an essential oil or synergy without a base product

Nervine: a substance that relaxes the nervous system; can reduce nervous disorders

Neuralgia: nerve pain; usually a sign or symptom of some other nervous system disorder or condition in which pain travels along a sensory peripheral nerve path

Neurogenesis: the ability to create new nerve tissue to replace the old

Olfaction: the sense of smell

Olfactory bulb: sits on top of the cribiform plate of the ethmoid bone and is continuous with the olfactory tract; the first site of odor recognition before it is passed along the olfactory tract

Olfactory epithelium: located at the top and on both sides of the superior nasal cavity; about the size of a small postage stamp, it is considered to be the "organ" of olfaction

Olfactory fading: occurs when our olfactory system adapts to a smell and ceases to register the aroma

Olfactory fatigue: occurs when our olfactory system is exposed to numerous odors within a short span of time

Olfactory receptor neurons: neurons that transduce the odor to electrical signals

Olfactory tract: a band of white matter that moves slightly upward and divides into two roots, the outer root that projects directly into the limbic system, specifically the amygdala and septum; and the inner root that projects into the olfactory cortex, which then connects to the temporal and frontal cerebral lobes

Organic chemistry: the study of carbon-based compounds

Oxides: organic compounds that have an oxygen molecule situated between two carbon molecules

Parosmia: a distortion of imagined odors

Parturient: a substance that helps to ease delivery in childbirth

Peng-Tzao-Kan-Mu: the earliest known publication on pharmacology, from China dated 2,700 BC, containing information on more than forty different kinds of salt and the processes of extraction

Percolation: similar to distillation however the steam comes in through the top rather than the bottom

Phagocytic cells: cells that ingest and destroys foreign matter such as microorganisms or debris

Phenols: organic compounds that contain an —OH group attached to the carbon of a benzene ring, also known as an aromatic ring

Phenylpropanoids: organic compounds having a basic 3-carbon chain attached to a benzene ring

Photoautotrophs: plants that depend on the sun in order for photosynthesis to occur thereby producing complex organic compounds necessary to sustain life

Photosensitizer: a substance that will cause burning or skin pigmentation changes, such as tanning, on exposure to sun or similar light (ultraviolet rays)

Plantar fasciitis: the pain and inflammation caused by injury to the plantar fascia of the foot

Point blend: an aromatherapy blend of essential oils and carrier oils for use on specific reflex or pressure points

Pre-blended synergies: a combination of two or more essential oils without a base, prepared in advance for common conditions or purposes

Primary metabolites: substances/nutrients that are vital to the plant's life, such as enzymes, protein, lipids, carbohydrates, and chlorophyll

Psoriasis: a skin disorder characterized by well-demarcated, raised red patches or thickening of the skin caused by rapid cell division

Raynaud's syndrome: defined by episodes of vasospasm of the arterioles, usually the fingers and toes

Receptor cells: cells in the olfactory epithelium that register chemical sensory input

Restorative: a substance that strengthens and revives the body systems

Rubefacient: a substance that increases cutaneous blood flow to a local area; causes reddening and warming of the skin

Saturated: when a carbon is bonded to other atoms only through single bonds, no double or triple bonds

Scent: a word derived from the French *"Sentir,"* which means to feel, smell

Sebaceous glands: oil glands in the skin which are attached to the hair follicle and produce oil called sebum

Secondary metabolites: constituents that are not considered necessary for life, such as alkaloids, flavonoids, and essential oils

Secretory cavities and ducts: large, intercellular spaces that are formed either by the separation of the walls of neighboring cells or by the disintegration of cells

Sedative: a substance that has a calming effect, relieving anxiety and tension

Sesquiterpene lactones: a subcategory of sesquiterpenes with a characteristic lactone ring structure derived ultimately from farnesyl pyrophosphate

Sesquiterpenes: compounds of fifteen carbon atoms; are based upon the joining of three isoprene units ($C_{15}H_{24}$)

Sodium chloride: salt

Solvent extraction: the use of solvents, such as petroleum ether, methanol, ethanol, or hexane to extract the odoriferous lipophilic material from the plant

Species: identifies the exact plant within a specific genus; has to do with direct characteristics of the plant, including leaf structure, flower structure, reproduction, and other characteristics within a family of plants

Stimulant: a substance that increases body or organ function and activity

Stomachic: digestive aid and tonic, improving appetite

Structure energy system: the system of attributing general properties to each chemical family

Styptic: a substance that helps control bleeding

Synergies: a combination of essential oils without a base carrier

Sudoriferous glands: sweat glands in the skin that help to maintain body temperature by secreting perspiration

Sudorific: a substance that causes sweating

Supporting cells: cells in the olfactory epithelium that protect the receptor neurons, secrete mucus, and remove mucus and dead sensory cells

Synergy: the combination of 3 to 5 essential oils without a carrier oil or other base product, such as a cream or lotion

Thalassotherapy: a type of hydrotherapy that refers specifically to the therapeutic use of seawater, seaweeds, or various other seawater extracts

Tempuromandibular joint disorder: refers to a multitude of problems in and around the jaw resulting from constant strain, stress, and malocclusion of the jaw

Terpenes: hydrocarbon chemical compounds classified according to the number of isoprene units that their molecules contain

Tonic: improves bodily performance

Undiluted: the use of essential oils applied directly to the skin without a carrier or base oil

Uterine relaxant: a substance that relaxes the uterus

Varicose eczema: commonly present in people with varicose veins and the elderly

Vasoconstrictor: a substance that decreases blood flow by narrowing the blood vessels

Vermifuge: a substance that expels worms from the intestines

Viscosity: the measurement of an essential oil's thickness

Volatility: refers to the ability of an essential oil to turn from liquid to vapor

Vulnerary: a substance that promotes wound healing, particularly skin wounds

Chapter One

1. c. Rene Maurice Gattefosse
2. b. lavender
3. Any of the following: arthritis, immune function disorders, asthma, bronchitis, insomnia, carpal tunnel syndrome, myofacial pain, chronic and acute pain, circulatory disorders, reduced range of motion, gastrointestinal disorders, sports injuries, stress, headache, TMJ dysfunction, spa therapy, cancer care, hospice care, or elderly care
4. True
5. a. individual
6. Any five of the following: stress/anxiety, headaches/migraines, insomnia, musculoskeletal problems, hormonal problems, respiratory problems, arthritis and rheumatism, skin problems, chronic fatigue, sinus problems
7. True
8. inhalation
9. True
10. False

Chapter Two

1. c. secondary metabolism
2. c. eucalyptol
3. b. aroma
4. c. allelopathy
5. d. glandular trichomes
6. b. tangerine
7. c. lime
8. a. an absolute
9. b. rose
10. c. distillation

Chapter Three

1. b. genus and species
2. c. specific chemotypes
3. d. the thickness of an oil
4. a. purity and chemical composition of an oil
5. a. in an immediate reaction to an essential oil
6. c. bergamot
7. b. cinnamon bark
8. False
9. False
10. False

Chapter Four

1. c. hydrocarbons
2. d. 10
3. b. geranial
4. d. an alcohol
5. a. benzene ring
6. d. lemongrass
7. c. photosensitizing
8. b. eucalyptol
9. c. thymol
10. b. photosensitizers

Chapter Five

1. a. current state of health, b. general lifestyle (including diet and exercise), c. emotional well-being, and d. current/past medical history
2. True
3. a. aromatic potency
4. Cypress   24 drops
   Eucalyptus   22 drops
   Rosemary   14 drops
5. c. together into glass first
6. a. chemistry and c. known therapeutic actions
7. b. pleasant
8. a. less potent
9. c. 3 to 5
10. d. 2.5 percent

Chapter Six

1. b. stratum corneum
2. c. immunity
3. Any of the following: temperature of the skin, hydration of the skin, lipophilic nature and molecular structure of the essential oil applied, skin integrity, hair follicles/thickness of skin, and/or occlusion.
4. d. Maury
5. b. cypress
6. c. lavender
7. d. vitamin A
8. b. oleic acid
9. c. calendula
10. d. free radicals

Chapter Seven

1. c. olfaction
2. Any of the following: • Reduce stress and anxiety • Relieve pain • Induce sleep or relaxation • Increase alertness and overall performance • Used for weight control or loss • Alleviate anxiety and distress • Balance and adjust sleep patterns • Help in alleviating nausea • Affect and improve mood and increase overall emotional well-being • Make treating phobias, depressions, sleep disorders, and addiction more effective • Affect the autonomic nervous system and used as tools for stress management • Ease physical ailments • Help shape our impressions of self and others
3. True
4. b. acute
5. a. chemoreceptors
6. False
7. d. neurogenesis
8. c. the emotional brain

9. True
10. True

Chapter Eight

1. b. lotions, gels, or oils
2. c. .5 to 1 percent
3. d. water
4. b. aloe vera
5. c. tea tree and lavender
6. c. scar therapy
7. b. only on reflex points
8. a. decrease stress and anxiety
9. d. enhance circulation
10. c. 1 percent

Chapter Nine

1. False
2. c. 75 percent
3. b. rose
4. c. nausea
5. b. Epsom salt and Dead Sea salt
6. a. a chronic muscle spasm
7. b. recent or acute injury
8. c. 105 to 110
9. a. always end with cold
10. False

Chapter Ten

1. b. German chamomile, helichrysum, lavender
2. a. black pepper, birch, clove bud
3. b. in the subacute or maturation phases
4. d. can include head and neck pain
5. c. fennel, ginger
6. c. can be successfully aided by essential oils and lymphatic massage techniques
7. d. lavender, geranium, clary sage
8. c. niaouli, tea tree, thyme
9. a. eucalyptus, ravensara, rosemary ct. cineole
10. b. rosemary, black pepper

Chapter Eleven

1. b. get the proper training
2. d. pennyroyal and wormwood
3. True
4. a. enjoy bodywork and human touch
5. b. gently and with care
6. False
7. d. tangerine and lavender
8. Any of the following: nausea, leg cramps, backache, anxiety, depression, stretch marks, varicose veins, edema, constipation, postpartum blues
9. False
10. a. need to learn self-care

Black pepper	German Chamomile
Roman Chamomile	Clary sage
Cypress	Eucalyptus
Fennel	Frankincense
Geranium	Ginger
Helichrysum	Juniper

Matricaria recutita

Anti-inflammatory, sedative, stress and anxiety relieving, wound/skin healer

BF: 1

Piper nigrum

Increases circulation, analgesic, warming, strengthening

BF: 3 to 4

Salvia sclarea

Feminine, euphoric, aphrodisiac, antidepressant, antispasmodic, Nervine, harmonal balancer

BF: 2 to 3

Chamaemelum nobile

Soothing, anti-inflammatory, anger, temper tantrums (children), wound healing, powerful antispasmodic

BF: 1

Eucalyptus globulus

Cooling, stimulating, clearing, antibacterial, expectorant

BF: 4 to 5

Cupressus sempervirens

Astringent, excessive perspiration, toning effect on vein

BF: 5

Boswellia carterii

Wound healing, all around healer, calming, meditation

BF: 3 to 4

Foeniculum vulgare

Digestive system, menstrual disorders, stimulating to digestion

BF: 3

Zingiber officinale

Analgesic, warming, digestive

BF: 4

Pelargonium graveolens

Balancing (particularly to hormones), harmonizing, uplifting, relaxing, refreshing, cleansing

BF: 3

Juniperus communis

Detoxifying, clearing, stimulating, strengthening, cleansing

BF: 4

Helichrysum italicum

Bruises, skin conditions, anti-inflammatory, wound healing

BF: 5

Lavender	Lemon
Mandarin/Tangerine	Marjoram
Sweet Orange	Patchouli
Peppermint	Rose
Rosemary	Tea Tree
Vetiver	Ylang ylang

Citrus limon

Cleansing, astringent, antiseptic, uplifting

BF: 4 to 5

Lavandula angustifolia

Balancing, nervous exhaustion, anxiety, wound healing, sedative

BF: 7

Origanum marjorana

Warming, antispasmodic, comforting, calming, sedative

BF: 3

Citrus reticulata

Calming yet uplifting, soothing, gentle

BF: 7

Pogostemon cablin

Grounding, centering, meditative, calming, skin care, antidepressant

BF: 5

Citrus sinensis

Uplifting, refreshing, warming, happy, cheerful, digestive

BF: 7

Rosa x damascena

Calming, soothing, female disorders, antidepressant

BF: 1

Mentha x piperita

Refreshing, cooling/warming, stimulating, digestive, pain relieving

BF: 1 to 2

Melaleuca alternifolia

Antibacterial, antifungal, antiviral, immune enhancing

BF: 3

Rosmarinus officinalis

Stimulating particularly for circulation, enhances memory, muscular system

BF: 2 to 3

Cananga odorata

Euphoric, aphrodisiac, antidepressant, calming, harmonizing

BF: 4

Vetiveria zizanioides

Calming, grounding, balancing

BF: 1

Angelica root	Bergamot
Birch	Cardamom
Carrot seed	Cedarwood
Cinnamon leaf	Clove bud
Grapefruit	Jasmine
Laurel	Lemongrass

Citrus bergamia

"Brings in the sunshine", uplifting, antidepressant, antiseptic, refreshing

BF: 7

Angelica archangelica

Balancing, strengthening, rejuvenating (especially after long illness), grounding

BF: 2 to 3

Elettaria cardamomum

Aphrodisiac, warming, stimulating yet comforting

BF: 4

Betula lenta

Pain relieving, stimulating, warming yet cooling

BF: 2

Cedrus atlantica

Antiseptic, preserving, soothing, spiritual

BF: 4

Daucus carota

Wound healing, digestive, stimulating

BF: 4 to 5

Syzygium aromaticum

Warming, pain relieving, aphrodisiac

BF: 3 to 4

Cinnamomum zeylanicum

Antimicrobial, antiviral, warming, stimulating, digestive

BF: 3 to 4

Jasminum grandiflorum

Nurturing, exotic, antidepressant

BF: 1

Citrus x paradisi

Uplifting, refreshing, cleansing, stimulating

BF: 6

Cymbopogon citratus

Antimicrobial, cleanses the air, strengthens connective tissue

BF: 1

Laurus nobilis

Immune supportive, stimulates lymphatic flow

BF: 2

Melissa	Myrrh
Neroli	Niaouli
Palmarosa	Petitgrain
Scots Pine	Ravensara
Sage	Sandalwood
Spearmint	Thyme

Commiphora molmol

Healing, rejuvenating, astringent

BF: 4 to 5

Melissa officinalis

Calming, soothing, tonic (heart, digestive, and nervous systems), revives and strengthens the spirit, antiviral (Herpes virus)

BF: 1

Melaleuca quinquenervia

Antiseptic, stimulating, immune enhancer

BF: 3

Citrus aurantium

Overwrought, sudden shock and fear, depression, lightly hypnotic, euphoric, aphrodisiac

BF: 2

Citrus aurantium

Pleasant, earthy, relaxing, soothing, delicate, refreshing

BF: 4 to 5

Cymbopogon martinii

Calming yet uplifting, inspiring, skin care, antimicrobial

BF: 3 to 4

Ravensara aromatica

Immune enhancing, antiviral, opens the lungs

BF: 7

Pinus sylvestris

Refreshing, antiseptic, energizing, opens up the lungs, breathing space

BF: 4 to 5

Santalum album or S. spicatum

Relaxing, soothing, meditative, dry conditions, emollient

BF: 6

Salvia officinalis

Restorative effect on the whole body, female reproductive system

BF: 3 to 4

Thymus vulgaris

Antimicrobial, immune enhancing, strengthening

BF: 1

Mentha spicata

Nausea, muscular system, digestive tonic

BF: 1 to 2